Etiology and Morphogenesis of Congenital Heart Disease:
Twenty Years of Progress in Genetics and Developmental Biology

Etiology and Morphogenesis of Congenital Heart Disease:
Twenty Years of Progress in Genetics and Developmental Biology

Edited by

Edward B. Clark, MD
Professor of Pediatrics,
University of Rochester Medical Center,
Rochester, NY

Makoto Nakazawa, MD
The Heart Institute of Japan,
Tokyo Women's Medical College,
Tokyo, Japan

Atsuyoshi Takao, MD
The Heart Institute of Japan,
Tokyo Women's Medical College,
Tokyo, Japan

**Futura Publishing
Company, Inc.**
Armonk, NY
2000

Library of Congress Cataloging-in-Publication Data

Etiology and morphogenesis of congenital heart disease : twenty years of progress in genetics and developmental biology / [edited by] Edward B. Clark, Makoto Nakazawa, Atsuyoshi Takao.
　　　p. ; cm.
　　Includes bibliographical references and index.
　　ISBN 0-87993-447-6 (alk. paper)
　　1. Congenital heart disease. I. Clark, Edward B. II. Nakazawa, Makoto, 1943- III. Takao, Atsuyoshi.
　　[DNLM: 1. Heart Defects, Congenital—genetics—Congresses. 2. Heart Defects, Congenital—embryology—Congresses. WG 220 E84 2000]
　　RC687 .E84 2000
　　616.1'2043—dc21

Published by
Futura Publishing Company, Inc.
135 Bedford Road
Armonk, NY 10504-0418

ISBN# 0-87993-447-6

Every effort has been made to ensure that the information in this book is as up to date and as accurate as possible at the time of publication. However, due to the constant developments in medicine, neither the author, nor the editor, nor the publisher can accept any legal or any other responsibility for any errors or omissions that may occur.

Printed in the United States of America.
This book is printed on acid-free paper.

Preface

This quinquennial series of symposia was started in 1978 with an aim to promote research on etiology and morphogenesis of congenital heart disease. It has been organized to facilitate the integration of basic science information for scientists and for its utilization by clinicians. One of the editors (A.T.), as a senior, enjoyed watching how fast our knowledge and understanding in this field of study have progressed.

The topics of the first symposium consisted of human genetics, segmental anatomy, embryology, physiology, pharmacology, pathology, teratology, and epidemiology. The second symposium held in 1983 included molecular cellular biology in addition to other basic science disciplines. From then on, in the succeeding symposia, tools of cutting edge science have been utilized in each discipline.

Such was the progress that the fundamental principles of the earliest stages of cardiovasculogenesis, being normal or abnormal, and functional maturation are beginning to be clarified at the molecular-cellular level. Spatiotemporal orderly pathways lead cardiac morphogenesis from appearance of the cardiac primordial cells to the primary heart tube, cardiac looping, visceroatrial disposition, chamber specification with septation, myocardial trabeculation, and compaction, its maturation and expansion, cushion formation, outflow septation, valve formation, endo-epicardial formation, coronaro-angiogenesis, conduction tissue specification resulting in eventual functional maturation.

At the clinical level, correlation of phenotype and genotype leads to discovery of new disease entity and to redefinition and/or subclassification of the already known pathology. Linkage analyses of families with multiple affected members and studies of patients with chromosome aberrations help us find responsible genes, identification of which leads to more causal approaches for diagnosis, management, and prevention.

Looking back over the years since 1978 when the first symposium was held, the progress made in this field of study has been so remarkable that our understanding of the mechanisms of cardiovascular morphogenesis and development, etiology and pathogenesis of congenital heart disease, although complexed, has become deeper and deeper.

However, at the turn of the century, we feel that we have just opened the door to more logical approach and in a sense we are still in the early stages of development.

By making the achievements we made during the past twenty years, a precious legacy to scientists and clinicians of the next century, we must go on with continuing effort to elucidate the mechanisms of how our cardiovascular system has developed.

Finally, we would like to express special thanks to the continuing generous support by the AKEMI fund of the Sankei Press and that by the Alumni Association of Department of Pediatric Cardiology, Tokyo Women's Medical University.

EBC, MN, AT

Contributors

Edward B. Clark, M.D.
Wilma T. Gibson Professor and Chairman, Department of Pediatrics, University of Utah, Salt Lake City, Utah, USA

Makoto Nakazawa, M.D.
Professor, Department of Pediatric Cardiology, The Heart Institute of Japan, Tokyo Women's Medical University, Tokyo, Japan

Atsuyoshi Takao, M.D.
Professor, Pediatric Cardiology, The Heart Institute of Japan, Tokyo Women's Medical University, Japan

Catherine A. Neill, M.D., FRCP
Professor Emeritus, Johns Hopkins Medical Center, Baltimore, Maryland, USA

Hitoshi Adachi, M.Sc.
Division of Molecular Biology, Institute for Molecular and Cellular Biology, Osaka University, Osaka, Japan

Kimio Akagawa, M.D.
Department of Physiology, Kyorin University School of Medicine, Mitaka, Tokyo, Japan

Kaoru Akimoto, M.D., Ph.D.
The Heart Institute of Japan, Tokyo Women's Medical University, Tokyo, Japan

Masahiko Ando, M.D.
The Heart Institute of Japan, Tokyo Women's Medical University, Tokyo, Japan

Shoichi Arai, B.Sc.
Department of Pediatric Cardiology, The Heart Institute of Japan, Department of Radiological Science, School of Health Science, International University of Health and Welfare, Tochigi, Japan

Orlando Aristizabal, Ph.D.
New York University Medical Center, New York, New York, USA

Michael Artman, M.D.
Department of Pediatrics, New York University Medical Center, New York, New York, USA

Stephanie Baer, B.S.
Department of Developmental Biology and Anatomy, University of South Carolina, Columbia, South Carolina, USA

H. Scott Baldwin, M.D.
Department Pediatrics (Cardiology), The University of Pennsylvania School of Medicine and Children's Hospital of Philadelphia, Philadelphia, Pennsylvania, USA

Gillian Barlow, Ph.D.
Cedars-Sinai Medical Center, University of California Los Angeles, Los Angeles, California, USA

Craig T. Basson, M.D., Ph.D.
Division of Cardiology, Weill Medical College of Cornell University, New York, New York, USA

Thomas K. Borg, Ph.D.
Department of Developmental Biology and Anatomy, University of South Carolina School of Medicine, Columbia, South Carolina, USA

Michael J. Bransby, B.S.
University of California Los Angeles, Los Angeles, California, USA

Martina Brueckner, M.D.
Department of Pediatrics/Cardiology, Yale School of Medicine, New Haven, Connecticut, USA

Marcia L. Budarf, M.D.
Divisions of Human Genetics and Molecular Biology, Department of Pediatrics, University of Pennsylvania School of Medicine, Philadelphia, Pennsylvania, USA

Phil Bullen, M.S., B.S.
Department of Fetal Medicine, University of Newcastle upon Tyne, United Kingdom

John Burn, M.D.
School of Biochemistry and Genetics, University of Newcastle, Newcastle upon Tyne, United Kingdom

Taj Burnside, B.S.
Department of Developmental Biology and Anatomy, University of South Carolina, Columbia, South Carolina, USA

J. Aidan Carney, M.D., Ph.D.
Department of Pathology, Mayo Clinic, Rochester, Minnesota, USA

Wayne Carver, Ph.D.
Department of Developmental Biology and Anatomy, University of South Carolina School of Medicine, Columbia, South Carolina, USA

Brett Casey, M.D.
Department of Pathology, Baylor College of Medicine and Texas Children's Hospital, Houston, Texas, USA

Mairead Casey, B.Sc.
Department of Medicine and Department of Cell Biology and Anatomy, Cornell University Medical College, New York, New York, USA

Settara C. Chandrasekharappa, Ph.D.
Genetics and Molecular Biology Branch, National Human Genome Research Institute, National Institutes of Health, Bethesda, Maryland, USA

Fuhua Chen, M.D.
University of California Los Angeles, Los Angeles, California, USA

Xiao–Ning Chen, M.D.
Cedars-Sinai Medical Center, University of California Los Angeles, Los Angeles, California, USA

Gang Cheng, M.D., Ph.D.
Department of Cell Biology and Anatomy, Medical University of South Carolina, Charleston, South Carolina, USA

Kenneth R. Chien, M.D., Ph.D.
Department of Medicine, University of California, San Diego, San Diego, California, USA

Emil Thomas Chuck, Ph.D.
Department of Pediatrics, Division of Cardiology, Case Western Reserve University School of Medicine, Cleveland, Ohio, USA

Edward B. Clark, M.D.
Department of Pediatrics, University of Utah, Salt Lake City, Utah, USA

Mark Clement-Jones, M.B., B.S.
Department of Fetal Medicine, University of Newcastle upon Tyne, United Kingdom

William A. Coetzee, D.Sc.
New York University Medical Center, New York, New York, USA

Simon Conway, Ph.D.
Department of Cell Biology and Anatomy, Medical University of South Carolina, Charleston, South Carolina, USA

Tony L. Creazzo, Ph.D.
Developmental Biology Program, Institute of Molecular Medicine and Genetics, Medical College of Georgia, Augusta, Georgia, USA

Andy Curtis, B.Sc.
School of Biochemistry and Genetics, University of Newcastle upon Tyne, United Kingdom

Fritz de Jong, M.D.
Department of Anatomy and Embryology, Academic Medical Centre, Amsterdam, The Netherlands

Maria Victoria de la Cruz, M.D.
Hospital Infantil de Mexico (Federico Gomez). Departamento de Biologia del Desarrollo y teratogenesis experimental, Mexico

Francesco J. Demayo, Ph.D.
Department of Cell Biology, Baylor College of Medicine, Houston, Texas, USA

Alfred E. Denio, M.D.
Center for Arthritis and Rheumatic Diseases, Virginia Beach, Virginia, USA

C.M. Diaz, M.D.
The Heart Institute of Japan, Tokyo Women's Medical University, Tokyo, Japan

Deborah A. Driscoll, M.D.
Division of Human Genetics and Molecular Biology, Departments of Pediatrics and Obstetrics and Gynecology, University of Pennsylvania School of Medicine, Philadelphia, Pennsylvania, USA

Diana M. Eccles, M.D.
University of Cambridge, Cambridge, United Kingdom

David A. Elliott, Ph.D.
The Victor Chang Cardiac Research Institute, Sydney, Australia

Beverly S. Emanuel, Ph.D.
Divisions of Human Genetics and Molecular Biology and Cardiology, The Children's Hospital of Philadelphia, Philadelphia, Pennsylvania, USA

Mitsuru Emi, M.D.
Department of Molecular Biology, Institute of Gerontology, Nippon Medical School, Kawasaki, Kanagawa, Japan

Michael Farrell, Ph.D.
Developmental Biology Program, Institute of Molecular Medicine and Genetics, Medical College of Georgia, Augusta, Georgia, USA

Steven A. Fisher, M.D.
Departments of Pediatrics and Medicine, Case Western Reserve School of Medicine, Cleveland, Ohio, USA

Timothy Fitzharris, Ph.D.
Department of Cell Biology and Anatomy, Medical University of South Carolina, Charleston, South Carolina, USA

Diego Franco, M.D.
Department of Anatomy and Embryology, Academic Medical Centre, Amsterdam, The Netherlands

Masahiko Fujinaga, M.D.
Department of Anesthesia, Stanford University School of Medicine, Palo Alto, California, USA

Hidetoshi Fujino, M.D.
Department of Pediatrics, Shiga University of Medical Science, Seta, Otsu, Shiga, Japan

Toshiro Fujita, M.D., Ph.D.
Fourth Department of Internal Medicine, School of Medicine, University of Tokyo, Tokyo, Japan

Yoshimitsu Fukushima, M.D.
Department of Hygiene and Medical Genetics, Shinshu University School of Medicine, Nagano, Japan

Michiko Furutani, B. Sc.
The Heart Institute of Japan, Tokyo Women's Medical University, Tokyo, Japan

Yoshiyuki Furutani, B.S.
The Heart Institute of Japan, Tokyo Women's Medical University, Tokyo, Japan

Adriana C. Gittenberger-de Groot, Ph.D.
Department of Anatomy and Embryology, Leiden University Medical Center, Leiden, The Netherlands

Laurie Glimcher, Ph.D.
Department of Cancer Biology, Harvard School of Public Health and Department of Medicine, Harvard Medical School, Boston, Massachusetts, USA

Robert E. Godt, Ph.D.
Developmental Biology Program, Institute of Molecular Medicine and Genetics, Medical College of Georgia, Augusta, Georgia, USA

Joshua I. Goldhaber, M.D.
University of California Los Angeles, Los Angeles, California, USA

Elizabeth Goldmuntz, M.D.
Division of Cardiology, Department of Pediatrics, University of Pennsylvania School of Medicine, Philadelphia, Pennsylvania, USA

Robert G. Gourdie, Ph.D.
Department of Cell Biology and Anatomy, Medical University of South Carolina, Charleston, South Carolina, USA

Paul D. Grossfeld, M.D.
Department of Medicine, University of California, San Diego, San Diego, California, USA

Hong Gu, Ph.D.
Department of Pediatric Cardiology, Heart Institute of Japan, Tokyo Women's Medical University, Tokyo, Japan

Peter S. Haddock, Ph.D.
New York University Medical Center, New York, New York, USA

Hiroshi Hamada, M.D., Ph.D.
Division of Molecular Biology, Institute for Molecular and Cellular Biology, Osaka University, Osaka, Japan

Takashi Hanato, M.D.
Department of Pediatrics, Shiga University of Medical Science, Seta, Otsu, Shiga, Japan

Neil Hanley, M.B., B.S.
School of Biochemistry and Genetics, University of Newcastle upon Tyne, United Kingdom

Richard P. Harvey, Ph.D.
The Victor Chang Cardiac Research Institute, Sydney, Australia

Cathy J. Hatcher, Ph.D.
Cardiology Division, Department of Medicine and Department of Cell Biology and Anatomy, Cornell University Medical College, New York, New York, USA

Chiaki Hidai, M.D.
Department of Cardiology, The Heart Institute of Japan, Tokyo, Japan

Eriko Hiratsuka, B. Sc.
The Heart Institute of Japan, Tokyo Women's Medical University, Tokyo, Japan

Hamao Hirota, M.D., Ph.D.
Medical Genetics, Cedars-Sinai Medical Center, University of California Los Angeles, Los Angeles, California, USA

Richard S. Houlston, M.D., Ph.D.
Institute of Cancer research, Surrey, United Kingdom

Anne Hughes, Ph.D.
Department of Medical Genetics, Queen's University, Belfast, Northern Ireland

Jeanette Hyer, Ph.D.
Department of Cell Biology, Cornell University Medical College, New York, New York, USA

Aritoshi Iida, Ph.D.
Department of Molecular Biology, Institute of Gerontology, Nippon Medical School, Kawasaki, Kanagawa, Japan

Kiyoshi Iida, M.D.
Department of Biochemistry, Akita University School of Medicine, Hondo, Akita, Japan

Hiromi Ikeda, M.D.
Department of Cardiology, The Heart Institute of Japan, Tokyo, Japan

Takashi Imai, Ph.D.
Laboratory of Human and Mouse Genome Mapping, Genome Research Group, National Institute of Radiological Sciences, Chiba, Japan

Shin-ichiro Imamura, D.V.M., Ph.D.
The Heart Institute of Japan, Tokyo Women's Medical University, Tokyo, Japan

Kyoko Imanaka-Yoshida, M.D.
Department of Pathology, Mie University School of Medicine, Tsu, Mie, Japan

Alan D. Irvine, M.D.
Department of Dermatology, Royal Victoria Hospital, Belfast, Northern Ireland

Shigeru Ishiyama, M.D.
Department of Pathology, Tokyo Women's Medical University, Tokyo, Japan

Seigo Izumo, M.D.
Cardiovascular Division, Beth Israel Deaconess Medical Center, Harvard Medical School, Boston, Massachusetts USA

Kunitaka Joh-o, M.D.
Kyushu Welfare Pension Hospital, Fukuoka, Japan

Hideaki Kakinuma, M.D.
Department of Biochemistry, Akita University School of Medicine, Hondo, Akita, Japan

Hiroshi Kasanuki, M.D.
Department of Cardiology, The Heart Institute of Japan, Tokyo, Japan

Naoko Kato, M.D.
Department of Biochemistry, Akita University School of Medicine, Hondo, Akita, Japan

Masatoshi Kawana, M.D.
Department of Cardiology, The Heart Institute of Japan, Tokyo, Japan

Bradley B. Keller, M.D.
Division of Pediatric Cardiology, University of Kentucky, Lexington, Kentucky, USA

Misa Kimura, M.S.
The Heart Institute of Japan, Tokyo Women's Medical University, Tokyo, Japan

Yuji Kira, M.D., Ph.D.
Division of Cardiology, Showa General Hospital, Kodaira City, Tokyo, Japan

Margaret L. Kirby, Ph.D.
Developmental Biology Program, Institute of Molecular Medicine and Genetics, Medical College of Georgia, Augusta, Georgia, USA

Sandra C. Klatt, B.A.
Department of Cell Biology and Anatomy, Medical University of South Carolina, Charleston, South Carolina, USA

Keiko Komatsu, B.Sc.
The Heart Institute of Japan, Tokyo Women's Medical University, Tokyo, Japan

Issei Komuro, M.D.
Department of Cardiovascular Medicine, University of Tokyo Graduate School of Medicine, Tokyo, Japan

Masanori Kondo, M.D.
Department of Pediatrics, Shiga University of Medical Science, Seta, Otsu, Shiga, Japan

Julie R. Korenberg, Ph.D., M.D.
Cedars-Sinai Medical Center, University of California Los Angeles, Los Angeles, California, USA

Haruhiko Koseki, M.D.
Chiba University School of Medicine, Chiba, Japan

Edward L. Krug, Ph.D.
Department of Cell Biology and Anatomy, Medical University of South Carolina, Charleston, South Carolina, USA

Tsutomu Kumazaki, Ph.D.
Department of Biochemistry and Biophysics, Research Institute for Radiation Biology and Medicine, Hiroshima University, Kasumi, Hiroshima, Japan

Yukiko Kurihara, M.D.
Department of Medicine III, The University of Tokyo, Tokyo, Japan

Wouter H. Lamers, M.D.
Department of Anatomy and Embryology, Academic Medical Centre, Amsterdam, The Netherlands

Joel A. Lawitts, M.D.
Transgenic Core Facility, Beth Israel Deaconess Medical Center, Harvard Medical School, Boston, Massachusetts USA

Linda Leatherbury, M.D.
Developmental Biology Program, Institute of Molecular Medicine and Genetics, Medical College of Georgia, Augusta, Georgia, USA

Ike W. Lee, M.D.
Cardiovascular Division, Beth Israel Deaconess Medical Center, Harvard Medical School, Boston, Massachusetts USA

Xuyang Li, B.Z., M.S.
Department of Cell Biology, Baylor College of Medicine, Houston, Texas, USA

Imad Libbus, M.D.
Department of Pediatrics, Division of Cardiology, Case Western Reserve University School of Medicine, Cleveland, Ohio, USA

Kersti K. Linask, Ph.D.
Department of Cell Biology, University of Medicine and Dentistry of New Jersey, Stratford, New Jersey, USA

Susan Lindsay, B.Sc., Ph.D.
School of Biochemistry and Genetics, University of Newcastle upon Tyne, United Kingdom

Wanda Litchenberg, Ph.D.
Department of Cell Biology and Anatomy, Medical University of South Carolina, Charleston, South Carolina, USA

Gary Lyons, Ph.D.
University of Wisconsin Medical School, Madison, Wisconsin, USA

Shuichi Machida, M.D.
Department of Pediatric Cardiology, The Heart Institute of Japan, Tokyo Women's Medical University, Tokyo, Japan

Caroline S. Mah, B.A.
Cardiology Division, Department of Medicine and Department of Cell Biology and Anatomy, Cornell University Medical College, New York, New York, USA

Roger R. Markwald, Ph.D.
Department of Cell Biology and Anatomy, Medical University of South Carolina, Charleston, South Carolina, USA

Rumiko Matsuoka, M.D.
Department of Pediatric Cardiology, The Heart Institute of Japan, Tokyo Women's Medical University, Tokyo, Japan

Donna McDonald-McGinn, M.S.
Division of Human Genetics and Molecular Biology, The Children's Hospital of Philadelphia, Philadelphia, Pennsylvania, USA

James McGrath, M.D., Ph.D.
Department of Comparative Medicine, Yale School of Medicine, New Haven, Connecticut, USA

Chikara Meno, DVM, Ph.D.
Division of Molecular Biology, Institute for Molecular and Cellular Biology, Osaka University, Osaka, Japan

Takashi Mikawa, Ph.D.
Department of Cell Biology, Cornell University Medical College, New York, New York, USA

Susumu Minamisawa, M.D., Ph.D.
Department of Medicine, University of California, San Diego, La Jolla, California, USA

Shinsei Minoshima, Ph.D.
Keio University School of Medicine, Tokyo, Japan

Vladimir Mironov, M.D., Ph.D.
Department of Cell Biology and Anatomy, Medical University of South Carolina, Charleston, South Carolina, USA

Laura Mitchell, Ph.D.
Division of Human Genetics and Molecular Biology, Department of Pediatrics, University of Pennsylvania School of Medicine, Philadelphia, Pennsylvania, USA

Naoyuki Miura, M.D., Ph.D.
Department of Biochemistry, Hamamatsu Medical College, Hamamatsu, Japan

Kohei Miyazono, M.D.
Department of Biochemistry, The Cancer Institute, Japanese Foundation for Cancer Research, Tokyo, Japan

Kensaku Mizuno, Ph.D.
Department of Biology, Kyushu University, Fukuoka, Japan

Takehiko Mizuno, M.D.
Department of Cardiovascular Medicine, University of Tokyo Graduate School of Medicine, Tokyo, Japan

Corey H. Mjaatvedt, Ph.D.
Department of Cell Biology and Anatomy, Medical University of South Carolina, Charleston, South Carolina, USA

Kazuo Momma, M.D.
Department of Pediatric Cardiology, The Heart Institute of Japan, Tokyo Women's Medical University, Tokyo, Japan

Antoon F.M. Moorman, Ph.D.
Department of Anatomy and Embryology, Academic Medical Centre, Amsterdam, The Netherlands

Masae Morishima, DVM, Ph.D.
The Heart Institute of Japan, Tokyo Women's Medical University, Tokyo, Japan

Touru Murakami, M.D.
Department of Surgery, Kidney Center, Tokyo Women's Medical University, Tokyo, Japan

Sachiko Miyagawa-Tomita, DVM, Ph.D.
Department of Pediatric Cardiology, The Heart Institute of Japan, Tokyo Women's Medical University, Tokyo, Japan

Hirotaka Nagashima, M.D.
Department of Cardiology, The Heart Institute of Japan, Tokyo, Japan

Masao Nakagawa, M.D.
Department of Pediatrics, Shiga University of Medical Science, Seta, Otsu, Shiga, Japan

Yuji Nakajima, M.D.
Department of Anatomy Saitama Medical School, Saitama, Japan

Hiroaki Nakamura, M.D.
Department of Anatomy Saitama Medical School, Saitama, Japan

Harukazu Nakamura, M.D.
Department of Molecular Neurobiology, Institute of Development, Aging, and Cancer, Tohoku University, Sendai, Myagi, Japan

Yusuke Nakamura, M.D.
Laboratory of Molecular Medicine, Human Genome Center, Institute of Medical Science, The University of Tokyo, Tokyo, Japan

Toshio Nakanishi, M.D.
Department of Pediatric Cardiology, Heart Institute of Japan, Tokyo Women's Medical University, Tokyo, Japan

Takashi Nakaoka,, M.D., Ph.D.
Department of Cell Biology and Anatomy, Medical University of South Carolina, Charleston, South Carolina, USA

Norio Nakatsuji, Ph.D.
Mammalian Development Laboratory, National Institute of Genetics, Mishimi, Shizuoka, Japan

Takahiro Nakayama, M.D.
Department of Physiology, Kyorin University School of Medicine, Tokyo, Japan

Makoto Nakazawa, M.D.
Department of Pediatric Cardiology, The Heart Institute of Japan, Tokyo Women's Medical University, Tokyo, Japan

Setsuko Nishijima, M.D.
Department of Pediatrics, Shiga University of Medical Science, Seta, Otsu, Shiga, Japan

Toshio Nishikawa, M.D.
Department of Surgical Pathology, Tokyo Women's Medical University, Tokyo, Japan

Setsuko Noda, Ph.D.
Department of Nursing School of Health Science, Tokai University, Isehara-city, Kanagawa prefecture, Japan

Shinji Oana, M.D., Ph.D.
Department of Pediatric Cardiology, The Heart Institute of Japan, Tokyo Women's Medical University, Tokyo, Japan

Takaya Oda, M.D., Ph.D.
Genetics and Molecular Biology Branch, National Human Genome Research Institute, National Institutes of Health, Bethesda, Maryland, USA

Teruhiko Ogita, M.D., Ph.D.
Fourth Department of Internal Medicine, Department of Pediatric Cardiology, University of Tokyo, Tokyo, Japan

Hirofumi Ohashi, M.D.
Saitama Children's Medical Center, Saitama, Japan

Masako Okada, M.D.
Department of Cardiology, The Heart Institute of Japan, Tokyo, Japan

Nobuhiko Okamoto, M.D.
Department of Pediatrics, Shiga University of Medical Science, Seta, Otsu, Shiga, Japan

Eric N. Olson, Ph.D.
Department of Molecular Biology and Oncology, University of Texas Southwestern Medical Center at Dallas, Dallas, Texas, USA

Zenshiro Onouchi, M.D.
Department of Pathology and Cell Regulation, Kyoto Prefectural University of Medicine, Kyoto, Japan

John M. Opitz, M.D.
Division of Medical Genetics, Department of Pediatrics, University of Utah, Salt Lake City, Utah, USA

Mark Pettenati, Ph.D.
Bowman Gray School of Medicine, Winston-Salem, North Carolina, USA

Colin Phoon, M.D.
New York University Medical Center, New York, New York, USA

Karen Piper, B.Sc.
School of Biochemistry and Genetics, University of Newcastle upon Tyne, United Kingdom

Robert E. Poelman, Ph.D.
Department of Anatomy and Embryology, Leiden University Medical Center, Leiden, The Netherlands

S. Steven Potter, Ph.D.
Divisions of Molecular and Developmental Biology, The Children's Hospital Research Foundation, Cincinnati, Ohio, USA

Gogieni Ranganayakulu, Ph.D.
Department of Molecular Biology and Oncology, University of Texas Southwestern Medical Center at Dallas, Dallas, Texas, USA

Ann Ranger, Ph.D.
Department of Cancer Biology, Harvard School of Public Health and, Department of Medicine, Harvard Medical School, Boston, Massachusetts, USA

James M. Reecy, M.D.
Department of Cell Biology, Baylor College of Medicine, Houston, Texas USA

Gail A. Robertson, Ph.D.
Department of Physiology, University of Wisconsin-Madison, Madison, Wisconsin, USA

Steven Robson, M.S., B.S., M.D.
Department of Fetal Medicine, University of Newcastle upon Tyne, United Kingdom

David S. Rosenbaum, M.D.
Department of Pediatrics, Division of Cardiology, Case Western Reserve University School of Medicine, Cleveland, Ohio, USA

Yukio Saijoh, M.D.
Division of Molecular Biology, Institute for Molecular and Cellular Biology, Osaka University, Osaka, Japan

Teruyo Sakakura, M.D.
Department of Pathology, Mie University School of Medicine, Tsu, Mie, Japan

Rui Sakuma, M.Sc.
Division of Molecular Biology, Institute for Molecular and Cellular Biology, Osaka University, Osaka, Japan

T. Kuber Sampath, Ph.D.
Creative BioMolecules, Inc., Hopkinton, Massachusetts, USA

Peter J. Scambler, Ph.D.
Institute of Child Health, London, England

Robert J. Schwartz, Ph.D.
Department of Cell Biology, Baylor College of Medicine, Houston, Texas, USA

Tamim Shaikh, Ph.D.
Division of Human Genetics and Molecular Biology, The Children's Hospital of Philadelphia, Philadelphia, Pennsylvania, USA

Toshimitsu Shibata, M.D.
The Heart Institute of Japan, Tokyo Women's Medical University, Tokyo, Japan, Department of Pediatrics, Yokohama City University, Yokohama, Kanagawa, Japan

Kazunori Shimada, M.D.
Department of Medical Genetics, Research Institute for Microbial Diseases, Osaka University, Osaka, Japan

Nobuyoshi Shimizu, Ph.D.
Keio University School of Medicine, Tokyo, Japan

Ichiro Shiojima, M.D.
Department of Cardiovascular Medicine, University of Tokyo Graduate School of Medicine, Tokyo, Japan

Manabu Shirai, Ph.D.
Department of Medical Genetics, Research Institute for Microbial Diseases, Osaka University, Osaka, Japan

Isao Shiraishi, M.D.
Division of Pediatrics, Children's Research Hospital, Department of Pathology and Cell Regulation, Kyoto Prefectural University of Medicine, Kyoto, Japan

Yasuaki Shirayoshi, D.Sc.
Department of Molecular and Cell Genetics, School of Life Sciences, Tottori University, Tottori, Japan

Bradley R. Smith, Ph.D.
Duke University Medical Center, Durham, North Carolina, USA

Patricia Soles-Rosenthal, M. Ed.
Department of Cell Biology and Anatomy, Medical University of South Carolina, Charleston, South Carolina USA

Shardha Srinivasan, M.D.
New York University Medical Center, New York, New York, USA

Deepak Srivastava, M.D.
Department of Pediatrics (Cardiology), Department of Molecular Biology and Oncology, University of Texas Southwestern Medical Center, Dallas, Texas, USA

Tom Strachan, B.Sc., Ph.D.
School of Biochemistry and Genetics, University of Newcastle upon Tyne, United Kingdom

Constantine A. Stratakis, M.D., Ph.D.
NICHD, National Institutes of Health, Bethesda, Maryland, USA

Toshihiro Sugiyama, M.D.
Department of Biochemistry, Akita University School of Medicine, Hondo, Akita, Japan

Hiroshi Sumida, Ph.D.
Department of Clinical Radiology, Faculty of Health Sciences, Hiroshima International University, Kurose, Hiroshima, Japan

Dorothy M. Supp, Ph.D.
Divisions of Molecular and Developmental Biology, The Children's Hospital Research Foundation, Cincinnati, Ohio, USA

Tetsuro Takamatsu, M.D.
Division of Pediatrics, Children's Research Hospital, Department of Pathology and Cell Regulation, Kyoto Prefectural University of Medicine, Kyoto, Japan

Atsuyoshi Takao, M.D.
Department of Pediatric Cardiology, The Heart Institute of Japan, Tokyo Women's Medical University, Tokyo, Japan

Kimiko Takebayashi-Suzuki, Ph.D.
Department of Cell Biology, Cornell University Medical College, New York, New York, USA

Takashi Takeuchi, Ph.D.
Mitsubishi Kasei Institute of Life Sciences, Tokyo, Japan

Yoshihiro Takihara, M.D.
Department of Medical Genetics, Research Institute for Microbial Diseases, Osaka University, Osaka, Japan

Makoto Tanaka, M.D.
Cardiovascular Division, Beth Israel Deaconess Medical Center, Harvard Medical School, Boston, Massachusetts USA

Mariko Tatsuguchi, M.D.
The Heart Institute of Japan, Tokyo, Japan

Louis Terracio, Ph.D.
Department of Developmental Biology and Anatomy, University of South Carolina School of Medicine, Columbia, South Carolina, USA

Robert P. Thompson, Ph.D.
Department of Cell Biology and Anatomy, Medical University of South Carolina, Charleston, South Carolina USA

Sachiko M. Tomita, DVM, Ph.D.
The Heart Institute of Japan, Tokyo Women's Medical University, Tokyo, Japan

Daihachiro Tomotsune, Ph.D.
Department of Medical Genetics, Research Institute for Microbial Diseases, Osaka University, Osaka, Japan

Jeffrey A. Towbin, M.D.
Departments of Pediatrics (Cardiology), Molecular & Human Genetics, and Cardiovascular Sciences, Baylor College of Medicine, Houston, Texas, USA

Matthew C. Trudeau, Ph.D.
Department of Physiology, Biophysics and HHMI, University of Washington, Seattle, Washington, USA

Takeshi Tsuda, M.D.
Department of Dermatology and Cutaneous Biology, Thomas Jefferson University, Jefferson Medical College, Philadelphia, Pennsylvania, USA

Daniel H. Turnbull, Ph.D.
New York University Medical Center, New York, New York, USA

Maurice J. B. van den Hoff, M.D.
Department of Anatomy and Embryology, Academic Medical Centre, Amsterdam, The Netherlands

Alexander J. VanRiper, M.S.
Permanente Medical Group, Sacramento, California, USA

Carl J. Vaughan, M.D.
Department of Medicine and Department of Cell Biology and Anatomy, Cornell University Medical College, New York, New York, USA

Mark Vekemens, M.D.
Hopital des Enfants-Malades, Paris, France

Mark-Paul Vrancken-Peeters, M.D., Ph.D.
Department of Anatomy and Embryology, Leiden University Medical Center, Leiden, The Netherlands

Karen Waldo, M.S.
Developmental Biology Program, Institute of Molecular Medicine and Genetics, Medical College of Georgia, Augusta, Georgia, USA

Jinling Wang, M.S.
Department of Physiology, University of Wisconsin-Madison, Madison, Wisconsin, USA

Michiko Watanabe, Ph.D.
Departments of Pediatrics and Medicine, Case Western Reserve School of Medicine, Cleveland, Ohio, USA

Stephanie Burns Wechsler, M.D.
Department of Pediatrics and Communicable Diseases, University of Michigan Medical Center, Ann Arbor, Michigan, USA

Yan Wei, Ph.D.
Department of Cell Biology, Cornell University Medical College, New York, New York, USA

Andy Wessels, Ph.D.
Department of Cell Biology and Anatomy, Medical University of South Carolina, Charleston, South Carolina, USA

Glenn T. Wetzel, M.D., Ph.D.
University of California Los Angeles, Los Angeles, California, USA

David I. Wilson, BA, MB.BS, Ph.D.
School of Biochemistry and Genetics, University of Newcastle upon Tyne, United Kingdom

Jordan Winter, B.A.
Department of Medicine and Department of Cell Biology and Anatomy, Cornell University Medical College, New York, New York, USA

Miho Yamada, M.D.
Department of Cell Biology, Baylor College of Medicine, Houston, Texas, USA

Hiroyuki Yamagishi, M.D.
Departments of Pediatrics and Molecular Biology and Oncology, University of Texas Southwestern Medical Center at Dallas, Dallas, Texas, USA

Toshiyuki Yamagishi, M.D.
Department of Anatomy Saitama Medical School, Saitama, Japan

Hideshi Yamamura, M.D.
Department of Cell Biology and Anatomy, Medical University of South Carolina, Charleston, South Carolina, USA

Naohito Yamasaki, M.D.
Cardiovascular Division, Beth Israel Deaconess Medical Center, Harvard Medical School, Boston, Massachusetts USA

Naohito Yamasaki, M.D.
Department of Geriatrics, Kochi Medical College, Kochi, Japan

Kenta Yashiro, M.D.
Division of Molecular Biology, Institute for Molecular and Cellular Biology, Osaka University, Osaka, Japan

Hiroshi Yasui, M.D.
Department of Pathology and Developmental Biology, Kyoto Prefectural Medical College, Tokyo, Japan

Takahiko Yokoyama, M.D.
Department of Anatomy and Developmental Biology, Tokyo Women's Medical University, Tokyo, Japan

Nobuaki Yoshida, M.D., Ph.D.
The Institute of Medical Science, University of Tokyo, Tokyo, Japan

H. Joseph Yost, Ph.D.
Department of Oncological Sciences, University of Utah, Salt Lake City, Utah, USA

Elaine H. Zackai, M.D.
Division of Human Genetics and Molecular Biology, Department of Pediatrics, University of Pennsylvania School of Medicine, Philadelphia, Pennsylvania, USA

Bin Zhou, M.D., Ph.D.
Department of Pediatrics (Cardiology), University of Pennsylvania School of Medicine and, Children's Hospital of Philadelphia, Philadelphia, Pennsylvania, USA

Contents

Section III

Section VI

Section VII

Color Appendix

Historical Overview

20 Years' Progress: Understanding the Heart of a Child

Catherine A. Neill, MD, FRCP

In the twenty years since the first Takao conference in 1978 there has been a dramatic growth in understanding some of the molecular biology of cardiac development. In many cases this growth in basic knowledge has been accompanied by advances in clinical management of children with severe cardiac syndromes.

These intertwining advances, growth in precise genotypic diagnosis combined with improved survival and better phenotypic assessment at all ages, have led to conceptual changes. For example, molecular biological advances in the 22q11 deletion syndrome, have led to a new way of analyzing the troubling developmental and psychological problems of some of these children. In the mid 1970s, when the spectrum of cardiac defects in DiGeorge and Shprintzen syndrome was first outlined, it was impossible to determine if developmental difficulties were due to genetic causes or postoperative sequelae. Although much still needs to be learned of genotypic-phenotypic correlation, it is already clear that the syndrome has major clinical implications for cardiologists and families.

Historic Perspective

The 1978 Takao symposium took place approximately 40 years after the publication of Maud Abbott's atlas in 1936, 35 years after the first Blalock Taussig shunt, 24 years after the dawn of open heart surgery, and less than 5 years after successful cardiac management in infancy became a reality (Fig. 1).

The clinical spectrum of many syndromes had already been described, and there was a beginning understanding of clinical genetic patterns. For example, the association of atrioventricular septal defect with trisomy 21 was already well recognized.

Over the past 20 years many genes involved in normal and abnormal cardiac development have been identified, and there is a growing list of mutations associated with congenital cardiac defects and with cardiomyopathies.

A number of investigative methods used to clarify understanding of cardiac development have been described in prior publications from these symposia. Building on the classic embryological studies of Mall and Streeter, dynamic embryology, electron microscopy, genetic and epidemiological studies have all made contributions. The late, beloved Tomas Pexieder, one of the most brilliant minds devoted to cardiac development, summarized the evolution of knowledge of conotruncal septation "at the advent of the molecular biology era."[2] He also tabulated some of

From Clark EB, Nakazawa M, Takao A (eds.): Etiology and Morphogenesis of Congenital Heart Disease: Twenty Years of Progress in Genetics and Developmental Biology. Armonk, NY: Futura Publishing Co., Inc.; © 2000.

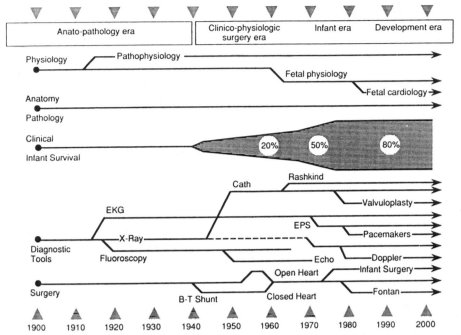

Figure 1. Landmarks in the development of pediatric cardiology: the rise of the developmental era. Reproduced with permission from Reference 1.

the genes then under study in cardiac development.

The genotypic-phenotypic correlations of many important cardiac disorders of childhood have been described.[3,4] In this brief discussion I will focus on the evolutionary pattern of understanding of a few syndromes. With rare exceptions this pattern has shown, at varying rates, the progression outlined in Table 1.

This evolutionary progression has occurred in hypertrophic cardiomyopathy, long QT syndrome, and other disorders, including nonsyndromic familial atrial septal defect with atrioventricular conduction abnormalities.[5]

Table 1
Pattern of Evolution of Syndrome Understanding

- Syndrome recognition
- Expanded clinical syndrome
- Studies clinical genetics, epidemiology, animal models, dynamic embryology, other
- Molecular biology studies, leading to genotypic phenotypic correlations, expanded understanding of natural history

---

By contrast, the study of vitamin A and retinoic acid began in 1949 with Warkany's experimental work on aortic arch development. Retinoic acid embryopathy was described almost 30 years later; the role of retinoic acid receptors in cardiac tissue remains under active investigation.[6]

Specific Syndromes

In the early years of therapy for cardiovascular malformations, the major emphasis was on isolated cardiac defects. However, long before the 20 years of progress discussed here, the association of cardiac and non-cardiac defects was recognized.

Marfan syndrome provides a model of the progressive understanding of an important disorder. First described in 1896, the clinical spectrum was elucidated and defined by McKusick in 1955, and the gene was assigned to a specific locus on chromosome 15 by Dietz and colleagues in 1991.[4] A molecular approach to the stratification of cardiovascular risk factors is now feasible,[7] and preimplantation diagnosis of an affected fetus has been reported.[8] This progression illustrates how molecular biological advances can be useful both in refining clinical diagnosis and prognosis, and in some preventive approaches.

Intertwined with these advances in molecular biology, clinical management has been improved by echocardiography, and by new medical and surgical therapies.

Down syndrome, the major cause of congenital heart disease in association with severe developmental delay, has the longest history. Described by Down in 1866, the frequent association with atrioventricular septal defect was known to Maud Abbott by 1936. Many contributions in the past 20 years including studies of animal models, have added to prior work by Lejeune, Rowe, and Uchida, and others.[1,9] In the Baltimore Washington Infant Study led by Dr. Charlotte Ferencz, 9% of all liveborn infants with cardiovascular malformations had Down syndrome.[10] This figure did not change over the nine year study period, despite the increasing availability of fetal echocardiography.

Molecular biological studies of chromosome 21 have been intensive,[11,12] genetic mapping is far advanced, and more effective screening procedures are in progress.[13]

Williams syndrome and supravalvar aortic stenosis (SVAS), though rare, have been of intense interest to cardiologists and behavioral psychologists since 1961. Although at first familial isolated SVAS was thought to be a separate disorder, some families with overlapping features were recognised early. Molecular biological analysis is continuing to elucidate this disorder of the elastin gene.[14]

22q11 deletion syndromes have brought new concepts to the practice of cardiology.[15–19] Until genotypic diagnosis was available, the sometimes subtle phenotypic variations in the syndrome were a source of great difficulty. Collaborative studies are now adding to knowledge of the clinical spectrum at all ages. Different conotruncal defects have a risk of the syndrome varying from 50% in interrupted

aortic arch, to between 5% and 12% in uncomplicated tetralogy with left aortic arch: the risk is minimal in compete transposition.[18] It will soon be possible to clarify in greater detail than at present the "syndrome load"[10] of individual cardiac defects.

Implications for Cardiologists and Families

The rapid pace of advance in molecular biological knowledge can be daunting to the clinical cardiologist. The recent American Heart Association position paper[4] is helpful in providing a consensus on the role of molecular biological studies in 3 major cardiac syndromes. The provision of timely authoritative updates on these and other syndromes will be of great value.

The advances have brought to vivid attention the value of careful clinical follow up into adult life. Only in this way can true assessment be made of long term quality of life. Some pediatric cardiac centers, almost all represented at this conference, are leading the way in collaboration between cardiologists, molecular biologists, clinical geneticists and behavioral psychologists. Such large scale networks are logistically challenging, but are essential to further understanding.

The cardiologist involved in fetal echocardiography confronts particularly difficult ethical issues.[20, 21] These issues have not yet been adequately discussed. It is clear that fetal echocardiographic diagnosis of a major conotruncal defect mandates amniocentesis and FISH studies for 22q11 deletions. There is, however, no current consensus on subsequent counseling. Many cardiologists believe that fetal diagnosis will help in preparatory guidance regarding speech therapy and schooling, but the risk factors for psychosis in adult life have yet to be determined.

The exciting, even dizzying, growth of basic knowledge at the dawn of the 21st century thus confronts cardiologists and families with unprecedented challenges in keeping abreast with information, in appropriate models of collaboration, and in ethical transmission of changing knowledge.

References

1. Neill CA, Clark EB. *The Developing Heart: A "History" of Pediatric Cardiology*. The Netherlands: Kluwer Academic Publishing; 1995.

2. Pexieder T. Conotruncus and its septation at the advent of the molecular biology era. In: Clark EB, Markwalld RR, Takao A, eds. *Developmental Mechanisms of Heart Disease*. Mount Kisco: Futura Publishing Co; 1995:227–247.

3. Johnson MC, Payne RM, Grant JW, et al. The genetic basis of pediatric heart disease. *Ann Med* 1995;27:289–300. Review.

4. Maron BJ, Moller JH, Seidman CE, et al. Impact of laboratory molecular diagnosis on contemporary diagnostic criteria for genetically transmitted cardiovascular diseases: Hypertrophic cardiomyopathy, long-QT syndrome, and Marfan syndrome. *Circulation* 1998;98:1460–1471.

5. Schott J-J, Benson DW, Basson CT, et al. Congenital heart disease caused by mutations in the transcription factor NKX2.5. *Science* 1998;281:108–111.

6. Sinning AR. Role of Vitamin A in the formation of congenital heart defects. *Anat Rec New Anat* 1998;253:147–153.

7. Pereira L, Levran O, Ramirez F, et al. A molecular approach to the stratification of cardiovascular risk in families with Marfan's syndrome. *N Engl J Med* 1994; 331:148–153.

8. Blaszczyk A, Tang YX, Dietz HC, et al. Preimplantation genetic diagnosis of human embryos for Marfan's syndrome. *J Assist Reprod Genet* 1998;15:281–284.

9. Marino B, DiCarlo D. Complete atrioventricular septal defect and Down syndrome. *Eur J Cardiothorac Surg* 1997;12:815.

10. Boughman JA, Neill CA, Ferencz C, et al. The genetics of congenital heart disease. In: Ferencz C, Rubin JD, Loffredo CA, et al., eds. *Epidemiology of Congenital Heart Disease: The Baltimore Washington Infant Study 1981–1998*. Mount Kisco: Futura Publishing Co; 1993:123–167.

11. Korenberg JR, Chen XN, Schipper R, et al. Down syndrome phenotypes: The consequences of chromosomal imbalance. *Proc Natl Acad Sci U S A* 1994;91:4997–5001.

12. Atonarakis SE. 10 years of Genomics, chromosome 21, and Down syndrome. *Genomics* 1998;51:1–16. Review.

13. Cuckle H. National Down syndrome screening policy. *Am J Pub Health* 1998; 88:972.

14. Wu YQ, Sutton VR, Nickerson E, et al. Delineation of the common critical region in Williams syndrome and clinical correlation of growth, heart defects, ethnicity, and parental origin. *Am J Med Genet* 1998;78:82–89.

15. Takao A, Momma K, Kondo C, et al. Conotruncal anomaly face syndrome. In: Clark EB, Markwald RR, Takao A, eds. *Developmental Mechanisms of Heart Disease*. Armonk, NY: Futura Publishing Co; 1995:555–558.

16. Ryan AK, Goodship JA, Wilson DJ, et al. Spectrum of clinical features associated with interstitial chromosome 22q11 deletions: A European collaborative study. *J Med Genet* 1997;34:798–804.

17. Goodship J, Cross I, LiLing J, et al. A population study of chromosome 22q11 deletions in infancy. *Arch Dis Child* 1998;79: 348–351.

18. Goldmuntz E, Clark BJ, Mitchell LE, et al. Frequency of 22q11 deletions in patients with conotruncal defects. *J Am Coll Cardiol* 1998;32:492–501.

19. Momma K, Kondo C, Ando M, et al. Tetralogy of Fallot associated with chromosome 22q11 deletion. *Am J Cardiol* 1995; 76:618–621.

20. Shinebourne EA, Carvallho JS. Ethics of fetal echocardiography. *Cardiol Young* 1996;6:261–263.

21. Bristow JD, Bernstein HS. Editorial comment: Counseling families with chromosome 22q11 deletions—the catch in CATCH-22. *J Am Coll Cardiol* 1998;32: 499–501.

Section I

1

Overview: Axes, Situs, and the Vertebrate Body Plan

H. Joseph Yost, PhD

A central step in the formation of a normal, functional heart is cardiac looping along the embryonic left-right axis. Because normal looping is essential for the subsequent formation of valves, septa, and outflow tract, there has been a long-standing interest in the genetic and developmental pathways that regulate cardiac loop morphogenesis. Recently, significant advances have been made in the understanding of the left-right orientation of cardiac looping in embryos of several vertebrate species. Four topics are reviewed: (1) Formation of the embryonic left-right axis is initiated early during embryogenesis, perhaps before gastrulation. (2) Embryonic cells that do not directly contribute to cardiac lineages regulate the formation of cardiac left-right orientation via cell-cell signaling. These lineages include lateral cells in the blastula-stage embryo, node, and midline cells. (3) Left-right orientation is specified in cardiac primordia long before looping morphogenesis occurs, as indicated by the asymmetric expression of both cell signaling and transcription regulation factors. (4) The part of the genetic pathway that is proximal to cardiac left-right specification is highly conserved in vertebrates. It is not yet clear whether the earliest steps in left-right axis formation are conserved. Each of these points, derived from basic research, has important clinical ramifications.

Embryonic Left-Right Axis Is Established Early During Embryogenesis

How and when in development are the orientations of left-right asymmetric morphogenetic events, such as the looping of the cardiac tube, coordinated with the mechanisms that regulate development along the dorsal-ventral and anterior-posterior axis? Clearly this coordination must occur in order to generate a well-organized, three-dimensional vertebrate organism. Advances during the last five years indicate that the genetic pathways and developmental mechanisms that direct cardiac orientation occur quite early in embryogenesis. Using *Xenopus* embryos as a model system, we have recently proposed that a group of cells on the left lateral side of blastula-stage embryos, called the left-right coordinator (LRC), breaks symmetry and begins the coordination of the left-right axis with the other body axes. Experimental results indicate that the LRC uses the Vg1 signaling pathway to establish left-sided identity. In the absence or repression of these signals, cells acquire right-sided identity.

Vg1 is a member of the TGFβ family. TGFβ are synthesized as latent, propro-

From Clark EB, Nakazawa M, Takao A (eds.): Etiology and Morphogenesis of Congenital Heart Disease: Twenty Years of Progress in Genetics and Developmental Biology. Armonk, NY: Futura Publishing Co., Inc.; © 2000.

teins that must be processed, usually by proteolysis, to release an active mature carboxy-terminal domain. The working hypothesis is that Vg1 protein processing is regulated along the left-right axis, so that it is processed into mature ligand on the left side but not on the right side. Ectopic production of mature Vg1 on the right side results in inversion of the left-right axis, so that the heart and gut are fully inverted. In embryos with an inverted left-right axis, downstream markers such as nodal, which is normally expressed on the left side, are turned off on the left and induced on the right. In these experiments, mature Vg1 ligand was generated using chimeric protein constructs containing the prepro-domains of other TGFβ family members (activin, BMP2 or BMP4) fused to the mature domain of Vg1. These chimeric proteins generate mature Vg1 ligand by utilizing the protein processing machinery that normally processes activin, BMP2 or BMP4. This allows experimental circumvention of the proposed block in Vg1 processing on the right side of the embryo. Results of a variety of experiments in which Vg1 ligand is ectopically expressed on the right side, or in which downstream signaling pathways are blocked on the left side, suggest that Vg1 protein processing and downstream signaling establishes the LRC on the left side of blastula-stage embryos.

Results from early tissue manipulations in chick embryos concur with the idea that signals from the lateral regions of the embryo impart left-right axial information on the node at the midline of the embryo. Experimental rotation of the node with respect to the lateral regions early in embryogenesis (stage 4), so that the right side of the node is in contact with the left side of the lateral regions, results in reorganization of left-right gene expression patterns within the node. This suggests that signals from the lateral regions are dominant and confer left-right patterning within the node. Rotation of the node a few hours later (stage 5/6) results in gene expression patterns that are consistent with the original orientation of the node. This suggests that at some point

in early development (between stages 4 and 6 in the chick), the ability of lateral regions to signal left-right information is diminished and the node becomes the dominant carrier of left-right information. It is likely that early interactions between lateral regions (including the LRC) and the node at the prospective embryonic midline serve to coordinate the three-dimensional arrangement of embryonic axes.

Cells That Do Not Directly Contribute to Cardiac Lineages Regulate the Formation of Cardiac Left-Right Orientation via Cell-Cell Signaling

Five years ago, the concept that noncardiac lineages could influence cardiac left-right development was just beginning to emerge.[1] Now, most of the genes that have been implicated in cardiac left-right development are known to be expressed in other cells in the embryo, not in cardiac progenitor cells (Fig. 1). The observation that many of these genes encode cell-cell signaling factors emphasizes the importance of interactions among several cell lineages to initiate cardiac left-right development. The above section outlined the interactions between the LRC region and cells in the node. Although cardiac progenitor cells transiently pass through the node during gastrulation,[2] cell lineages derived from the LRC region, the node and the midline (notochord and neural floorplate) do not contribute cells directly to the developing heart.

The node appears to play a central role in the development of the embryonic axes, as exemplified by classic experiments in which transplanted nodes are capable of organizing an embryonic axis de novo.[3] This powerful group of cells, called the Organizer, expresses a variety of signaling molecules.[4,5] The node is the point at which cells ingress into the embryo during gastrulation, forming the an-

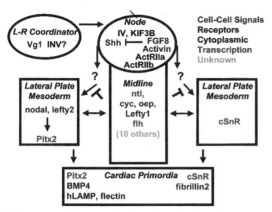

Figure 1. Summary of the proposed embryonic tissue interactions and some of the genes involved in establishing cardiac left-right orientation. Black labels and boxes or ovals indicate the embryonic regions that have roles in left-right development, diagrammed with left-sided regions on the left side of the figure and midline regions in the center. These regions include the Left-Right coordinator, the node (with monocilia) and midline (notochord and floorplate) regions, left and right lateral plate mesoderm, and cardiac primordia. Early genes are placed at the top of the figure, late genes at the bottom. Genes are color-coded by their actions and cell locations, as cell-cell signaling proteins (purple), transmembrane receptors for cell-cell signaling proteins (blue), cytoplasmic proteins (green), transcription factors (red), or unknown functions (orange). For references to individual genes, see review by Ramsdell and Yost.[56]

teroposterior axis. Cells from the node give rise to the notochord, ventral floorplate of the neural tube, hypochord and roof of the archenteron at the embryonic midline. Subsequently, these midline cells have central roles in dorsoventral axis formation, such as patterning of the neural tube and somites, as well as anteroposterior patterning in neural development.

Recent studies implicate the node as a pivotal player in left-right axis formation. In the chick, several genes are asymmetrically expressed in the node. Sonic hedgehog, a cell-cell signaling protein, is expressed on the left.[6] RNAs encoding a subunit of the activin transmembrane receptor, cActRIIa,[6] and the cell-signaling protein FGF8[7] are expressed on the right. There is strong evidence that the hedgehog signaling pathway instructs subsequent left-right development in avian embryos. Experiments that place sonic hedgehog signals on the right side, opposite the normal expression, or that inhibit sonic hedgehog signaling with a blocking antibody, result in altered left-right.[6,8] Disappointingly, the asymmetric gene expression patterns seen in nodes of chick embryos have not been found in nodes of other vertebrates. This could be due to limits of detection or could reflect the possibility that similar pathways are regulated at post-transcriptional levels in other vertebrates, such asymmetric protein distribution or function could arise from symmetrically expressed RNA.

In *Xenopus*, experimental induction of conjoined twins also suggests a role for the organizer in left-right development.[9-11] In conjoined twins, typically the twin on the left has normal laterality development and the twin on the right has complex anomalies. It is not known whether this is due to influences of the organizers or midlines during early development.[12]

In mice, mutants of left-right dynein (LRD)[13] or kinesin KIF3B have left-right developmental defects.[14] RNAs from these genes are expressed symmetrically in the node, as well as in some other locations during early development. These genes are members of families of multifunctional molecular motor proteins. While neither LRD or KIF3B RNAs have been reported to have asymmetric expression patterns along the prospective left-right axis, the distributions of these motor proteins within cells has not been described. Other members of the dynein and kinesin families have been shown to move in opposite directions along microtubules,[15,16] suggesting that intracellular movement of LRD or KIF3B proteins could result in left-right asymmetric distribution within cells, if microtubules are consistently aligned within the node cells.

There are at least two possible roles for motor proteins in left-right development. First, they could move vesicles along cytoskeleton within cells or enable cells to exocytose vesicles that contain signaling molecules. Vesicle movement could provide an asymmetric distribution of information within cells or could transmit, via motor-dependent transcytosis, information to neighboring cells. LRD RNA is present before gastrulation and could redistribute information along the left-right axis by an intracellular mechanism.[13] If these motor molecules are involved in exocytosis, information could be transmitted to other cells, including lateral mesoderm and cardiac mesoderm progenitors, as they transiently pass through the node during gastrulation. Second, the roles of kinesin and dynein motor molecules in the node could be to move cilia at the surface of cells. A specialized monocilium has been described on node cells in chick and mice embryos.[14,17,18] Monocilia within the node appear to be capable of moving extracellular particles in an asymmetric direction and are defective in KIF3B mutants.[14] Monocilia movement could either asymmetrically distribute extracellular signaling information or serve as a barrier, preventing dispersal of information across the midline. The identity of this extracellular information is unknown, but it is clear that it is subcellular in size. There appears to be very little movement of cells across the midline, from one side of the embryo to the contralateral side.[19,20] The issues of the roles of motor molecules, vesicle transport and monocilia function, will be addressed by analysis in mouse embryos that have mutations in other early genes such as IV (LRD) and INV, which encodes a ankyrin-domain protein of unknown function.[21–23] inv/inv mutants have inverted left-right axis orientation,[21] and it might be predicted that monocilia movement is reversed in these mutants. Furthermore, analysis of node cells in other vertebrates will assess whether these mechanisms are conserved. With any of these proposed mechanisms, it would not be surprising if additional members of protein motor families are found to have roles in left-right development.

Through the process of gastrulation, node cells give rise to embryonic midline structures including notochord, prospective ventral floorplate of the neural tube, and hypochord. Observations in several vertebrate systems indicate that cells in the embryonic midline are crucial for maintaining normal left-right patterning after gastrulation is complete. Removal of midline cells at the open neural plate stages in *Xenopus* results in bilateral expression of Xnr-1 (nodal) in the lateral plate mesoderm and randomization of heart left-right orientation.[24–26] Removal of midline cells after neural tube closure does not perturb left-right development, suggesting the midline cells are necessary for left-right development only during open neural plate stages.[24]

Outstanding genetic evidence confirms the embryological evidence for midline regulation of left-right development. In zebrafish, a large number of mutant lines that have defects in midline development also have defects in cardiac left-right gene expression patterns[27] and loop morphogenesis.[24,27] Two of the genes, *no tail* and *floating head*, implicated in left-right development[24] encode transcription regulation factors expressed in the midline.[28,29] Many of the zebrafish genes identified by mutation await additional molecular analysis and will provide a superb system for discovering the epistatic relationships of a large number of genes in the pathway common to midline and laterality development.

In mice, Lefty1, a member of the TGFb superfamily, is expressed on the left side of the prospective ventral floorplate.[30] Targeted mutagenesis of Lefty1 results in bilateral expression of downstream genes that are normally expressed on the left side and in thoracic left isomerism.[31] Other mice mutants, such as *no turning* and *brachyury*, also show a link between midline defects and perturbed left-right development.[32,33] In humans, some X-linked laterality anomalies result from mutation of ZIC3.[34] ZIC3 is a member of the odd-paired family of zinc-finger transcription factors, is expressed in the midline in mice and Xenopus embryos, and has roles in early neural development.[35,36]

The linkage of specific stages of midline development with cardiac left-right development has important clinical implications.[12] Examination of clinical records found that there are statistically significant associations between laterality anomalies and midline anomalies in humans.[37] These findings open for consideration the possibility that maternal nutritional supplementation that alleviates some midline developmental defects might also help promote normal left-right cardiac development.

Left-Right Orientation Is Specified in Cardiac Primordia Long Before Looping Morphogenesis Occurs

Two complementary approaches, explantation and assessment of asymmetric gene expression patterns, indicate that left-right specification occurs early both in lateral plate mesoderm (LPM) and in the cardiac progenitor fields. Nodal and lefty, members of the TGFβ family of cell-signaling proteins, are expressed in left sided LPM. Explants of LPM, from either frog[25,26,38] or chick,[8,38] can express nodal asymmetrically, depending on what other tissues, including midline and pre-somitic tissues, are co-cultured with the LPM explants. In *Xenopus*, explants of cardiac primordia shortly after gastrulation result in formation of a cardiac tube, but the orientation of the cardiac tube is random. Explants of cardiac primordia taken a few hours later, as the neural tube is closing, form a cardiac tube that is looped in the normal left-right orientation.[24] In *Xenopus* explants, co-culture with midline cells results in suppression of nodal expression in LPM, suggesting that signals from the midline can actively suppress specification in the lateral plate mesoderm.[26] Together, these results indicate that left-right orientation is specified during the stages of neural tube closure by signals from the midline and intervening tissues, long before the cardiac primordia form a cardiac tube.

Expression of nodal in the left LPM occurs during analogous developmental stages in chick, mouse, frog and zebrafish.[6,39–42] Lefty2, another member of the TGFβ family, is expressed in similar patterns in mouse and zebrafish lateral plate mesoderm.[30,43–45] Apparently downstream of these asymmetric expression patterns, the putative transcription factor Pitx-2 is induced and asymmetrically expressed in the left mesoderm, including the left side of some of the precardiac mesoderm, in all vertebrate embryos examined to date.[31,46–51] Another putative transcription factor, cSnR, a member of the Snail family of zinc finger proteins, is expressed in the right LPM in the absence of Nodal signaling.[52] Within the heart fields, cell-matrix or cell signaling proteins are expressed asymmetrically, perhaps in response to these upstream transcription regulatory factors. In chick, JB3 (a fibrillin-related protein) is expressed on the right and hLAMP1 (heart-specific lectin-associated matrix protein-1) on the left.[53] Flectin, a large extracellular matrix protein, is expressed on the left side in the chick heart primordia throughout looping[54] and has a distinct and dynamic asymmetric expression pattern during murine cardiac tube looping.[55]

To What Extent Is the Genetic Pathway to Cardiac Left-Right Specification Conserved in Vertebrates?

It is becoming clear that gene expression patterns (e.g., Nodal, Lefty2, and Pitx-2) are highly conserved in LPM or in cardiac primordia during the developmental period of cardiac left-right specification. Thus, it is likely that the developmental mechanisms immediately preceding specification of cardiac left-right orientation, and the mechanisms that occur during early morphogenesis of cardiac left-right asymmetry, are conserved in vertebrates. However, it is unclear whether earlier events in the establishment of the left-right body plan, which eventually impinge upon specification of left-right orientation in the cardiac primordia, are conserved. It is quite plausible that diverse mechanisms early in vertebrate development converge upon common themes of specifying left-right orientation in lateral plate and precardiac mesoderm. The question of the early developmental pathways that establish the left-right body axis will be the target of significant research activity in the next five years.

References

1. Yost HJ. Regulation of vertebrate left-right asymmetries by extracellular matrix. *Nature* 1992;357:158–161.
2. Garcia-Martinez V, Schoenwolf GC. Primitive-streak origin of the cardiovascular system in avian embryos. *Dev Biol* 1993;159:706–719.
3. Spemann, H. *Embryonic Development and Induction.* New York: Hafner; 1938.
4. Lemaire P, Kodjabachian L. The vertebrate organizer—Structure and molecules. *Trends Genet* 1996;12:525–531.
5. Smith JL, Schoenwolf GC. Getting organized: New insights into the organizer of higher vertebrates. *Curr Top Dev Biol* 1998;40:79–110.
6. Levin M, Johnson RL, Stern CD, et al. A molecular pathway determining left-right asymmetry in chick embryogenesis. *Cell* 1995;82:803–814.
7. Boettger T, Wittler L, Kessel M. FGF8 functions in the specification of the right body side of the chick. *Curr Biol* 1999;9:277–280.
8. Pagan-Westphal SM, Tabin CJ. The transfer of left-right positional information during chick embryogenesis. *Cell* 1998;93:25–35.
9. Hyatt BA, Lohr JL, Yost HJ. Initiation of vertebrate left-right axis formation by maternal vg1. *Nature* 1996;384:62–65.
10. Nascone N, Mercola M. Organizer induction determines left-right asymmetry in Xenopus. *Dev Biol* 1997;189:68–78.
11. Hyatt BA, Yost HJ. The left-right coordinator: The role of Vg1 in organizing left-right axis formation. *Cell* 1998;93:37–46.

12. Yost HJ. The genetics of midline and cardiac laterality defects. *Curr Opin Cardiol* 1998;13:185–189.
13. Supp DM, Witte DP, Potter SS, et al. Mutation of an axonemal dynein affects left-right asymmetry in inversus viscerum mice. *Nature* 1997;389:963–966.
14. Nonaka S, Tanaka Y, Okada Y, et al. Randomization of left-right asymmetry due to loss of nodal cilia generating leftward flow of extraembryonic fluid in mice lacking KIF3B motor protein. *Cell* 1998;95:829–837.
15. Vallee RB, Gee MA. Make room for dynein. *Trends Cell Biol* 1998;8:490–494.
16. Hirokawa N. Kinesin and dynein superfamily proteins and the mechanism of organelle transport. *Science* 1998;279:519–526.
17. Sulik K, Dehart DB, Iangaki T, et al. Morphogenesis of the murine node and notochordal plate. *Dev Dyn* 1994;201:260–278.
18. Bellomo D, Lander A, Harragan I, et al. Cell proliferation in mammalian gastrulation: The ventral node and notochord are relatively quiescent. *Dev Dyn* 1996;205:471–485.
19. Schoenwolf GC, Garcia-Martinez V, Dias MS. Mesoderm movement and fate during avian gastrulation and neurulation. *Dev Dyn* 1992;193:235–248.
20. Levy V, Khaner O. Limited left-right cell migration across the midline of the gastrulating avian embryo. *Dev Genet* 1998;23:175–184.
21. Yokoyama T, Copeland NG, Jenkins NA, et al. Reversal of left-right asymmetry: A situs inversus mutation. *Science* 1993;260:679–682.
22. Mochizuki T, Saijoh Y, Tsuchiya K, et al. Cloning of inv, a gene that controls left/right asymmetry and kidney development (in process citation). *Nature* 1998;395:177–181.
23. Morgan D, Turnpenny L, Goodship J, et al. Inversin, a novel gene in the vertebrate left-right axis pathway, is partially deleted in the inv mouse [published erratum appears in *Nat Genet* 1998;20:312]. *Nat Genet* 1998;20:149–156.
24. Danos MC, Yost HJ. Role of notochord in specification of cardiac left-right orientation in zebrafish and *Xenopus. Dev Biol* 1996;177:96–103.
25. Lohr JL, Danos MC, Yost HJ. Left-right asymmetry of a nodal-related gene is regulated by dorsoanterior midline structures

during *Xenopus* development. *Development* 1997;124:1465–1472.

26. Lohr JL, Danos MC, Groth TW, et al. Maintenance of asymmetric nodal expression in *Xenopus laevis*. *Dev Genet* this issue, 1998.

27. Chen JN, van Eeden FJ, Warren KS, et al. Left-right pattern of cardiac BMP4 may drive asymmetry of the heart in zebrafish. *Development* 1997;124:4373–4382.

28. Schulte-Merker S, van Eeden FJM, Halpern ME, et al. *no tail (ntl)* is the zebrafish homologue of the mouse *T (Brachyury)* gene. *Development* 1994;120:1009–1015.

29. Talbot WS, Trevarrow B, Halpern ME, et al. A homeobox gene essential for zebrafish notochord development. *Nature* 1995;378:150–157.

30. Meno C, Saijoh Y, Fujii H, et al. Left-right asymmetric expression of the tgf-beta-family member lefty in mouse embryos. *Nature* 1996;381:151–155.

31. Meno C, Shimono A, Saijoh Y, et al. lefty-1 is required for left-right determination as a regulator of lefty-2 and nodal. *Cell* 1998; 94:287–297.

32. Melloy PG, Ewart JL, Cohen MF, et al. No turning, a mouse mutation causing left-right and axial patterning defects. *Dev Biol* 1998;193:77–89.

33. King T, Beddington RSP, Brown NA. The role of the brachyurany gene in heart development and left-right specification in the mouse. *Mech Dev* 1998;79:29–37.

34. Gebbia M, Ferrero GB, Pilia G, et al. X-linked situs abnormalities result from mutations in ZIC3. *Nat Genet* 1997;17:305–308.

35. Nagai T, Aruga J, Takada S, et al. The expression of the mouse Zic1, Zic2, and Zic3 gene suggests an essential role for Zic genes in body pattern formation. *Dev Biol* 1997;182:299–313.

36. Nakata K, Nagai T, Aruga J, et al. *Xenopus* Zic3, a primary regulator both in neural and neural crest development. *Proc Natl Acad Sci U S A* 1997;94:11980–11985.

37. Goldstein AM, Ticho BS, Fishman MC. Patterning the heart's left-right axis: From zebrafish to man. *Dev Genet* 1998; 22:278–287.

38. Levin M, Mercola M. Evolutionary conservation of mechanisms upstream of asymmetric Nodal expression: Reconciling chick and *Xenopus*. *Dev Genet* 1998; 23:185–193.

39. Lowe LA, Supp DM, Sampath K, et al. Conserved left-right asymmetry of nodal expression and alterations in murine situs inversus. *Nature* 1996;381:158–161.

40. Lustig KD, Kroll K, Sun E, et al. A *Xenopus* nodal-related gene that acts in synergy with noggin to induce complete secondary axis and notochord formation. *Development* 1996;122:3275–3282.

41. Erter CE, Solnica-Krezel L, Wright CV. Zebrafish nodal-related 2 encodes an early mesendodermal inducer signaling from the extraembryonic yolk syncytial layer. *Dev Biol* 1998;204:361–372.

42. Feldman B, Gates MA, Egan ES, et al. Zebrafish organizer development and germ-layer formation require nodal-related signals. *Nature* 1998;395:181–185.

43. Meno C, Ito Y, Saijoh Y, et al. Two closely-related left-right asymmetrically expressed genes, lefty-1 and lefty-2: Their distinct expression domains, chromosomal linkage and direct neuralizing activity in *Xenopus* embryos. *Genes Cells* 1997;2: 513–524.

44. Thisse C, Thisse B. Antivin, a novel and divergent member of the TGFbeta super-family, negatively regulates mesoderm induction. *Development* 1999;126:229–240.

45. Bisgrove B, Essner J, Yost HJ. Regulation of midline development by antagonism of *lefty* and *nodal* signaling. *Development* 1999 (in press).

46. St Amand TR, Ra J, Zhang Y, et al. Cloning and expression pattern of chicken Pitx2: A new component in the SHH signaling pathway controlling embryonic heart looping. *Biochem Biophys Res Commun* 1998;247:100–105.

47. Piedra ME, Icardo JM, Albajar M, et al. Pitx2 participates in the late phase of the pathway controlling left-right asymmetry. *Cell* 1998;94:319–324.

48. Ryan AK, Blumberg B, Rodriguez-Esteban C, et al. Pitx2 determines left-right asymmetry of internal organs in vertebrates. *Nature* 1998;394:545–551.

49. Yoshioka H, Meno C, Koshiba K, et al. Pitx2, a bicoid-type homeobox gene, is involved in a lefty-signaling pathway in determination of left-right asymmetry. *Cell* 1998;94:299–305.

50. Logan M, Pagan-Westphal SM, Smith DM, et al. The transcription factor Pitx2 mediates situs-specific morphogenesis in response to left-right asymmetric signals. *Cell* 1998;94:307–317.

51. Campione M, Steinbeisser H, Schweickert A, et al. The homeobox gene Pitx2: Mediator of asymmetric left-right signaling in vertebrate heart and gut looping. *Development* 1999;126:1225–1234.
52. Isaac A, Sargent MG, Cooke J. Control of vertebrate left-right asymmetry by a snail-related zinc finger gene. *Science* 1997;275:1301–1304.
53. Smith SM, Dickman ED, Thompson RP, et al. Retinoic acid directs cardiac laterality and the expression of early markers of precardiac asymmetry. *Dev Biol* 1997;182:162–171.
54. Tsuda T, Philp N, Zile MH, et al. Left-right asymmetric localization of flectin in the extracellular matrix during heart looping. *Dev Biol* 1996;173:39–50.
55. Tsuda T, Majumder K, Linask KK. Differential expression of flectin in the extracellular matrix and left-right asymmetry in mouse embryonic heart during looping stages. *Dev Genet* 1998;23:203–214.
56. Ramsdell AF, Yost HJ. Molecular mechanisms of vertebrate left-right development. *Trends Genet* 1998;14:459–465.

2

Motor Proteins and the Development of LR Asymmetry

Dorothy M. Supp, MD, S. Steven Potter, MD,
James McGrath, MD, and Martina Brueckner, MD

The development of handed asymmetry across the left-right (LR) axis is an essential and unique process in vertebrate development. Especially the heart is dependent on correct LR positional cues for normal morphogenesis. The first connection between motor proteins and the development of LR asymmetry was made by Bjorn Afzelius,[1] when he observed several male patients with immotile sperm, non-functional tracheal cilia and complete situs inversus. This triad is called Kartagener syndrome, and ultrastructural analysis of cilia in patients with Kartagener syndrome demonstrated an absence of outer dynein arms. These patients appear to have a defect in one of the components of the minus-end directed microtubule motor, dynein. This provided an obvious explanation for the infertility and ciliary dysfunction: in the absence of outer dynein arms, the motive force required to directionally bend tracheal or sperm cilia cannot be generated, and the cilia are immotile. This results in the inability to effectively clear respiratory secretions and in immotile sperm. Several hypotheses on the connection between absent dynein arms and situs inversus were

made, including that there are directionally motile cilia during early embryogenesis that actually move developing organs to one side of the embryo or the other.

Two independent mouse mutations also point to a pivotal role for motor proteins in the development of LR asymmetry. A targeted mutation of a plus-end directed microtubule motor, KIF3B, in the mouse also results in defective development of LR asymmetry, indicating that dynein is not the only microtubule-associated motor involved in the development of LR asymmetry.[2] Unlike patients with Kartagener syndrome, the KIF3B $-/-$ mice die at embryonic day 9.5. They have multiple abnormalities including severe pericardial swelling and growth failure, suggesting that KIF3B has important developmental functions beyond the generation of LR asymmetry. The molecular marker *lefty*, that is normally localized on the left in the developing embryo, is found on both sides of the KIF3 $-/-$ embryos, suggesting a complete failure to generate asymmetry across the LR axis. KIF3B, along with a second motor protein KIF3A and a non-motor protein comprise the heterotrimeric kinesin complex that has been shown to be important in intraflagellar transport and ciliary assembly in sea urchin and Chlamydomonas.[3] In the KIF3B $-/-$ mice, the monocilia normally found on the ventral node cells are absent.[2]

The mouse *iv* mutation, which results in random orientation of organs across

From Clark EB, Nakazawa M, Takao A (eds.): Etiology and Morphogenesis of Congenital Heart Disease: Twenty Years of Progress in Genetics and Developmental Biology. Armonk, NY: Futura Publishing Co., Inc.; © 2000.

the LR axis in otherwise normal liveborn mice[4,5] is also a mutation in a motor protein: left-right dynein (lrd), a member of the axonemal dynein heavy chain family.[6] Dyneins are microtubule-based motors that motor toward the microtubule minus end. They are large proteins comprising 1 to 3 heavy chains and many medium and light chains that determine cargo specificity and may serve to regulate motor function. The heavy chains each contain four force-generating ATPase domains and are responsible for dynein motor function itself. The iv mutation is a point mutation affecting the motor domain of lrd between the 2nd and 3rd ATPase domains. A significant number of iv/iv homozygous mice die of unknown causes between e7.5 and e8.5, or of congenital cardiac defects associated with abnormal LR development between e14 and e18.[7] In contrast to the KIF3B defective mice, iv/iv mice do however develop asymmetry of normally asymmetric markers such as nodal and lefty. This asymmetry in iv/iv mice is randomly oriented relative to the anteroposterior and dorsoventral axes, reflecting the random asymmetry of LR organ position observed in liveborn iv/iv mice.[8,9]

In order to further define the role of cilia and motor proteins in the establishment of LR asymmetry, we have generated an additional mutation in lrd by targeted mutagenesis in mice and examined the phenotype and cilia of both mutations.

Results

Targeted Mutagenesis of LR Dynein

A targeting construct to create the lrd Δ^{P1} allele was created by replacing the two exons encoding the first ATPase domain (P-Loop) of lrd with the neomycin resistance gene. This construct permitted in-frame splicing across the deleted exons to produce a mutant RNA deleted only of the first P-loop (Supp et al, unpublished results). As the first P-loop is essential for dynein motor function, the targeted lrd gene would encode a protein unable to catalyze ATP hydrolysis and without motor function. Three independent ES cell lines that had demonstrated homologous recombination by PCR and Southern blotting were used to generate homozygous targeted mice by standard techniques.

Gross Anatomic Ohenotype of lrd Δ^{P1}/Δ^{P1} Mice

Intercrosses of heterozygous lrd $\Delta^{P1}/+$ mice produced 11.9% liveborn offspring with situs inversus. This does not differ significantly from the expected 12.5%, and indicates the absence of any embryonic lethality, in marked contrast to that observed with the iv mutation. Anatomic analysis of 31 liveborn lrd Δ^{P1}/Δ^{P1} mice revealed that 15 demonstrated complete situs solitus, 12 had mirror-image situs inversus and 4 had varying degrees of heterotaxy. Notably, no anatomic defects outside of defects of LR organ positioning were noted in any of the lrd Δ^{P1}/Δ^{P1} mice examined.

Microscopic Analysis of Cilia in iv/iv and lrd Δ^{P1}/Δ^{P1} Mice

Neither iv/iv or lrd Δ^{P1}/Δ^{P1} mice suffer from respiratory illnesses or male infertility. Consistent with the absence of ciliary symptoms, examination of tracheal cilia of mice with both lrd mutations showed normal ultrastructure and motility. The single cilium found on the ventral cells of the node at e7.5 was studied by scanning electron microscopy and immunohistochemistry with an anti-acetylated tubulin antibody. This antibody specifically decorates stable microtubule structures such as cytoplasmic bridges and monocilia. Both methods demonstrated normal size and distribution of monocilia on the ventral node cells of iv/iv and lrd Δ^{P1}/Δ^{P1} mice (Fig. 1). The node monocilia of e7.5 wild-type and lrd Δ^{P1}/Δ^{P1} mice were observed by videomicroscopy. While the wild-type cilia moved in a vortical motion, the lrd Δ^{P1}/Δ^{P1} node monocilia were

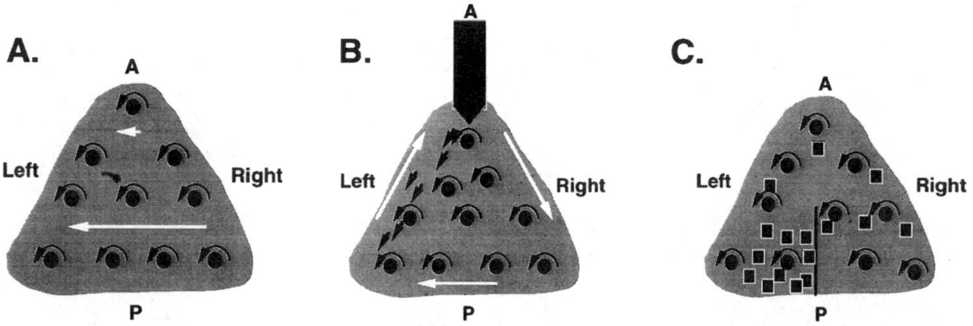

Figure 1. Three models for the generation of organismal LR asymmetry by counterclockwise motion of the node monocilia. **A.** A net leftward flow is generated by the currents produced by a gradient of cilia extending from the anterior apex of the triangular node to the posterior base. **B.** A factor that diffuses from the anterior end of the node is initially moved to the left side by counterclockwise flow. **C.** A factor accumulates at the left side by the interaction of counterclockwise flow and an impermeable midline barrier.

rigid, with even very little Brownian motion (Supp et al, unpublished results).

Discussion

The lrd Δ^{P1}/Δ^{P1} mutation is unique among mutations that affect the development of LR asymmetry in that it represents a pure defect of LR development. There is no associated embryonic lethality such as that observed with the *iv* mutation. In addition, lrd Δ^{P1}/Δ^{P1} mice have no defects of antero-posterior or midline development such as those observed with many other mutations that also affect LR development. This indicates that lrd motor function is essential for LR development alone, and that the LR axis defect in lrd Δ^{P1}/Δ^{P1} mice is not secondary to defective AP or midline development. There is only a single observable defect in the lrd Δ^{P1}/Δ^{P1} mice: rigor of the node monocilia. This observation lends strong support to the hypothesis that vortical motion of node monocilia is essential to the development of LR asymmetry.[2] Therefore, bilateral symmetry is broken at the node at the time of gastrulation. Handedness is provided to the organism by the chirality of the cilium itself, which is oriented relative to the antero-posterior and dorsoventral axes. Assembly of the node mono-

cilia requires heterotrimeric kinesin KIF3A. The macromolecular chirality of the cilium is then converted to organismal asymmetry by the *lrd* driven ciliary motility. Several models can be proposed to explain how counterclockwise motion of the peri-nodal fluid results in downstream asymmetry (Fig. 2). The first of these invokes the antero-posterior asymmetry of the node itself to create net leftward flow of fluid.[2] In the second, a factor is secreted from the anterior end of the node; counterclockwise flow then moves this factor to cells on the left side of the node first.[10] Finally, an impermeable midline barrier coupled with counterclockwise flow could lead to accumulation of a soluble factor on the left side of node.

Node monocilia are not classical motile cilia with nine outer microtubule doublets and two inner microtubule doublets; they lack the inner microtubule doublet and thereby more closely resemble nonmotile monocilia.[11] Their vortical motion also differs strikingly from the bending movements of 9+2 microtubules found in ciliated epithelium. The mechanism by which an outer-arm axonemal dynein such as *lrd* drives node monociliary motility remains unclear. It is possible that these cilia represent a unique class of cilia, "embryonic cilia," which use vortical

A.   **B.**

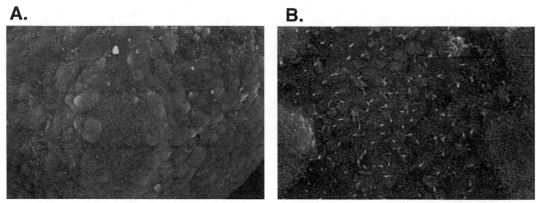

Figure 2. Scanning electron microscopy of the node of an e7.5 *iv/iv* embryo. **A.** (500X) The node is triangular in shape with a population of central pit cells. **B.** (2,000X) There is a monocilium on each of the pit cells.-

motion to drive directed movement of extracellular substances during embryogenesis.

References

1. Afzelius BA. A human syndrome caused by immotile cilia. *Science* 1976;193:317–319.
2. Nonaka S, Tanaka Y, Okada Y, et al. Randomization of left-right asymmetry due to loss of nodal cilia generating leftward flow of extraembryonic fluid in mice lacking KIF3B motor protein. *Cell* 1998;95:829–837.
3. Morris RL, Scholey JM. Heterotrimeric kinesin-II is required for the assembly of motile 9+2 ciliary axonemes on sea urchin embryos. *J. Cell Biol* 1997;138:1009–1022.
4. Hummel KP, Chapman DB. Visceral inversion and associated anomalies in the mouse. *J Hered* 1959;50:9–13.
5. Layton WM. Random determination of a developmental process. *J Hered* 1976;67:336–338.
6. Supp DM, Witte DP, Potter SS, et al. Mutation of an axonemal dynein affects left-right asymmetry in inversus viscerum mice. *Nature* 1997;389:963–966.
7. Icardo JM, Sanchez de Vega MJ. Spectrum of heart malformations in mice with situs solitus, situs inversus, and associated visceral heterotaxy. *Circulation* 1991;84:2547–2558.
8. Lowe LA, Supp DM, Sampath K, et al. Conserved left-right asymmetry of *nodal* expression and alterations in murine situs inversus. *Nature* 1996;381:158–161.
9. Collignon J, Varlet I, Robertson EJ. Relationship between asymmetric *nodal* expression and the direction of embryonic turning. *Nature* 1996;381:155–158.
10. Vogan KJ, Tabin CJ. A new spin on handed asymmetry. *Nature* 1999;397:295–298.
11. Wheatley DN, Wang AM, Strugnell GE. Expression of primary cilia in mammalian cells. *Cell Biol Int* 1996;20:73–81.

3

Expression of the inv Gene During Development and Intracellular Localization of the inv Protein

Takahiko Yokoyama, MD, Yasuaki Shirayoshi, MD,
Touru Murakami, MD, and Norio Nakatsuji, MD,

Though the left and the right side of the vertebrate body are externally symmetrical, almost all internal structures show marked left/right (L/R) asymmetry such as left sided stomach and heart, and more lung lobes in the right side than that in the left side. In mice and humans, several mutants in which these asymmetries are reversed have been known.

The inv mutation was found in a family of transgenic mice carrying tyrosinase minigene.[1,2] The inv mouse is unique because homozygous inv mice show a consistent reversal of L/R polarity.[2-5] The inv mutant is caused by insertional mutation that destroyed an essential gene or genes to establish handed asymmetry. We have identified a novel gene located at the transgenic integration site. Furthermore, the introduction of the gene under a ubiquitous promoter (β-actin promoter) completely cures all abnormalities associated with the inv mouse, providing the evidence that the cloned gene is responsible for all the inv phenotypes including inversion of L/R asymmetry and cyst formation of the kidney.[6] The inv protein encodes 1062 amino acids and 15 successive repeats of about 33 amino ac-

ids (Ank/swi 6) motif in its N-terminus and two bipartite nuclear localization signals in C-terminus.[6,7]

To understand its role in establishment of L/R polarity, we studied a pattern of the inv gene expression during development by whole mount in situ hybridization. We also studied intracellular localization of the inv protein.

Mouse embryos were collected at day 7.5 and 8.5 after mating. Whole-mount in situ hybridization[8] at embryonic day 7.5 shows that the inv gene expresses embryo proper but not extraembryonic tissue (Fig. 1A, B). [Whole-mount in situ hybridization was performed in the following manner: Embryos were collected from randomly bred ICR mice. For stages of pregnancy, the day of vaginal plug detection was designated as embryonic day 0.5. Digoxigenin-labeled (Boehringer, Mannheim, Germany) probe was generated with SP6 RNA polymerase (anti-sense) or T7 RNA polymerase (sense) from a 2.5-kb EcoRI-HindIII fragment of clone 28. Whole-mount in situ hybridizations were performed at high stringency.] Area that is to be the future neural plate does not show strong staining (Fig. 1B). At day 8.5, the staining is symmetrically observed in the whole embryo (Fig. 1C, D). No asymmetric expression was observed in embryos examined.

From Clark EB, Nakazawa M, Takao A (eds.): Etiology and Morphogenesis of Congenital Heart Disease: Twenty Years of Progress in Genetics and Developmental Biology. Armonk, NY: Futura Publishing Co., Inc.; © 2000.

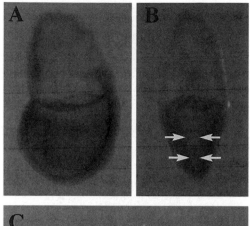

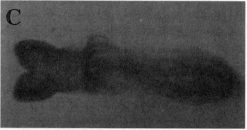

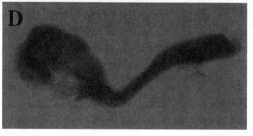

Figure 1. Whole-mount in situ hybridization. **A, B.** Day 7.5 embryos (**A:** side view; **B:** frontal view). White arrows indicate the area that shows weak staining. **C, D.** Day 8.5 embryos (**C:** ventral view; **D:** side view)

Because the inv protein does not have any signal peptide, it is thought to be intracellular protein. To study intracellular localization of the inv protein, we made green fluorescent protein (GFP)-inv fusion construct. [Construction of GFP-inv fusion construct: N-terminal region of the mouse inv gene between nucleotide 58 and 824, was amplified by PCR to generate *Bam*HI site at the N-terminus. The fragment was inserted into pGEX2 (Pharmacia & Upjohn, Kalamzoo, MI, USA). The resultant clone was digested with *Pst*I and *Xba*I and this region was replaced with *Pst*I-*Xba*I fragment of clone

28–17. Next, this clone (named Ex-inv 1) was digested with *Xba*I and *Eco*RI. A 2.0-kb *Xba*I-*Eco*RI fragment of clone 28 was inserted into *Xba*I-*Eco*RI sites of Ex-inv1 and named Ex-inv3. Approximately 3.0 kb *Bam*HI-*Eco*RI fragment of Ex-inv3 was inserted into *Bgl*II-*Eco*RI site of EGFP-C1 (Clontech Palo Alto, CA) and named GFP-inv3. The ggs-inv[6] was digested with *Apa*I and *Bam*HI. *Apa*I-*Bam*HI fragment of ggs-inv was inserted into *Apa*I-*Bam*HI sites of GFP-inv 3. The resultant clone was named GFP-inv 5. A junction between GFP and inv gene was sequenced and confirmed to have a correct reading frame.] The advantage to using GFP is that we can observe fusion protein localization under fluorescent microscopy without any treatment.

We transfected GFP-inv fusion construct into cos-7 cells with lipofectin (GibcoBRL, Sparks, MD, USA). (The cos-7 cells are maintained in minimal essential medium supplemented with 5% FCS. Transfection was performed according to a manufacture provided protocol.) Fluorescent signals were observed the next day under fluorescent microscopy. Signals were localized in the cytoplasm, especially surrounding the nucleus (Fig. 2). Although the deduced amino acid sequence of the inv gene product predicts two bipartite nuclear localization signals, we hardly observed signals in the nucleus. In the cytoplasm, we observed two patterns of signals, granular (Fig. 2A, B) and fibrous (Fig. 2C, D).

Up to now, a variety of genes have been found to be involved in establishment of L/R asymmetry. These genes could be classified into two groups. One group is genes that are expressed asymmetrically or work at one side. In mice, this group includes lefty, nodal and PitX2.[9–12] Genes in this group work at late stages of L/R establishment. The other includes genes that are expressed or work at midline structure. Genes that belong to this group are iv and KIF3B. In mice, iv is shown to be located upstream of nodal, lefty and Pitx2 in a genetic pathway to determine the L/R asymmetry. The iv gene has been cloned and shown to

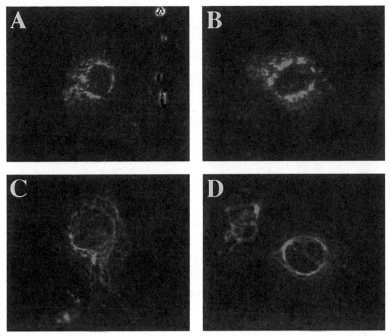

Figure 2. Intracellular localization of GFP-inv fusion protein in cos-7 cells. Two types of GFP signals: granular (**A, B**) and fibrous (**C, D**).

encode a member of dynein named left-right dynein (lrd).[13] The iv gene is expressed in the node, therefore, it is thought to work at the node. The other gene, KIF3B, which encodes kinesin family, is also involved in establishment of L/R asymmetry[14] and works upstream of lefty gene. A KIF3B knockout mouse shows abnormality in node cilia. Abnormal node cilia are suggested to cause abnormal L/R asymmetry.

In the present study, we did not detect asymmetrical expression of the inv. Combined with the rescue experiment result in which a ubiquitous β-actin promoter was used,[6] we concluded that the inv gene does not need asymmetric expression to establish left/right asymmetry. The pattern of the inv expression is unique because it is expressed uniformly in the embryos. The inv is shown to be located upstream of nodal, lefty, and Pitx2-like lrd and KIF3B. It is entirely unknown how the inv protein interacts with lrd and KIF3B, which work at the node. Recent chick experiments suggested that the node does not create the initial left/right information, rather the surrounding tissue gives the initial left/right information to the node.[15] It is possible that the inv protein works at tissue surrounding the node and gives some signal to the node.

There are two other possibilities. First, the inv works at the node together with iv and KIF3B. The other possibility is that the inv receives some signals from iv and KIF3B. In this situation, the inv is expected to work at tissue surrounding the node. Because inv expression was observed almost uniformly in the embryo, we are unable to exclude these possibilities.

Cell transfection results indicate that the GFP-inv fusion protein is localized in the cytoplasm, suggesting that the protein may work at the cytoplasm. It is unclear what two types of signals means. A fibrous signal pattern may suggest the interaction between the inv protein and cytoskeleton. We could not exclude a possibility that the inv protein works at the nucleus. In this experiment, we use cos-7 cell that is SV40 transformed kidney epithelial-like cells. The protein may localize in different places in different cell types. In addition, localization of the protein may change according to cell cycles.

Although the inv gene is essential to establish normal left/right asymmetry, it is still a mystery how the inv gene functions.

References

1. Yokoyama T, Silverside DW, Waymire KG, et al. Conserved cysteine to serine mutation in tyrosinase is responsible for the classical albino mutation in laboratory mice. *Nucl Acids Res* 1990;18:7293–7298.
2. Yokoyama T, Copeland NG, Jenkins NA, et al. Reversal of left-right asymmetry: A situs inversus mutation. *Science* 1993;263:679–681.
3. Lowe LA, Supp DM, Sampath K, et al. Conserved left-right asymmetry of nodal expression and alterations in murine situs inversus. *Nature* 1996;381:158–161.
4. Meno C, Saijoh H, Fujii H, et al. Left-right asymmetric expression of the TGFb-family member in mouse embryos. *Nature* 1996;381:151–155.
5. Collignon J, Varlet I, Robertson EJ. Relationship between asymmetric nodal expression and the direction of embryonic turning. *Nature* 1996;381:155–158.
6. Mochizuki T, Saijoh Y, Tsuchiya K, et al. Cloning of inv, a gene that controls left/right asymmetry and kidney development. *Nature* 1998;395:177–181.
7. Morgan D, Turnpenny L, Goodship J, et al. Inversin, a novel gene in the vertebrate left-right axis pathway, is partially deleted in the inv mouse. *Nature Genetics* 1998;20:149–155.
8. Wilkinson DG. *In Situ Hybridization: A Practical Approach*. Oxford: IRL Press; 1992:75–84.
9. Piedra ME, Icardo JM, Albajar M, et al. Pitx2 participates in the late phase of the pathway controlling left-right asymmetry. *Cell* 1998;94:319–324.
10. Logan M, Pagan-Westphal M, Smith DM, et al. The transcription factor pitx2 mediates situs specific morphogenesis in response to left-right asymmetric signals. *Cell* 1998;94:307–317.
11. Yoshioka H, Meno C, Koshiba K, et al. Pitx2, a bicoid-type homeobox gene, is involved in a left-right signaling pathway in determination of left-right asymmetry. *Cell* 1998;94:299–305.
12. Ryan AK, Blumberg B, Rodriguez-Esteban C, et al. Pitx2 determines left-right asymmetry of internal organs in vertebrates. *Nature* 1998;394:545–551.
13. Supp DM, Witte DP, Potter SP, et al. Mutation of an axonemal dynein affects left-right asymmetry in inversus viscerum mice. *Nature* 1997;389:963–966.
14. Nonaka S, Tanaka Y, Okada Y, et al. Randomization of left-right asymmetry due to loss of nodal cilia generating leftward flow of extraembryonic fluid in mice lacking KIF3B motor protein. *Cell* 1998;95:829–837.
15. Pagan-Westphal SM, Tabin CJ. The transfer of left-right positional information during chick embryogenesis. *Cell* 1998;93:25–35.

4

Molecular Basis of Left-Right Asymmetry: Role of *Lefty* Genes and Their Transcriptional Regulation

Hiroshi Hamada, MD, PhD, Chikara Meno, DVM, PhD, Yukio Saijoh, MD, Rui Sakuma, MSc, Kenta Yashiro, MD, and Hitoshi Adachi, MSc

Role of *lefty* Genes in L-R Determination

The murine *lefty* locus is composed of two highly conserved genes, *lefty-1* and *lefty-2,* that are tightly linked on mouse chromosome 1. Although both genes are expressed in a left-right (L-R) asymmetric manner on embryonic day 8.0 (E8.0), their expression patterns differ: *lefty-1* is expressed predominantly in the left half of the prospective floor plate (PFP), whereas *lefty-2* is strongly expressed on the left side of lateral plate mesoderm (LPM).[1,2] To examine the role of *lefty-1* in L-R asymmetry, we generated mutant mice deficient in *lefty-1* and analyzed their phenotype.[3] When we examined the phenotype of *lefty-1*$^{-/-}$ mice, a variety of positional defects (heterotaxia) was apparent in visceral organs. Although the precise phenotype varied among individual animals, the most common feature of the *lefty-1*$^{-/-}$ mice was thoracic left isomerism associated with malpositioning of

the cardiac outflow tracts, the inferior vena cava (IVC), and the azygos vein.

Positional defects were apparent in the heart and cardiac outflow tracts. In the *lefty-1*$^{-/-}$ mice, the shape of the right atrium was abnormal and resembled that of the left atrium suggestive of bilateral left atrial appendages. The pulmonary artery was located dorsal to the aorta or the two great arteries were positioned side by side. The mutant mice also showed abnormal ventriculo-arterial alignment, such as transposition of the great arteries (TGA) in which the pulmonary artery connects to the left ventricle and the aorta connects to the right ventricle, and double-outlet right ventricle (DORV) in which both the pulmonary artery and aorta connect to the right ventricle. Abnormal atrioventricular connections, such as atrioventricular canal (CAVC) and tricuspid atresia (TAt), were also observed. These defects were always associated with additional malformations such as ventricular septal defect (VSD) and atrial septal defect (ASD). Reversed arching of the aorta was detected in one animal. It is likely that such combined defects of the heart and cardiac outflow tracts were responsible for the neonatal lethality.

From Clark EB, Nakazawa M, Takao A (eds.): Etiology and Morphogenesis of Congenital Heart Disease: Twenty Years of Progress in Genetics and Developmental Biology. Armonk, NY: Futura Publishing Co., Inc.; © 2000.

It appeared paradoxical that deficiency of *lefty-1,* a gene expressed in the left half of the PFP, caused thoracic left isomerism rather than the predicted right isomerism. To gain insight into the molecular basis of the positional defects, we examined expression of *lefty-1, lefty-2,* and *nodal.* The *lefty-1*$^{-/-}$ embryos recovered at E8.0 appeared morphologically normal. However, expression of *lefty-2* and *nodal* was affected in the mutant embryos. In *lefty-1*$^{-/-}$ embryos *lefty-2* expression in the PFP was not only upregulated but also bilateral. Furthermore, ectopic *lefty-2* expression was apparent on the right side of LPM. The lack of *lefty-1* also affected *nodal* expression. In *lefty-1*$^{+/+}$ and *lefty-1*$^{+/-}$ embryos, *nodal* expression was confined to left LPM. However, in *lefty-1*$^{-/-}$ embryos, *nodal* expression in LPM was apparent on the left side, right side, or both sides, depending on developmental stage. At a relatively early stage (two to three somite pairs), most (8 of 9) of the homozygous mutant embryos expressing *nodal* showed left-sided expression. At a later stage (five somite pairs), however, most (5 of 6) showed bilateral or right-sided expression. Also, Pitx2, a transcription factor that is normally expressed in the left LPM, was bilaterally expressed in the mutant embryos.

The phenotype of *lefty-1*$^{-/-}$ mice confirms the role of *lefty-1* in L-R asymmetry and places *lefty-1* directly within a molecular pathway that includes *iv.* Bilateral expression of *lefty-2* and *nodal* in the mutant embryos suggest that *lefty-1* regulates these two genes. It is likely that *lefty-2* and/or *nodal* rather than *lefty-1* encodes a determinant for leftness, which would explain why the *lefty-1* mutant mice showed the paradoxical left isomerism in the thorax. Although it is not clear how *lefty-1* regulates *lefty-2* and *nodal,* one possibility is that the Lefty-1 protein serves as (or induces) a midline barrier to prevent the diffusion of a molecule that regulates expression of these two genes (Fig. 1).

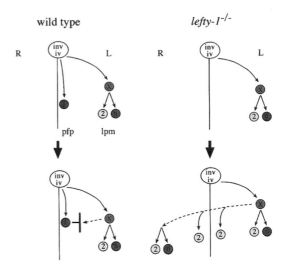

Figure 1 Diagram showing possible mechanism whereby *Lefty-1* regulates expression of *lefty-2* and *nodal* genes.

Transcriptional Regulation of Asymmetric Expression of *lefty* Genes

We examined the transcriptional activity of upstream regions of *lefty-1* and *lefty-2.*[4] For *lefty-1,* the 9.5-kb upstream region containing the TATA box was linked to *lacZ,* yielding *L1-9.5.* For *lefty-2,* the 5.5-kb upstream region including the TATA box was fused to *lacZ,* yielding *L2-5.5.* *L1-9.5* and *L2-5.5* were injected separately into the pronuclei of fertilized embryos at the one-cell stage. The embryos were allowed to develop in utero until embryonic day 8.2 (E8.2), when they were recovered and the expression of the *lacZ* transgene was examined by staining with X-Gal (5-bromo-4-chloro-3-indoyl-β-D-galactoside). *L1-9.5* and *L2-5.5* were able to recapitulate the expression patterns of *lefty-1* and *lefty-2,* respectively. These results also indicate that *lefty-1* and *lefty-2* are regulated independently, even though they are tightly linked on the same chromosome.

To locate *cis*-elements responsible for the asymmetric expression of *lefty-2,* we tested two sets of deletion mutants from *L2-5.5.* The results indicated the presence

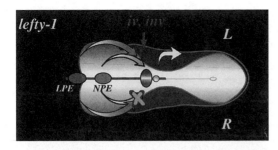

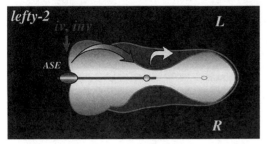

Figure 2. Diagram showing the results of an asymmetric enhancer on the expression of *lefty-2*.

that ASE is essential and sufficient for the asymmetric expression of *lefty-2* (Fig. 2).

To localize the transcriptional regulatory elements of *lefty-1,* we tested various restriction fragments derived from the 9.5-kb upstream region for the ability to confer asymmetric expression. Two enhancers were found in the upstream region, but they were bilateral enhancers. L-R specificity was determined not by these enhancers but by a silencer (RSS: right side-specific silencer) located in the proximal promoter region that can repress transcription on the right side when combined with the bilateral enhancers (Fig. 2).

of a left side-specific enhancer referred to as asymmetric enhancer (ASE) in a 380-bp region between −4.1 and −3.7 kb. Internal deletion of the 380-bp region containing ASE from *L2-5.5* abolished asymmetric expression. The *ASE-lef2p* construct, in which the 380-bp ASE fragment is linked to the minimal promoter region of *lefty-2* (from −300 to +90 bp), yielded left-sided X-Gal staining in left LPM and PFP. Finally, constructs in which the 380-bp fragment was linked to the *hsp68* promoter instead of the *lefty-2* promoter gave rise to X-Gal staining in left LPM and left PFP. These results demonstrate

References

1. Meno C, Saijoh Y, Fujii H, et al. Left-right asymmetric expression of the TGFβ-family member *lefty* in mouse embryo. *Nature* 1996;381:151–155.
2. Meno C, Ito Y, Saijoh Y, et al. Two closely-related left-right asymmetrically-expressed genes, *lefty-1* and *lefty-2:* Their distinct expression domains, chromosomal linkage and direct neuralizing activity in *Xenopus* embryos. *Genes Cells* 1997;2:513–524.
3. Meno C, Shimono A, Saijoh Y, et al. *lefty-1* is required for left-right determination as a regulator of *lefty-2* and *nodal. Cell* 1998;94: 287–297.
4. Saijoh Y, Adachi H, Hirao A, et al. Distinct transcriptional regulatory mechanisms underlie left-right asymmetric expression of *lefty-1* and *lefty-2. Genes Dev* 1999;13(3): 259–269.

5

Search for the Mechanism of Nitrous Oxide-Induced Situs Inversus

Masahiko Fujinaga, MD

Nitrous oxide (N_2O), so-called "laughing gas," has been used as an anesthetic in clinical practice for more than 100 years, and is considered as one of the least toxic inhalational anesthetics. However, N_2O is known to cause reproductive toxicity in experimental animals. In 1967, Shepard's group at the University of Washington first reported teratogenic effects of N_2O in a mammalian species, the rat,[1] although several earlier studies reported embryonic toxicity in chicks. In 1987, we found that N_2O caused a high incidence of right-sided (inverted) aortic arch in rats[2] in addition to other abnormalities that had been reported previously, e.g., early postimplantation loss, and rib and vertebral abnormalities.[3] In subsequent studies, we demonstrated that N_2O caused situs inversus, including both partial and complete types, as well as isolated right-sided aortic arch.[4-6]

To further investigate this unique effect of N_2O, we used an in vitro rat whole embryo culture model[7] based on the system that was originally developed by New and colleagues in the 1970s.[8] Because N_2O is clinically known to have sympathomimetic properties, we hypothesized that adrenergic stimulation was the cause of situs inversus, and we demonstrated that phenylephrine, an $\alpha1$ adrenergic agonist, caused situs inversus in the rat whole embryo culture model.[9,10] Stimulation of $\alpha2$ or β adrenoceptors did not cause situs inversus.[10] The maximum incidence of phenylephrine-induced situs inversus was approximately 50%, and no other abnormalities were seen. In addition, we showed that prazosin, an $\alpha1$ adrenergic antagonist, blocked phenylephrine-induced situs inversus, but prazosin alone did not cause situs inversus. These results suggested that $\alpha1$ adrenergic stimulation interfered with signal transduction pathways that are involved in normal development of left-right sidedness, leading to a random determination of sidedness. In a subsequent experiment, we demonstrated that N_2O-induced situs inversus is indeed blocked by prazosin.[11]

In later experiments, we found that the critical period for induction of situs inversus by $\alpha1$ adrenergic stimulation was stage 11a[12] (using a modified Theiler staging system[13]), the so-called "early neural plate stage" of gestational day 9 (gestational day 0 = the day when the copulatory plug was observed). We also found that at least four hours of $\alpha1$ adrenergic stimulation was needed to cause situs inversus.[12] In the mouse, $\alpha1$ adrenergic stimulation also caused situs inversus.[14] However, the significance of the effect was less than in the rat because of the high background incidence of situs inversus that occurs under in vitro conditions in control embryos. Furthermore, mouse embryos show susceptibility to $\alpha1$ adren-

From Clark EB, Nakazawa M, Takao A (eds.): Etiology and Morphogenesis of Congenital Heart Disease: Twenty Years of Progress in Genetics and Developmental Biology. Armonk, NY: Futura Publishing Co., Inc.; © 2000.

ergic stimulation until stage 11b, whereas rat embryos are much less susceptible at the same stage.[14]

In other experiments, we demonstrated that gene expression of α1 adrenoceptor subtypes, at least α1A and α1B subtypes (genetic classification), was detected in the embryo at stage 11a using RNase protection assays.[15] In addition, we found that gene expression of catecholamine synthesizing enzymes was present in the embryo at a much earlier stage than previously was thought. For example, mRNA of tyrosine hydroxylase, the rate limiting enzyme for catecholamine synthesis, was detected as early as at stage 10a (so-called "early amnion stage").[16] This

stage is much earlier than the beginning of neurulation or the differentiation of neural crest cells. Thus, our findings suggest that catecholamine synthesizing capability is not limited to the cells of nervous system or of sympathoadrenal lineage which originates from neural crest cells. In addition, our findings suggest the possibility that N_2O induces catecholamine release from catecholamine synthesizing cells, which results in stimulation of α1 adrenoceptors to cause situs inversus.

To date, α1 adrenoceptors are known to activate at least two types of protein kinases, Ca^{2+}/calmodulin dependent protein kinase II and protein kinase C, which

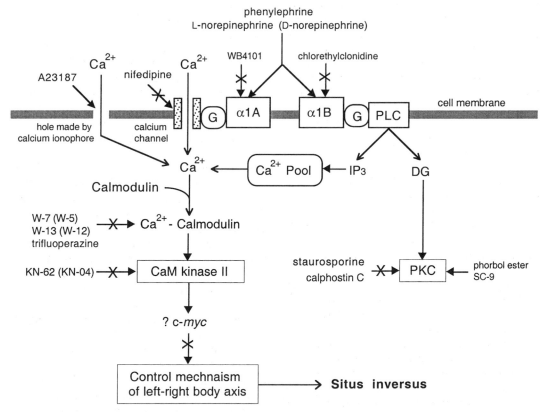

Figure 1. Signal transduction pathways related to α1 adrenoceptors and the chemicals that are known to activate or inhibit different sites of the pathways; the chemicals in parenthesis are negative controls. (Modified with permission from Reference 25.) Abbreviations: α1A, α1A adrenoceptor subtype; α1B, α1B adrenoceptor subtype; CaM kinase II, Ca^{2+}/calmodulin dependent protein kinase II; DG, diacylglycerol; G, guanosine nucleotide-binding protein; IP3, inositol triphosphate; PKC, protein kinase C; PLC, phospholipase C.

are associated with different intracellular signal transduction pathways.[17] Using various chemicals which are known to activate or inhibit different sites of signal transduction pathways (Fig. 1), we subsequently demonstrated that the effect was mediated by the α1A but not the α1B adrenoceptor subtype (pharmacological classification), and by Ca^{2+}/calmodulin dependent protein kinase II but not protein kinase C.[17,18] Interestingly, KN-62, a Ca^{2+}/calmodulin dependent protein kinase II antagonist alone also caused situs inversus at higher concentrations.[17] In another experiment, we also found that lidocaine, a local anesthetic that is known to have an effect on Ca^{2+} mobilization in relation to the effects on muscle contraction, caused situs inversus.[19] These findings suggest that changes in intracellular Ca^{2+} concentration at the critical time of development interfere with normal development of left-right sidedness and result in situs inversus.

As a next step, we searched for a transcriptional factor mediating α1 adrenergic stimulation induced situs inversus. Until recently, several early immediate genes are known to be induced by adrenergic stimulation in other experimental models, i.e., c-*fos*, c-*jun*, *jun*-b, *egr*-1, and c-*myc*. We cultured rat embryos at stage 11a with 100 μM phenylephrine, and total RNA was isolated and was subjected to Northern blot assays for above genes. We found that expression of c-*myc* but not c-*fos*, c-*jun*, *jun*-b or *egr*-1 was induced by phenylephrine.[20] In other experiments, we found that phenylephrine induced early ectopic expression of c-*myc* gene compared with untreated embryos (Fig. 2). However, we could not detect any specific region of c-*myc* gene expression in embryos induced by phenylephrine (unpublished data).

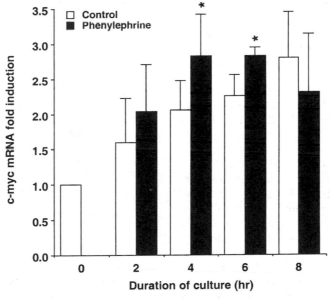

Figure 2. Time course of c-*myc* gene expression in rat embryos cultured from stage 11a with 100 μM phenylephrine (closed bar) or without phenylephrine (open bar). The c-*myc* mRNA values were analyzed by Northern blot assays using human c-*myc* cDNA probe (0.4 kb; Cat. No. HP111, Oncogene, Cambridge, Mass). Glyceraldehyde-3-phosphate dehydrogenase (G3PDH) mRNA was used as an internal control; human G3PDH cDNA probe (1.1 kb; Cat. 9805–1, Clontech, Palo Alto, Calif). Data, expressed as fold increase over the embryo at stage 11a, are mean ± SD of 5 separate experiments. A total of 3295 embryos were used for the entire study, and 20 to 30 μg of total RNA was used for each assay of Northern blot analysis.

In recent years, various genes have been shown to be expressed asymmetrically during embryogenesis in chicks and mice, and were thought to be involved in development of left-right sidedness. We have examined the expression pattern during rat embryogenesis of one such gene, *nodal*, a member of the TGF-β gene family, and the effects of $\alpha1$ adrenergic stimulation.[21] Using reverse transcription-polymerase chain reaction (RT-PCR) and whole mount in situ hybridization assays, we found the *nodal* gene is expressed in rats during embryogenesis in a pattern similar to that in mouse embryos.[22,23] Namely, *nodal* gene expression was detected in the embryo between stage 9 and stage 12/s6 (6 somite pairs) but not from older embryos. Furthermore, *nodal* gene expression in the lateral plate is limited to the left side between stage 12/s3 and 12/s5. When rat embryos were treated with 100 μM phenylephrine at stage 11a, *nodal* gene expression was detected by RT-PCR assay from both sides of the lateral plates at stages 12/s6 and 12/s7, but not from either side of younger embryos. These results indicate that $\alpha1$ adrenergic stimulation delays *nodal* gene expression as well as randomizes its sidedness.

In summary, we have demonstrated that N_2O-induced situs inversus is mediated by stimulation of $\alpha1$ adrenoceptors in the embryo at stage 11a, the so-called "early neural plate stage." This results in interference with signal transduction pathways that are involved in normal development of the left-right sidedness, leading to random determination of sidedness. It is likely that a change in intracellular Ca^{2+} concentration is the underlying mechanism of situs inversus affecting normal activity of Ca^{2+}/calmodulin dependent protein kinase II and perhaps gene expression of c-*myc*. We also have found that $\alpha1$ adrenergic stimulation delays *nodal* gene expression as well as randomizes its sidedness. The mechanisms whereby N_2O stimulates $\alpha1$ adrenoceptors and the precise manner and site of $\alpha1$ adrenergic stimulation interferes with signal transduction pathways remain to be further elucidated.

Acknowledgments: The author wishes to thank Dr. Richard Mazze for editing the manuscript.

References

1. Fink BR, Shepard TH. Teratogenic activity of nitrous oxide. *Nature* 1967;214;146–148.
2. Fujinaga M, Baden JM, Yhap EO, et al. Reproductive and teratogenic effects of nitrous oxide, isoflurane, and their combination in Sprague-Dawley rats. *Anesthesiology* 1987;67:960–964.
3. Shepard TH, Fink BR. Teratogenic activity of nitrous oxide in rats. In: Fink BR, ed. *Toxicity of Anesthetics*. Baltimore, Md: Williams & Wilkins; 1968:308–325.
4. Fujinaga M, Baden JM, Mazze RI. Nitrous oxide alters body laterality in rats. *Teratology* 1990;41:131–135.
5. Fujinaga M, Baden JM, Suto A, et al. Preventive effects of phenoxybenzamine on nitrous oxide induced reproductive toxicity in Sprague-Dawley rats. *Teratology* 1991;43:151–157.
6. Fujinaga M, Baden JM, Mazze RI. Susceptible period of nitrous oxide teratogenicity in Sprague-Dawley rats. *Teratology* 1989; 40:439–444.
7. Fujinaga M, Mazze RI, Baden JM, et al. Rat whole embryo culture: An in vitro model for testing nitrous oxide teratogenicity. *Anesthesiology* 1988;69:401–404.
8. New DAT. Whole embryo culture and the study of mammalian embryos during organogenesis. *Biol Rev* 1978;53:81–122.
9. Fujinaga M, Baden JM. Evidence for an adrenergic mechanism in the control of body asymmetry. *Dev Biol* 1991;143:203–205.
10. Fujinaga M, Maze M, Hoffman BB, et al. Activation of α-1 adrenergic receptors modulates the control of left/right sidedness in rat embryos. *Dev Biol* 1992;150: 419–421.
11. Fujinaga M, Baden JM. Methionine prevents nitrous oxide-induced teratogenicity in rat embryos grown in culture. *Anesthesiology* 1994;81:184–189.
12. Fujinaga M, Baden JM. Critical period of rat development when sidedness of body asymmetry is determined. *Teratology* 1991; 44:453–462.
13. Fujinaga M, Brown NA, Baden JM. Comparison of staging systems for the gastrulation and early neurulation period in ro-

dents: A proposed new system. *Teratology* 1992;46:183–190.

14. Fujinaga M, Hu Z-W, Okazaki M, et al. Expression of mRNA for α1-adrenoceptor subtypes at the beginning of neurulation in rat embryos. *Toxicol In Vitro* 1995;9:601–606.

15. Fujinaga M. Development of sidedness of asymmetric structures in vertebrates. *Int J Dev Biol* 1997;41:153–186.

16. Fujinaga M, Scott JC. Gene expression of catecholamine synthesizing enzymes and β adrenoceptor subtypes during rat embryogenesis. *Neurosci Lett* 1997;231:108–112.

17. Exton JH. The roles of calcium and phosphoinositides in the mechanisms of α1-adrenergic and other agonists. *Rev Physiol Biochem Pharmacol* 1988;111:117–231.

18. Fujinaga M, Hoffman BB, Baden JM. Receptor subtype and intracellular signal transduction pathway associated with situs inversus induced by α1 adrenergic stimulation in rat embryos. *Dev Biol* 1994; 162:558–567.

19. Fujinaga M, Park HW, ShepardTH, et al. Staurosporine does not block adrenergic-induced situs inversus, but causes a unique syndrome of defects in rat embryos

grown in culture. *Teratology* 1995;50:261–274.

20. Fujinaga M. Assessment of teratogenic effects of lidocaine in rat embryos cultured in vitro. *Anesthesiology* 1998;89:1553-1558.

21. Fujinaga M, Okazaki M, Baden JM, et al. Gene expression of transcriptional factor induced by α1 adrenoceptor stimulation in rat embryos at the beginning of neurulation. Abstract. *Dev Biol* 1995;170:744.

22. Fujinaga M, Lowe L, Kuehn MR. Expression pattern of *nodal* during rat embryogenesis and the effects of α1 adrenergic stimulation in relation to the left-right body axis development. Abstract. *Dev Biol* 1997;186:326.

23. Lowe L, Supp D, Sampath K, et al. Conserved left-right asymmetry of nodal expression and alterations in murine situs inversus. *Nature* 1996;381:158–161.

24. Collignon J, Varlet I, Robertson EJ. Relationship between asymmetric *nodal* expression and the direction of embryonic turning. *Nature* 1996;381:155–158.

25. Fujinaga M. Anesthetics. *Handbook Exp Pharmacol* 1997;124/II:295–331.

6

Left, Left, Left-Right-Left: The Genetics of Human Laterality Malformations

Brett Casey, MD

Rightward looping of the midline heart tube is the first overt manifestation of anatomic left-right (LR) differences that eventually come to include the lungs and most of the unpaired organs of the abdomen. Heart malformations associated with abnormal looping, therefore, usually occur as one manifestation of a more global abnormality of LR-axis development. The typical case presents with complex structural heart anomalies, abnormalities of spleen position and/or number, and some degree of gut malrotation. The overall LR anatomy of this individual might be described as "situs ambiguus," or indeterminate sidedness, in contrast to "situs solitus" (normal sidedness) and "situs inversus" (complete LR reversal). Manifestations are quite variable, however, even among affected individuals from the same family. For example, heart looping and other abnormalities can occur in the absence of visceral malformations, as can R-sided stomach and intestinal malrotation without associated cardiovascular malformations.[1]

Heart malformations attributable to abnormal laterality occur uncommonly, with a prevalence of 1.44 of 10,000 live births and accounting for 3.4% of all cardiac defects reported in the recent Baltimore-Washington Infant Study.[2] Males and females appear to be affected equally. Many familial cases have been reported. Of these, multiple affected sibs is the most common scenario, and occasionally the parents are consanguineous. Affected individuals in more than one generation have been described, including inheritance in a small number of these families that is (or appears to be) X-linked.[1]

Complete LR reversal (situs inversus), which imparts no functional abnormality, probably occurs with about the same prevalence as situs ambiguus. Approximately 25% of situs inversus individuals have immotile cilia syndrome (ICS), a disorder of cilia and flagella function.[3] Curiously, only approximately half of ICS individuals are situs inversus whereas the others are usually situs solitus (situs ambiguus has been described in some ICS cases). Until recently, the relationship between abnormal cilia and LR-axis development has remained a mystery (see below).

Ascertainment of familial cases, characterization of several murine situs mutants,[4–7] and identification of genes with LR asymmetric expression has led to the conclusion that genetics contributes significantly to the pathogenesis of human situs abnormalities. Molecular genetic studies have yielded some support for this hypothesis. Previously a locus for situs defects was mapped to Xq26.2.[8] A zinc-finger transcription factor, *ZIC3*, was positionally cloned from this region, and mutations were identified among sporadic

From Clark EB, Nakazawa M, Takao A (eds.): Etiology and Morphogenesis of Congenital Heart Disease: Twenty Years of Progress in Genetics and Developmental Biology. Armonk, NY: Futura Publishing Co., Inc.; © 2000.

Table 1
Mutation Analysis of Situs Ambiguus Cases

Gene	Patient	Clinical Features	Mutation	Present in Control Chromosomes	Parental Carrier
NODAL	66	Situs ambiguus	R183Q	No	M
	262	L-TGA, vent inv	V284F	No	P
	347	Situs ambiguus	M339V	No	P
	141	Situs ambiguus	G262R	1/120	M
HNF-3b	141	Situs ambiguus	P419T	4/110	M
	148	Situs ambiguus	P419T	4/110	?
LEFTY-A	143	Situs ambiguus	R314X	No	P
	137	Situs ambiguus	S342K	No	M
ACVR2B	314	Situs ambiguus	R40H	No	?
	414	Situs ambiguus	R40H	No	P
	415	Situs ambiguus	V494I	No	M
INV	329	L-TGA, VSD, PA	S371G	No	?

Abbreviations: L-TGA, levo transposition of great vessels; vent inv, ventricular inversion; VSD, ventricular septal defect; PA, pulmonary artery atresia; M, maternal; P, paternal.

and familial cases.[9] *ZIC3* mutations, however, have been found in only a small percentage of affected individuals (K. Kosaki and B. Casey, unpublished data), which is not surprising given the relatively equal incidence of disease among males and females, the variety of inheritance patterns seen among familial cases, and the presumed genetic complexity of the developmental process.

In an effort to identify other genes involved in situs abnormalities, we have performed a search for linkage in an extended pedigree with autosomal dominant transmission of LR axis malformations. We evaluated 35 members of a four generation kindred in which seven individuals manifest abnormal situs. Four obligate gene carriers are normal, and two individuals have only complex heart malformations. Linkage to known candidate genes was excluded. Subsequently a genome-wide screen was performed utilizing 350 short-tandem-repeat polymorphisms separated by an average distance of approximately 12 cM. By multipoint analysis we obtained a maximum lod score of 3 with marker D6S426, which maps to chromosome 6p21.1. The remainder of the genome was excluded from linkage by negative lod scores.

Studies in other vertebrates are yielding additional candidate genes for human LR abnormalities (for recent review see Reference 10). For example, several genes are asymmetrically expressed along the LR axis in chick prior to the development of anatomic LR asymmetry.[11] Some (but not all) of these genes are also asymmetrically expressed in mouse, including *nodal* and *pitx2*, as well as *lefty-1* and *lefty-2*, two TGFβ family members whose chick orthologues have yet to be identified.[12–15] Genetic studies in mice have also implicated several additional genes in LR axis development in which asymmetric expression has not been detected, including *HNF3β*, *ActrIIb*, and *Smad2*.[12,16,17] Mutation analysis has been carried out on a large panel of situs ambiguus cases for human homologues of *nodal*, *HNF3β*, *ActRIIb* and *lefty-1* and *-2*. A small number of mutations has been detected in each (see Table 1).[10,18,19] Although preliminary, these studies also suggest the possibility of a complex contribution of mutations or polymorphisms in those loci in a subset of patients.

References

1. Casey B. Two rights make a wrong: Human left-right malformations. *Hum Mol Genet* 1998;7(10 Review):1565–1571.
2. Ferencz C, Loffredo C, Correa-Villasenor A, et al. *Genetic & Environmental Risk Factors of Major Cardiovascular Malfor-*

mations: The Baltimore-Washington Infant Study 1981–1989. Armonk, NY: Futura Publishing Co, Inc; 1997.

3. Afzelius B, Mossberg B. In: Scriver C, Beaudet A, Sly W, et al., eds. *The Metabolic and Molecular Basis of Inherited Disease.* New York: McGraw-Hill; 1995:3943–3954.

4. Melloy PG, Ewart JL, Desmond ME, et al. No turning, a mouse mutation causing left-right and axial patterning defects. *Dev Biol* 1998;193:77–89.

5. Supp DM, Witte DP, Potter SS, et al. Mutation of an axonemal dynein affects left-right assymetry in inversus viscerum mice. *Nature* 1997;389:963–966.

6. Yokoyama T, Copeland NS, Jenkins NA, et al. Reversal of left-right asymmetry: a situs inversus mutation. *Science* 1993;260:679–682.

7. van der Hoeven F, Schimmang T, Volkmann A, et al. Programmed cell death is affected in the novel mouse mutant Fused toes (Ft). *Development* 1994;120:2601–2607.

8. Casey B, Devoto M, Jones KL, et al. Mapping a gene for familial situs abnormalities. *Nature Genet* 1993;5:403–407.

9. Gebbia M, Ferrero GB, Pilia G, et al. X-linked situs abnormalities result from mutations in ZIC3. *Nature Genet* 1997;17:305–308.

10. Harvey RP. Links in the left/right axial pathway. *Cell* 1998;94:273–276.

11. Levin M. Left-right asymmetry in vertebrate embryogenesis. *BioEssays* 1997;19:287–296.

12. Collignon J, Varlet I, Robertson EJ. Relationship between asymmetric nodal expression and the direction of embryonic turning. *Nature* 1996;381:155–158.

13. Lowe LA, Supp DM, Sampath K, et al. Conserved left-right asymmetry of nodal expression and alterations in murine situs inversus. *Nature* 1996;381:158–161.

14. Meno C, Shimono A, Saijoh Y, et al. Lefty-1 is required for left-right determination as a regulator of lefty-2 and nodal. *Cell* 1998;94:287–297.

15. Yoshioka H, Meno C, Koshiba K, et al. Pitx2, a bicoid-type homeobox gene, is involved in a lefty-signaling pathway in determination of left-right asymmetry. *Cell* 1998;94:299–305.

16. Oh SP, Li E. The signaling pathway mediated by the type IIB activin receptor controls axial patterning and lateral asymmetry in the mouse. *Genes Dev* 1997;11:1812–1826.

17. Nomura M, Li E. Smad2 role in mesoderm formation, left-right patterning and craniofacial development. *Nature* 1998;393:786–790.

18. Bassi MT, Kosaki K, Belmont J, et al. *Am J Hum Genet* 1997;61:8A.

19. Kosaki K, et al. Characterization and mutation analysis of human LEFTY A and LEFTY B, homologues of murine genes implicated in left-right axis development. *Am J Hum Genet* 1999;64(3):712–21.

7

Positional Cloning of the Inversion Breakpoints of inv(11)(q13,q25) Found in a Patient with Heterotaxy

Aritoshi Iida, PhD, Mitsuru Emi, MD, Takashi Imai, PhD, Hirofumi Ohashi, MD, Rumiko Matsuoka, MD, Yoshimitsu Fukushima, MD, and Yusuke Nakamura, MD

Heterotaxy (OMIM 208530, 306955) is characterized by a variable group of congenital anomalies that include complex cardiac defects, situs inversus or situs ambiguus, altered lung lobation, splenic abnormalities (asplenia, polysplenia). The occurrence is usually sporadic, but familial cases (autosomal dominant, autosomal recessive, X-linked) have been described (Reviews 1, 2). In addition, ten heterotaxy cases with chromosomal abnormalities have been reported.[1]

We studied an interesting family in which the heterotaxy phenotype was associated with chromosomal abnormalities. Cytogenetical analysis revealed that the patient with heterotaxy had a paracentric inversion of chromosome 11 [46, XY, inv(11)(q13,q25)].[3] The rearrangement was also detected in the patient's phenotypically normal father. We called these regions "*DHTX (disrupted in heterotaxy)-A*" at 11q13 and "*DHTX-B*" at 11q25, respectively. In the present study, based on a hypothesis that one or more of the putative heterotaxy genes are disrupted at a breakpoint of the inversion,

we constructed a physical map and isolated the breakpoints in a patient.

First of all, Fluorescent *in situ* hybridization (FISH) was performed to map the *DHTX-A* region. Eighteen cCI11-cosmids,[4] from localization throughout chromosome 11q13-q14, and a cZNF6 cosmid clone, containing the ZNF6 gene, were localized on metaphase chromosomes of patient cell line 1005 (CL1005) to determine whether each was located proximally or distally to the *DHTX-A* breakpoint at 11q13. The closest flanking markers identified by FISH analysis were cZNF6 and cCI11–404, which were proximal and distal to the *DHTX-A*, respectively. To localize the *DHTX-A* breakpoint more precisely, several 11q13–11q14 CEPH mega YACs were identified by electronically accessing the CEPH YAC physical mapping database. FISH was used to determine whether any of the YACs spanned the *DHTX-A* breakpoint from CL1005. Subsequently, the *DHTX-A* breakpoint in the CL1005 was spanned by YAC, y775-h-1 (380 Kb), as hybridization signals from the YACs were visible at both breakpoint sites of the inversion. This result implied the chromosomal breakage with 380 Kb (Fig. 1). To further characterize the *DHTX-A* breakpoint, we constructed a cosmid library from this YAC clone. FISH signals of labeled mixed

From Clark EB, Nakazawa M, Takao A (eds.): Etiology and Morphogenesis of Congenital Heart Disease: Twenty Years of Progress in Genetics and Developmental Biology. Armonk, NY: Futura Publishing Co., Inc.; © 2000.

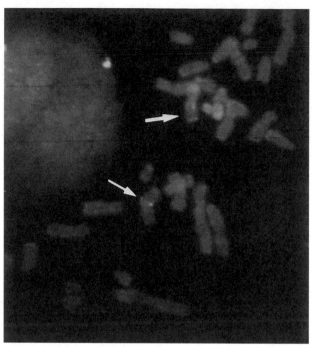

Figure 1. Metaphase spread of a cell derived from the heterotaxy patient, probed with y775-h-1 mapped on 11q13. Bold arrow and the thin arrow indicate inv(11)(q13,q25) and normal chromosome 11, respectively. FISH analysis was carried out, as described previously.[5] See color Appendix.

clones (cIS1, cIS2, and cIS3) were detected at both the *DHTX-A* and *DHTX-B* region at 11q25 of the inv(11) and at the *DHTX-A* region of the normal chromosome 11. We confirmed that the cosmid clones, cIS1 and cIS2, mapped proximally while clone cIS3 mapped distally to the breakpoint respectively. Hence, the cIS1 and cIS3 were chosen as the anchor-point for the cosmid contig of the *DHTX-A* breakpoint region. We achieved bi-directional chromosome walking from these anchor-points by means of cosmid-cosmid hybridization method. Moreover, P1 derived artificial chromosome (PAC) library was screened with D11S1321. The PAC ends were also sequenced to generate new STSs, which were used for further STS content mapping and in walking experiments to identify further PAC clones. A subset of PACs and cosmids was used to construct the contig spanning the *DHTX-A* breakpoint shown in Fig. 2.

The patient's DNA was examined by Southern hybridization using the walking clones as probes. This result implied that the *DHTX-A* breakpoint occurred within a 1.8 Kb *Bam*HI fragment, p21BA, derived from a cosmid cIH-21. Moreover, FISH analysis confirmed that two cosmids clones from the contig, cIH4 and cIH21, span the breakpoint. To examine the mechanism of the inversion breakpoint, we constructed a cosmid library from patient DNA and isolated a cosmid, c1005BP2.1, clone containing the breakpoint using the 1.8 Kb *Bam*HI fragment as a probe. The regions of the breakpoint from the inversion chromosome and corresponding to the normal chromosomes were sequenced and compared.

In the present study, we first constructed a high-resolution physical map of the *DHTX-A* region at 11q13. The map of the *DHTX-A* region was assembled by the integration of three contig levels, together with the localization of new 11 STSs within

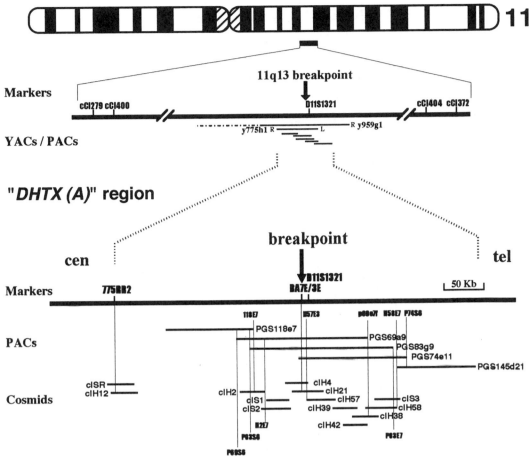

Figure 2. The PAC/Cosmid contig spanning the *DHTX-A* breakpoint at 11q13. A vertical arrow marks the position of the *"DHTX-A"* breakpoint. Genomic clones are represented by horizontal bars. Cosmid clones and PAC clones noted by "c" and "P" prefixes, respectively.

the contig. Moreover, we cloned and identified the breakpoints in a patient with inv(11)(q13,q25). The detailed map and cloned DNA resources should allow for multiple simultaneous approaches for identification of the putative heterotaxy gene(s).

Acknowledgments: This work was supported by grants from the Ministry of Education, Science, Sports, and Culture of Japan and by the Kanagawa Academy of Science and Technology Research Grants (AI).

References

1. Kosaki K, Casey B. Genetics of human left-right axis malformations. *Cell Dev Biol* 1998;9:89–99.

2. Casey B. Two rights make a wrong: Human left-right malformations. *Hum Mol Genet* 1998;7:1565–1571.

3. Fukushima Y, Hoovers J, Mannens M, et al. Detection of a cryptic paracentric inversion within band 11p13 in familial aniridia by fluorescence in situ hybridization. *Am J Hum Genet* 1993;53(suppl):203–209.

4. Hori T, Takahashi E, Tanigami A, et al. A high-resolution cytogenic map of 168 cosmid DNA markers for human chromosome 11. *Genomics* 1992;13:129–133.

5. Inazawa J, Saito H, Ariyama T, et al. High-resolution cytogenic mapping of 342 new cosmid markers including 43 RFLP markers on human chromosome 17 by fluorescence in situ hybridization. *Genomics* 1993;17:153–162.

8

Left-Right Asymmetry Regulation and Heart Looping: The Expression Pattern of the Extracellular Matrix Protein, Flectin, During Early Heart Development in the Mouse Embryo

Takeshi Tsuda, MD and Kersti K. Linask, PhD

Introduction

One of the earliest morphogenetic indications of left-right axis formation in the vertebrate embryos is seen at the heart looping stage. The process of heart looping is a critical step in determining the subsequent structural development of the heart. During this heart looping stage, a primitive tubular heart develops into a highly differentiated four chambered heart. The exact mechanism of looping is, however, not clearly understood.

A novel extracellular matrix protein flectin is expressed asymmetrically prior to and during heart looping in the avian embryo.[1] We hypothesized that the specific asymmetric organization of flectin in the extracellular matrix may be related to the morphogenesis of heart looping in the avian models. In this chapter, the relationship between left-right asymmetry regulation and heart looping in the mouse embryo is discussed in association with asymmetric flectin expression in the extracellular matrix of the heart.

Materials and Methods

Mouse Embryos

C57Bl/6J mice (Jackson Labs) were used in this study. The *inv/inv* mouse embryos have been genotyped and been provided by Dr. Overbeek (Baylor College of Medicine, Houston, Tex).

Antibodies

The monoclonal antibody F-22 (mouse anti-chick flectin) has been provided by Dr. Nancy Philp (Pennsylvania College of Optometry, Philadelphia, Pa, also see References 2 and 3).

Immunohistochemistry and Microscopy

Microanatomy of the embryonic mouse heart was examined in 1 to 2 μm

From Clark EB, Nakazawa M, Takao A (eds.): Etiology and Morphogenesis of Congenital Heart Disease: Twenty Years of Progress in Genetics and Developmental Biology. Armonk, NY: Futura Publishing Co., Inc.; © 2000.

plastic section at every 5- to 10-μm interval.[4,5]

Results

Here we propose the following stages for the developmental assessment of mouse heart looping based upon differential flectin expression.[6]

Prelooping Stage (ED 8.0)

At this stage, when the heart is a short, straight tubular structure, flectin shows increased expression in the ECM of cardiac jelly, basal myocardium, and endocardial endothelium in a symmetric fashion (Fig. 1A).

Early Looping Stage (ED 8.0–8.25)

The heart starts to loop to the right side initially from the anterior portion of the round-shape tubular heart. The initiation of heart looping in mouse embryos begins with the reshaping of the wide based heart into a narrow tubular heart in an anterior-posterior direction, almost simultaneously followed by the rightward deviation of the outflow tract from the midline. Throughout the heart, flectin expression continues to show the same symmetric pattern as the previous stage.

Mid Looping Stage (ED 8.5–8.75)

The tubular heart has fully looped in an antero-posterior direction; the entire length of the heart has become narrowed and has become a looped tubular struc-

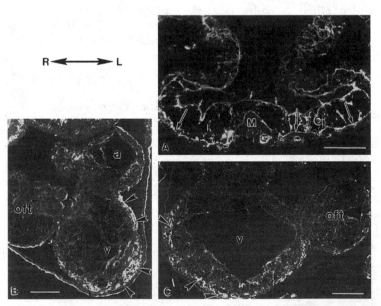

Figure 1. A. In ED 8.0 mouse embryonic heart (prelooping stage), flectin expression is seen within the cardiac jelly, basal myocardium (black arrows), and endocardium in a symmetric manner. Magnification bar = 50 μm. **B.** Flectin localization in ED 9 mouse embryonic heart (advanced looping stage). Flectin is predominantly localized at the left side of common ventricle (v; also see black arrowheads). Magnification bar = 100 μm. **C.** Flectin localization in *inv/inv* mouse at ED 9.0. Flectin expression pattern is mirror image of that of normal mouse embryo with an equivalent stage. Magnification bar = 100 μm. M, myocardium; Cj, cardiac jelly; R, right side; L, left side.

ture (i.e., reshaping). During this period, flectin begins to show increased localization in a differential pattern: flectin is seen on the inner curvature of the tubular heart and a mild increase is apparent on the left side of the ventricular region.

Advanced Looping Stage (ED 9.0–9.5)

At the advanced looping stage, morphological looping is more advanced in terms of the progress in chamber specification inside the tubular heart. Each cardiac compartment is more differentiated from the simple looped tubular structure seen at the previous stage, i.e., specific extracellular matrix (ECM) remodeling of the cardiac jelly is observed in association with the differentiation of the different cardiac compartments (Fig. 1B). Asymmetric expression of flectin is most prominently seen at this stage. Flectin is more localized in the left outer curvature of the common ventricle. Flectin is also expressed diffusely in the thin subendocardium of the common atrium.

Post-Looping Stage/Chamber Specification (ED 10–11)

At this stage, the tubular heart shows advanced chamber specification. Flectin expression is diffusely diminished, but still seen in the extracellular matrix in the atrial wall and subepicardial ECM of the ventricles.

inv/inv Mouse Embryos

In ED 9.0 inv/inv mice, flectin localization pattern appears as a mirror image to that of the wild type at the equivalent stage and the same differential organization pattern is maintained (Fig. 1C).

Discussion

Molecular determination of left-right asymmetry is made prior to embryonic heart looping. In the mouse embryo, asymmetric expression of nodal[7,8] and lefty[9] are shown to be downstream of the inv and the iv genes, although neither nodal nor lefty is specifically expressed in the heart-forming area. Many studies on determination of laterality in the embryo have used the downstream event of heart looping as an end-point marker of upstream left-right asymmetry determination in the embryo. It is important, however, to understand that left-right asymmetry regulation is only an initial signal of the whole developmental sequence that rules normal heart looping (Fig. 2). The downstream events need to be more emphasized in early heart organogenesis in correlation with upstream regulatory factors.

Flectin is an ECM protein that is expressed asymmetrically prior to heart looping and its asymmetric localization persists throughout the looping stages in avian embryos.[1] In the mouse embryo, flectin is expressed in a specific asymmetric pattern but is spatiotemporally expressed differently from that seen in the avian embryo.[6] The differing flectin expression patterns between chick and mouse may reflect a fundamental differ-

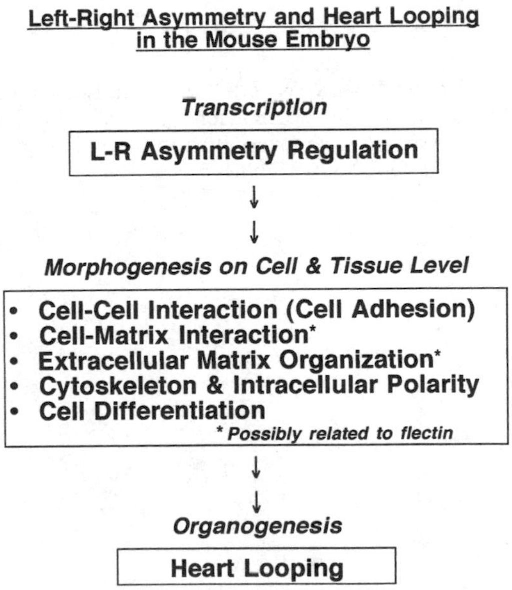

Left-Right Asymmetry and Heart Looping in the Mouse Embryo

Transcription

| L-R Asymmetry Regulation |

↓
↓

Morphogenesis on Cell & Tissue Level

- **Cell-Cell Interaction (Cell Adhesion)**
- **Cell-Matrix Interaction***
- **Extracellular Matrix Organization***
- **Cytoskeleton & Intracellular Polarity**
- **Cell Differentiation**

* Possibly related to flectin

↓
↓

Organogenesis

| Heart Looping |

Figure 2.

ence in heart development between the two species. The analysis of embryonic hearts of the *inv/inv* mutant (ED 9.0) indicates that asymmetric localization of flectin is the mirror image of that of wild type with conserved differential expression in relation to chamber.[6] The asymmetric flectin expression pattern both in wild type and its mirror image expression in *inv/inv* embryonic hearts indicates that flectin's regulation is downstream of the *inv* gene. Determination of the direct upstream regulators of flectin expression and of its matrix-binding partners will provide information on regulation of flectin expression and asymmetric localization.

The process of looping is extremely important in aligning components of the heart tube so that the inflow and the outflow tracts are brought into proximity for the compartments of the heart to be connected and aligned in the correct fashion.[10] Flectin appears to be related to extracellular matrix assembly organization and cell-matrix interaction (Fig. 2) during heart looping in both mouse and chick embryos and thus to be an important marker to address morphoregulation of heart looping.

References

1. Tsuda T, Philp N, Zile MH, et al. Left-right asymmetric localization of flectin in the extracellular matrix during heart looping. *Dev Biol* 1996;173:39–50.

2. Mieziewska K, Szel A, Van Veen T, et al. Redistribution of insoluble interphotoreceptor matrix components during photoreceptor differentiation in the mouse retina. *J Comp Neurol* 1994;345:115–124.

3. Mieziewska KE, Devenny J, van Veen T, et al. Characterization of a developmentally regulated component of ocular extracellular matrix that is evolutionarily conserved. *Invest Ophthalmol Vis Sci* 1994;35:1608.

4. Davis CA. Whole-mount immunohistochemistry. *Methods Enzymol* 1993;225:502–516.

5. Linask KK, Tsuda T. Application of plastic embedding for sectioning whole-mount immunostained early vertebrate embryos. In: Tuan R, Lo CW, eds. *Developmental Biology Protocols*. Humana Press, In press.

6. Tsuda T, Majumder K, Linask KK. Differential expression of flectin in the extracellular matrix and left-right asymmetry in mouse embryonic heart during heart looping. *Dev Genet* 1998;23:203–214.

7. Lowe LA, Supp DM, Sampath K, et al. Conserved left-right asymmetry of nodal expression and alterations in murine situs inversus. *Nature* 1996;381:158–161.

8. Collignon J, Varlet I, Robertson EJ. Relationship between asymmetric nodal expression and the direction of embryonic turning. *Nature* 1996;381:155–158.

9. Meno C, Saijoh Y, Fujii H, et al. Left-right asymmetric expression of the TGF-fl-family member lefty in mouse embryos. *Nature* 1996;381:151–155.

10. Fishman MC, Chien KR. Fashioning the vertebrate heart: Earliest embryonic decisions. *Development* 1997;124:2099–2117.

Section II

9

Molecular Genetics of Congenital Heart Disease

Paul D. Grossfeld, MD and Kenneth R. Chien, MD, PhD

Molecular Basis of Cardiovascular Disease

Congenital heart disease (CHD) has been considered to arise from a combination of environmental and/or genetic (i.e., multifactorial) causes.[1-9] Through advances in molecular biology, researchers have begun to identify several genes that are associated with congenital heart defects.[10-14] Aberrant expression of these genes may lead to the development of congenital heart defects. Familial forms of most human congenital cardiac lesions have been described. In addition, many congenital heart defects have been found to be associated with specific chromosomal abnormalities, which suggests the presence of causative genes that reside within the implicated chromosomal regions. For this review, a new classification scheme of congenital heart defects related to genetic mechanism has been adopted. This reclassification is based on the growing body of evidence that underlying genetic defects affecting a variety of congenital cardiovascular disorders are functionally related, as in the obstructive cardiomyopathies and the long QT syndromes (see later discussion). Accordingly, in this review we will discuss the genetic basis of congenital heart defects

(Fig. 1), focusing on the current understanding of genetic etiologies and emphasizing genetic mechanisms and principles as they apply to CHD.

Cardiomyopathies

The cardiomyopathies are a heterogeneous group of disorders, in which myocardial structure is altered, leading to systolic and/or diastolic dysfunction. The cause of death in children with cardiomyopathies is usually arrhythmias or congestive heart failure.[15] Cardiomyopathies associated with known genes are classified into four categories: hypertrophic, dilated, metabolic, and mitochondrial. The basis for the relationship between gene function and the clinical class of cardiomyopathy (e.g., dilated, hypertrophic, restrictive) is unclear. Single gene defects have been found in association with sporadic and familial cardiomyopathies, including some previously classified as "idiopathic" (Table 1).

Hypertrophic Obstructive Cardiomyopathy

Hypertrophic obstructive cardiomyopathy (HOCM) is characterized by asym-

From Clark EB, Nakazawa M, Takao A (eds.): Etiology and Morphogenesis of Congenital Heart Disease: Twenty Years of Progress in Genetics and Developmental Biology. Armonk, NY: Futura Publishing Co., Inc.; © 2000.

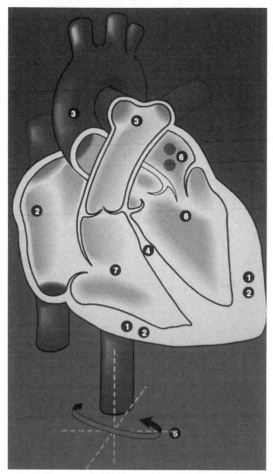

Figure 1. Congenital cardiac defects with a probable genetic etiology. 1, cardiomyopathy; 2, arrhythmias; 3, connective tissue disorders; 4, defects of septation; 5, defects of laterality; 6, defects in pulmonary venous connections; 7, defects of right-sided structures; 8, defects of left-sided structures

metric septal hypertrophy. In histologic study, cardiac myocytes demonstrate myofibrillar disarray and interstitial fibrosis, and the global cardiac hypertrophy phenotype gives rise to dynamic outflow obstruction and an increased incidence of sudden death.[14,15] HOCM occurs with a prevalence of 1 to 10 per 10,000, and 60% of cases are familial with an autosomal dominant pattern of inheritance.[16–19] The identification of seven genes associated with HOCM suggests that HOCM is the common endpoint phenotype for defects in genes that encode the structural components of the sarcomere (Fig. 2).[20–25]

Dilated Cardiomyopathy

The dilated cardiomyopathies are a heterogeneous group of disorders characterized by an increased ventricular dimension and decreased systolic ventricular function.[15] Of all cases of idiopathic dilated cardiomyopathy, 20% are familial. Autosomal dominant, autosomal recessive, and X-linked forms have been reported.[26–37]

Arrhythmogenic Right Ventricular Dysplasia

Arrhythmogenic right ventricular dysplasia (ARVD) is predominantly a disorder of the right ventricle in which the myocardium is significantly reduced in thickness with patchy, fibrofatty replacement. On pathologic study, it appears to mimic most closely a progressive, degenerative disease similar to Duchenne muscular dystrophy. There is a wide variety of clinical manifestations, thereby reflecting the anatomic heterogeneity of this disorder. Interestingly, the disease rarely involves the left ventricle, although it may occasionally involve the interventricular septum. Ventricular arrhythmias, usually monomorphic with left bundle branch block or anterior T-wave inversion, are common.[38] The disease occurs more commonly among certain subsets of patients, especially those who are young and otherwise healthy. The gold standard for diagnosis is endomyocardial biopsy. Familial forms of ARVD have been reported,[39–42] and at least 2 loci have been identified.[43,44]

Other Syndromes of Ventricular Dysplasia

Hypoplasia of the compact zone of the heart is distinct from other ventricular dysplasias in which there is essentially a genesis of all muscle layers of the developing myocardial wall (i.e., the compact zone, spongy layer, and trabecular layer). The first of these rare

Table 1
Primary Cardiomyopathies

Disease	Gene	Locus	Transmission
Cardiomyopathies:			
HOCM	β-MHC	14q11-q12	AD
HOCM	Troponin T	1q32	AD
HOCM	α tropomyosin	15q22	AD
HOCM	MBP-C	11p11.2	AD
HOCM	MELC	3p	?
HOCM	MRLC	12q	?
Dilated:			
Duchenne, Becker	Dystrophin	X	X-L
Barth	G4.5 (Tafazzins)	Xq28	X-L
—	Adhalin	17q21	AR
Myotonic Dystrophy	55Kd PK	19q13.3	AD
—	Connexin 40	1p1-1q1	AD
—	?	1q32	AD
—	?	3p25-p28	AD
—	?	9q13-q22	AD
—	?	10q21-q23	AD
ARVD	α-Actinin?	1q42-q43	AD
ARVD	α-Actinin?	14q23-q24	AD

HOCM, hypertrophic obstructive cardiomyopathy; MBP-C, myosin binding protein-C; MELC, myosic essential light chain; MRLC, myosin regulatory light chain; AD, autosomal dominant; X-L, X-linked; AR, Autosomal recessive; ARVD, Arrhythmogenic Right Ventricular Dysplasia.

clinical entities was described by Osler in 1905 as dramatic thinning and dilatation of both the right and left ventricular chambers, termed *parchment heart*. In 1952, Uhl described a syndrome restricted to the right ventricular chamber and sparing the interventricular septum,[45] distinct from the patchy, fibrofatty replacement seen in ARVD. As in ARVD, there are rarely associated congenital abnormalities, with the exception that it is usually diagnosed at a much earlier age. Although familial forms of Uhl syndrome have been reported,[46] a careful reanalysis of these and other cases shows that in the past, Uhl syndrome and ARVD were frequently confused in diagnosis, and that, in fact, familial occurrence of true Uhl syndrome has not been convincingly reported.

Cardiomyopathies Caused by Metabolic Disorders

A large number of cardiomyopathies are secondary to systemic metabolic disorders (Table 2).[47] Many of these are the result of defects in specific genes encoding enzymes involved in fatty acid oxidation, glycogen metabolism, lysosomal storage, iron metabolism, and collagen metabolism. These disorders may cause restrictive, dilated, or hypertrophic cardiomyopathies and are usually inherited in an autosomal recessive pattern.

Cardiomyopathies Caused by Mitochondrial DNA Defects

Researchers have found an association between certain cardiomyopathies and mutations in mitochondrial genes[47-49] (Table 2). The human mitochondrial genome is 16 kilobases in length and encodes mitochondrial transfer and ribosomal RNAs. Mitochondria are maternally inherited, and genetically identical or different copies of the mitochondrial genome may exist in an individual cell, resulting in homoplasmy or heteroplasmy, respectively. The relative distribution of the wild-type

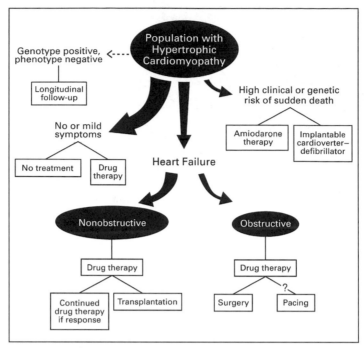

Figure 2. Sarcomeric proteins are mutated in hypertrophic cardiomypathy.

and mutant genomes can change over generations as a result of differences in the rates of replication and stability of the different genomes. The clinical expression of mitochondrial mutations depends on the extent of heteroplasmy and the tissue threshold for which normal function cannot be maintained by the relative amount of wild-type mitochondrial genomes. Human mitochondrial diseases display a wide range of clinical variability. Mitochondrial diseases have been associated with hypertrophic and dilated cardiomyopathies, and a number of other organ systems can be involved, most commonly skeletal muscle. Mutations have been found in mitochondrial genes that encode enzymes involved in oxidative phosphorylation.

Arrhythmias

Long QT Syndrome

Long QT syndrome is a significant cause of sudden cardiac death in children (Table 3).[50–64] The hallmark feature of long QT syndrome is delayed repolarization of the cardiac myocyte. As many as 50% of all cases of long QT syndrome are familial. Two inherited forms have been described: Romano-Ward, which is autosomal dominant, and Jervell and Lange-Nielsen, which is autosomal recessive and associated with congenital neural deafness. Between 5% and 20% of patients die of cardiac arrhythmias within 1 year of the time of diagnosis. A large number of patients are asymptomatic before death and many cases are diagnosed retrospectively after study of relatives.

Studies in families with long QT syndrome have led to the identification of four genetic loci on chromosomes 3, 4, 7, and 11. Three genes have been identified. Identification of the genetic defect in long QT syndrome may ultimately guide therapy in these patients.[64–66] For example, mexiletine, a sodium channel blocker, was shown to preferentially decrease the QT interval in patients with SCN5A (sodium channel) mutations.[65] In patients with mutations in the HERG gene, potassium

Table 2
Cardiomyopathies Secondary to Metabolic Disorders

Infiltrative (storage)
Disorders of glycogen metabolism
  Glycogen storage disease type II (Pompe disease: acid maltase deficiency)
  Glycogen storage disease type III (Cori disease: debranching enzyme deficiency)
  Glycogen storage disease type IV (Andersen disease: branching enzyme deficiency)
  Glycogen storage disease type IX (cardiac phosphorylase kinase deficiency)
  Glycogen storage disease with normal acid maltase
Disorders of mucopolysaccharide degradation
  Mucopolysaccharidosis type I (Hurler syndrome)
  Mucopolysaccharidosis type II (Hunter syndrome)
  Mucopolysaccharidosis type III (Sanfillippo syndrome)
  Mucopolysaccharidosis type IV (Morquio syndrome)
  Mucopolysaccharidosis type VI (Maroteaux-Lamy syndrome)
  Mucopolysaccharidosis type VII (Sly syndrome)
Disorder of glycosphingolipid degradation (Fabry disease)
Disorder of glucosylceramide degradation (Gaucher disease)
Disorder of phytanic acid oxidation (Refsum disease)
Disorders of combined ganglioside/mucopolysaccharide and oligosaccharide degradation
  G_{M1} gangliosidosis
  G_{M2} gangliosidosis (Sandhoff disease)
Disorders of glycoprotein metabolism
  Carbohydrate-deficient glycoprotein syndrome (neonatal olivopontocerebellar syndrome)
Disorder of oxalic acid metabolism (oxalosis)
  Diminished energy production
Disorders of pyruvate metabolism
  Pyruvate dehydrogenase complex deficiency (Leigh disease)
Disorders of oxidative phosphorylation
  Complex I deficiency
  Complex II deficiency
  Complex III deficiency (histiocytoid CM)
  Complex IV deficiency (muscle and Leigh disease forms)
  Complex V deficiency
  Combined respiratory chain deficiencies
    Mitochondrial transfer RNA mutations
    MELAS syndrome
    MERRF syndrome
      Others
    Mitochondrial DNA deletions and duplications
      Kearns-Sayre syndrome
    Others
    Barth syndrome (3-methylglutaconic aciduria type II)
      Sengers syndrome
      Others
Disorders of fatty acid metabolism
Primary or systemic carnitine deficiency (carnitine uptake deficiency)
  Muscle carnitine deficiency
  Carnitine palmitoyl transferase type II deficiency
  Carnitine acylcarnitine translocase deficiency
  Very-long-chain acyl-CoA dehydrogenase deficiency
  Long-chain acyl-CoA dehydrogenase deficiency
  Long-chain 3-hydroxyacyl-CoA dehydrogenase deficiency
  Short-chain 3-hydroxyacyl-CoA dehydrogenase deficiency
  Multiple acyl-CoA dehydrogenase deficiency (glutaric acidemia type II)
Toxic intermediary metabolites
Disorders of amino acid of organic acid metabolism
  Propionic acidemia
  Methylmalonic acidemia
    Malonic acidemia
    β-Ketothiolase deficiency
    Mevalonic acidemia
    Tyrosinemia

Table 3
Arrhythmias

Long QT Syndromes: Disease	Gene	Locus	Transmission
LQT-1	KVLQT-1 (Potassium Channel ?)	11p15.5	AD
LQT-2	HERG (Potassium Channel)	7q35-q36	AD
LQT-3	SCN5A (Sodium Channel)	3p21-p24	AD
LQT-4	?	4q25-q27	AD
Jervell and Lange-Nielsen	KVLQT-1	11p15.5	
Progressive familial Heartblock, type I	Kallikrein-1(?)	19q13.2-q13.3	AD
Supraventricular Tachycardia (WPW)	?	7q3	AD
Familial atrial fibrillation	ADRB1, ADRA2, GPRK5 (?)	10q22-q24	AD

AD, autosomal dominant.

supplementation seemed to decrease the frequency of the arrhythmias.[66]

Familial Atrial Fibrillation

Atrial fibrillation, the most common arrhythmia in adults, is rare in children. Familial cases have been reported (Fig. 3),[67] and chromosomal linkage to 10q22-q24 has been demonstrated.[68] Two genes

encoding adrenergic receptors reside at this locus, and whether mutations in these genes are responsible for this disorder remains to be determined.

Progressive Familial Heart Block, Type I

Progressive familial heart block type I is an autosomal dominant disease char-

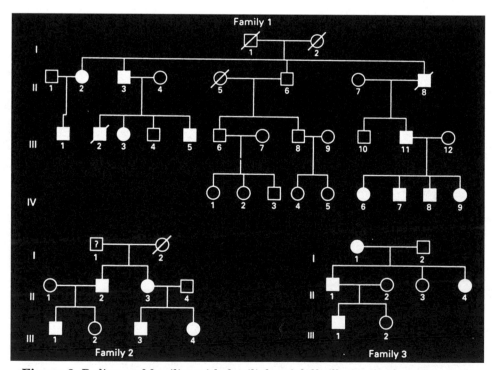

Figure 3. Pedigree of families with familial atrial fibrillation (with permission).

Table 4
Connective Tissue Disorders

Disease	Gene	Locus	Transmission
Marfan syndrome	fibrillin-1	15q15-q21	AD
CCA	fibrillin-2	5q23-q31	AD
SVAS	elastin	7q11.23	AD

CCA, congenital contractural arachnodactyly; AD, autosomal dominant; SVAS, supravalvar aortic stenosis.

acterized by progression from a normal conduction pattern to bundle branch block and subsequently to complete heart block with wide QRS complexes.[69] Sudden death may occur, and treatment with pacemaker placement is required. A study of 86 family members of three pedigrees, in which 34 members were affected, led to the demonstration of genetic linkage to chromosome 19 (19q13.2-q13.3). Several candidate genes reside within this region; one such gene is Klk-1, which encodes a member of the kallikrein family.

Supraventricular Tachycardia

Supraventricular tachycardia is the most common arrhythmia affecting infants and adolescents. Wolff-Parkinson-White (WPW) syndrome is a disorder of preexcitation of the ventricle by an accessory conduction pathway, which predisposes affected persons to the development of supraventricular tachycardia. Numerous familial cases of WPW have been described, which is suggestive of autosomal dominant inheritance. In a single pedigree of 25 living members with either WPW or hypertrophic cardiomyopathy, or both, the disorder was linked to chromosome 7.[70]

Connective Tissue Disorders

Marfan Syndrome

Marfan syndrome is an autosomal dominant disease characterized by skeletal, cardiovascular, skin, and ocular defects, and occurs with a frequency of 1 to 2 in 20,000 (Table 4). Premature death occurs from progressive dilation of the aortic root, which leads to dissection and aortic insufficiency. A neonatal form of Marfan syndrome is associated with a high rate of mortality from severe congestive heart failure resulting from multiple dysplastic valves. In patients with Marfan syndrome, tissues affected by the disease have been found to have decreased fibrillin due to mutations in the fibrillin gene.[71]

Williams Syndrome and Supravalvar Aortic Stenosis

Williams syndrome is an autosomal dominant disorder that is characterized by supravalvar aortic stenosis, peripheral pulmonary stenosis, obstructive coronary lesions, abnormal facies, and mental retardation. Williams syndrome was found to be associated with a deletion of a region on chromosome 7 (7q11.23) that includes the elastin gene and is thought to be a contiguous gene disorder caused by the deletion of multiple adjacent genes (Fig. 4).[72]

Supravalvar aortic stenosis (SVAS) occurs with a frequency of 1 of 25,000. A

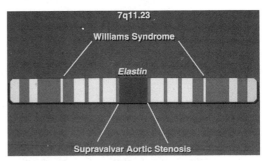

Figure 4. Contiguous gene disorder.

familial pattern of SVAS with autosomal dominant inheritance has been reported. SVAS has been linked to chromosome 7 and results from a defect in the elastin gene.[72]

Defects of Septation

Atrial Septal Defects

Familial cases of atrial septal defects in association with limb defects and cardiac conduction abnormalities have been reported (Table 5).[73] Holt-Oram syndrome, with an incidence of approximately 0.95 per 100,000 births, is characterized by cardiac defects, most commonly secundum atrial septal defects, occasionally ventricular septal defects, in association with upper arm defects, ranging from subclinical radiographic abnormalities of the radial or thenar bones to frank absence of the limb. HOS-1, which encodes a transcription factor that corresponds to the mouse Tbx5 gene, was found to be mutated in patients with familial or sporadic forms of Holt-Oram syndrome.[74,75] Another study of 14 family members with autosomal dominant transmission of atrial septal defects and first-degree heart block excluded linkage to 12q.2.[76] Most recently, mutations in another transcription factor (NKX2–5), which is expressed in the developing heart, were found in patients with an atrial septal defect.[77] Genetic linkage to chromosome 4p16 has been established for Ellis-van Creveld syndrome, an autosomal reces-

sive disorder characterized by dwarfism and a high frequency of atrial septal defects.[78] Thus, atrial septal defects are associated with mutations in at least four different genes, three with autosomal dominant and one with autosomal recessive inheritance.

Conotruncal Lesions and DiGeorge Syndrome

DiGeorge syndrome is characterized by mental retardation, dysmorphic facies, cleft palate, hypoparathyroidism, thymic hypoplasia, and cardiac defects.[79] This syndrome is caused by a defect in the development of the third and fourth embryonic branchial pouches (Fig. 5). The cardiac defects result from abnormalities in the development of the conotruncus, presumably as a result, at least in some cases, of aberrant development of the aortic arches. These defects include tetralogy of Fallot with pulmonary atresia, truncus arteriosus, type B interruption of the aortic arch, right aortic arch, D-transposition of the great arteries, and absence of the pulmonary valve.[80, 81]

DiGeorge syndrome, along with the velocardiofacial syndrome (Shprintzen syndrome) and CATCH-22 (cardiac defects, abnormal facies, thymic hypoplasia, cleft palate, and hypocalcemia) are linked to a chromosome 22 (22q11) deletion.[82–92] It is estimated that as many as 30% of patients with isolated conotruncal lesions may carry a 22q11 microdeletion.[84] Fine mapping of the 22q11 deletions has led to

	Table 5		
	Defects of Septation		
Disease	Gene	Locus	Transmission
ASD	HOS-1 (Tbx5)	12q2	AD
(Holt-Oram)			
(Ellis-van Creveld)	?	4p16	AR
Conotruncal Defects	?	22q11	AD(?)
(DiGeorge)		(300kb CR)	
Atrioventricular canal	?	21q22.3	AD(?)
		(4Mb MR)	

ASD, atrial septal defect; AD, autosomal dominant; AR, adrenergic receptor.

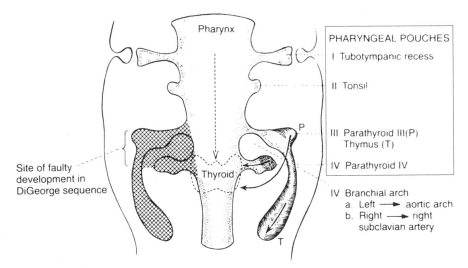

Figure 5. Developmental field defect in the 3rd and 4th branchial arches in DiGeorge syndrome (Reproduced with permission).

the identification of a DiGeorge critical region, an approximately 300-kb sequence within the 22q11 region (Fig. 6).[84, 85] Numerous genes reside within or near this region, and several reports have identified potential candidate genes (Table 6),[93–107] but no single candidate gene has been found to be consistently deleted in patients with DiGeorge syndrome and a deletion in 22q11.

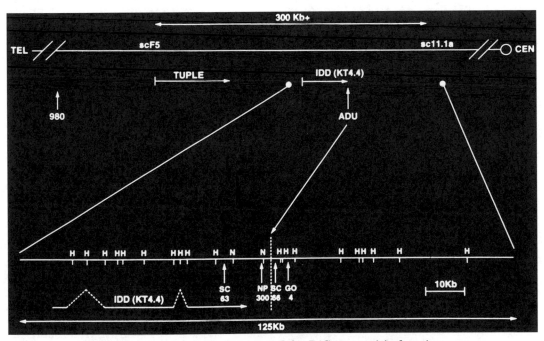

Figure 6. Schematic diagram of the DiGeorge critical region.

Table 6
DiGeorge Critical Region (22q11)
Candidate Genes

Tuple 1 (*Saccharomyces cerevisiae*)
IDD (Transmembrane protein)
Zinc-finger DNA binding protein
LZTR (DNA binding protein)
Adhesion receptor protein
Clathrin heavy chain protein
Serine/threonine kinase
Citrate mitochondrial transport protein
ES2 (*Caenorhabditis elegans*)
UFD1L

Atrioventricular Canal Defects and Down Syndrome

Down syndrome is the most common trisomy identified in newborns.[108] Although recognized in artistic representations as early as the first century B.C.,[109] it was first formally described in 1866 by John Langdon Down. The clinical features of Down syndrome show a high degree of penetrance and include characteristic facial features, such as low-set ears, a short and narrow palate, epicanthal folds, unusual palm creases, short stature, and muscular flaccidity. Associated defects include an Alzheimer's-like organic brain syndrome, hearing loss, disorders of purine metabolism, duodenal stenosis, susceptibility to infection, ocular lens defects, and a predilection for acute leukocytic and megakaryocytic leukemias.[110–113] Although never mentioned by Down, 40% of children with Down syndrome have an associated cardiac defect,[114,115] and 40% of these defects are endocardial cushion defects; other defects affecting the remaining 60% of patients with Down syndrome and heart disease include tetralogy of Fallot, truncus arteriosus, and double-outlet right ventricle.

The molecular basis of Down syndrome as trisomy 21 was first described by Lejeune as a maternal trisomy in 1959.[116] Approximately 95% of persons with trisomy 21 have an extra copy of chromosome 21; in approximately 5% of affected persons, a single copy is translocated from another chromosome. Although the precise gene or genes responsible for the phenotypes of Down syndrome are not known, considerable progress has been made in defining a down syndrome critical region. Mapping the chromosomal region that gives rise to the phenotypic characteristics of Down syndrome has been facilitated by the existence of partial human trisomies of chromosome 21. Studies of three generations in a family with Down syndrome, in which affected members had an atrioventricular canal defect and a chromosome 21 translocation, led to the identification of a 9-megabase Down syndrome critical region located at 21q22.1–22.3. Duplication of the distal region of 21q22 near D21S55 produces CHD with the same probability and phenotypic variation as full trisomy 21, which strongly suggests that single gene or locus in this region is responsible for the heart defects.[117, 118]

In one case, a patient with an atrioventricular canal-like ventricular septal defect was found to be mosaic for trisomy 21; most cells from lung and heart tissue displayed trisomy 21, whereas most skin cells and peripheral blood lymphocytes did not.[119] Thus, tissue-specific trisomy 21 mosaicism may cause isolated atrioventricular canal defects in patients who do not otherwise have the Down syndrome phenotype. In addition, several families with atrioventricular canal defects and autosomal dominant inheritance did not show genetic linkage to chromosome 21.[120,121]

Defects of Laterality

Several disorders involve abnormal spatial positioning of the heart or of structures within the heart (heterotaxy),[122] and there is strong evidence for a genetic etiology (Table 7).[123–132] These disorders include abnormal relationships between visceral organs (situs), atria, ventricles, and great arteries. One of these disorders, dextrocardia (abdominal organs in the correct location with the heart in the right side of the chest) has a high association with congenital heart defects.

Table 7
Disorders of Laterality

Disease	Gene	Locus	Transmission
Heterotaxy	Connexin 43 (GJA1)	6q21-q23.2	?
Kartagener	Microtubulin (?)	?	AD
Kartagener-like	?	?	AD, AR, Mt
Heterotaxy	?	?	AD
Heterotaxy	?	Xq24-q27.1	X
Heterotaxy	Int-1? Hox-3?	t(12,13)	?
Heterotaxy	?	Deln 10	?
Heterotaxy	?	Deln 13	?

AD, autosomal dominant; AR, adrenergic receptor; Mt, mitochondrial.

Ciliary Dyskinesia

Kartagener syndrome, an autosomally recessive disorder, is characterized by situs inversus, sinusitis, bronchiectasis, and male infertility. The disease is caused by a defect in the dynein arms of the microtubules, which are required for ciliary motility. Families with a Kartagener-like syndrome have been identified with autosomal dominant, X-linked, and mitochondrial forms of inheritance. In one case, all affected family members were missing dynein arms in their nasal cilia. Additional defects that affect the radial spokes and alter ciliary motion have been found. Thus, defects in many genes may lead to a final common phenotype as a result of ciliary dyskinesia.

Connexin 43

Mutations in the connexin 43 gene were found in a group of patients with heterotaxy. The connexin 43 protein comprises gap junctions, which function to mediate ion exchange between adjacent cells. Of 30 patients with a variety of congenital heart defects, 7 had mutations in the connexin 43 gene; 6 of those 7 had visceroatrial heterotaxy with pulmonary atresia.

Other Familial Cases or Chromosomal Abnormalities Associated With Defects in Laterality

An autosomal dominant form of heterotaxy has been reported in six families, and another family with heterotaxy demonstrated X-linked recessive inheritance. Thirty-nine family members were studied, and the locus was mapped to Xq24-q27.1. Other families or individuals with heterotaxy have been found to carry a translocation between chromosomes 12 and 13. Human counterparts to two fruitfly genes, transcription factors that regulate early pattern formation (Int-1 and Hox-3), are located near the site of this translocation breakpoint. In addition, deletions in chromosomes 10 and 13 have been found. Therefore, defects in laterality appear to be a heterogeneous group of disorders.

Table 8
Defects in Pulmonary Venous Connections

Disease	Gene	Locus	Transmission
TAPVR	VEGFR(?)	4p13.q12	AD
PAPVR (Scimitar syndrome)	?	?	AD

TAPVR, total anomalous pulmonary venous return; PAPVR, partial anomalous pulmonary venous return; AD, autosomal dominant.

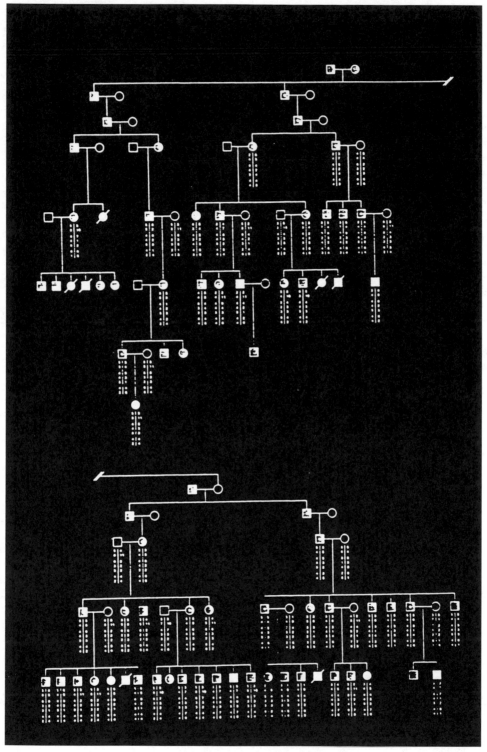

Figure 7. Eight-generation pedigree of family with isolated total anomalous pulmonary venous return.

Defects in Pulmonary Veins

Total Anomalous Pulmonary Venous Return

Total anomalous pulmonary venous return is present in approximately 1 in 10,000 live births (Table 8).[133] Many affected patients have associated syndromes, and multiple familial cases have been reported. In one report, 14 individuals over eight generations had isolated total anomalous pulmonary venous return, suggestive of autosomal dominant inheritance with low penetrance and variable expression (Fig. 7). Linkage analysis demonstrated an association with chromosome 4 (4p13.q12). One candidate gene at this locus encodes a vascular endothelial growth factor receptor, which is thought to have a role in vasculogenesis.[134]

Partial Anomalous Pulmonary Venous Return and Scimitar Syndrome

Scimitar syndrome is characterized by anomalous pulmonary venous drainage of the right lung (partial anomalous pulmonary venous return), in association with right lung hypoplasia, dextrocardia, right pulmonary artery malformation and hypoplasia, anomalous systemic arterial supply to the right lower lung, and malformation of the tracheobronchial tree. Twenty-five percent of infants have other associated cardiac defects, most commonly atrial septal defects. Three familial cases have been described.[135]

Left-Sided Obstructive Lesions

Hypoplastic Left Heart Syndrome

Hypoplastic left heart syndrome comprises approximately 2% of structural heart defects seen in liveborn children and is responsible for 10% to 25% of all neonatal deaths from CHD in the first few weeks of life (Table 9).[136] There are multiple examples suggesting a genetic etiology. Numerous familial occurrences of hypoplastic left heart syndrome have been reported and have demonstrated autosomal dominant and recessive inheritance. A recurrence rate of up to 14% has been reported.[137] In addition, in a study of first-degree relatives of infants with hypoplastic left heart syndrome, 5 of 41 (12.2%) had a bicommissural aortic valve,[138] approximately 10 times the frequency of the general population.

Patients with hypoplastic left heart syndrome have been reported to have as high as a 28% frequency of associated chromosomal defects or other syndromes.[139] One such syndrome, Jacobsen syndrome, is characterized by dysmorphic facies, growth and developmental delay, and mental retardation.[140] Approximately 70 such cases have been described,[141–143] and half of these patients have had hemodynamically significant cardiac defects, including 7 with hypoplastic left heart syndrome and 2 with left-sided obstructive lesions (Table 10). Thus, hypoplastic left heart syndrome occurs in patients with Jacobsen syndrome at a frequency about 625 times that of the general population. All patients with Jacobsen syndrome carry a deletion in the distal end of the long arm of chromosome 11 (Fig. 8). Most of these deletions are terminal; the remainder either are interstitial or are the consequence of the formation of a ring chromosome. A trinucleotide repeat sequence, which has been

Table 9
Defects in Left-Sided Structures

Disease	Left-Sided Lesions Locus	Transmission
HLHS	11q23	AD(?)
CoA	XO, XY−	AD/AR
BAV	—	AD
AS	—	AD
SubAS	—	AD/AR
AbCoAr	—	AD

HLHS, hypoplastic left heart syndrome; AD, autosomal dominant; CoA, coarctation of the aorta; BAV, Bicuspid Aortic Valve; AS, Aortic Stenosis; SubAS, Sub Aortic Stenosis; AbCoAr, aberrant coronary arteries.

Table 10
Heart Defects in Jacobsen Syndrome

VSD	12
HLHS	7
Coarctation	1
Shone	1
ASD	2
VSD/1° ASD	1
TA	2
TOF	1
TA/single ventricle	1
ECD	1
MISC	9
TOTAL:	40/72

VSD, ventricular septal defect; HLHS, hypoplastic left heart syndrome; ASD, atrial septal defect; VSD, ventricular septal defect; TA, tricuspid atresia; TOF, tetralogy of Fallot; ECD, endocardial cushion defect.

implicated in the pathogenesis of other human genetic diseases, has been identified in this region.[144] A comparison of the deleted regions of patients with or without heart defects, by karyotype analysis and/or physical mapping with molecular probes, has led to the identification of an approximately 20-megabase minimal (critical) region for the heart defects, located at 11q23.3-q24.1 (Fig. 9). Thus Jacobsen syndrome may be a contiguous gene disorder involving multiple genes at 11q23-q24, within which may lie a gene that can give rise to isolated hypoplastic left heart syndrome in the absence of other associated features of Jacobsen syndrome.

Subvalvar Aortic Stenosis

Subvalvar aortic stenosis is a relatively common lesion in the pediatric population that usually results from the development of a discrete subvalvar fibromuscular ridge, or long segment left ventricular outflow tract narrowing. It is usually not observed in newborns. Familial occurrences demonstrating autosomal recessive and autosomal dominant inheritance have been reported.[145, 146]

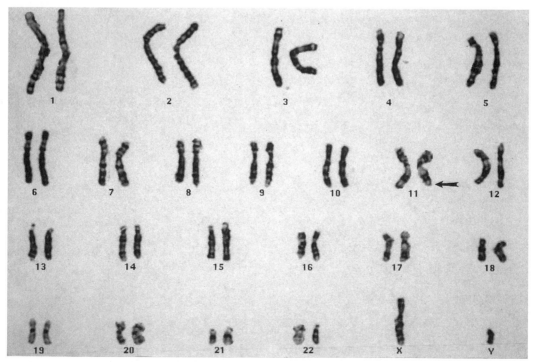

Figure 8. Karyotype of patient with Jacobsen syndrome and 11q-terminal deletion (Reproduced courtesy of Dr. Oliver William Jones, UCSD, School of Medicine)

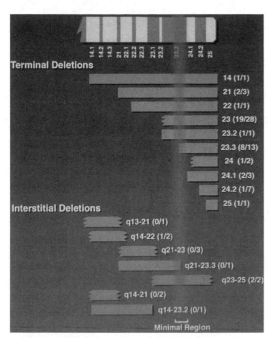

Figure 9. Genotype/phenotype relationship of 11q-patients. Shaded region indicates hypothetical minimal region for cardiac defects. Numbers in parentheses refer to number of patients with a cardiac defects, divided by total number of patients with the specific deletion. Jagged deletion indicates subband boundary is not defined.

Defects of the Aortic Valve

Bicommissural aortic valve occurs in about 1% to 2% of the general population and can be a predisposing factor for the development of aortic stenosis.[147] Familial cases with autosomal dominant inheritance have been reported.[148]

Aortic stenosis is a common lesion in children. Familial cases demonstrating autosomal dominant inheritance have been reported.[149] In one familial case, there was calcification of the valve and ascending aorta and no evidence of a bicommissural aortic valve in the affected members. At least three affected members also had immunologic abnormalities and no history or evidence of a previous syphilitic infection. One hypothesis is that aortic calcification may have been the consequence of an autoimmune disorder in these patients.[150]

Coarctation of the Aorta

Coarctation of the aorta is present in approximately 2 of 10,000 live births.[151] As many as one third of patients with Turner syndrome (the absence of one X chromosome), which is characterized by short stature, gonadal dysgenesis, and multiple somatic defects,[152] may have aortic anomalies, most commonly coarctation of the aorta and aortic stenosis.[153, 154] It has been hypothesized that cystic hygroma and distended thoracic lymph ducts compress the aortic arch and lead to the development of coarctation. Other sex chromosome disorders (for example, 46X,Yp-) with Turner-like features have also been found to have a high frequency (18%) of aortic anomalies. One possibility is that aortic arch anomalies in Turner syndrome may be secondary to defects in genes that interfere with the development of adjacent structures. However, several familial cases of coarctation of the aorta in patients without Turner syndrome have also been reported with autosomal dominant and recessive inheritance.[155–157]

Aberrant Coronary Arteries

Anomalous origin of the left coronary artery from the right sinus of Valsalva is one of the most common coronary artery anomalies. In one family, a father, son, and daughter were affected, which is suggestive of autosomal dominant inheritance.[158]

Right-Sided Lesions

Tricuspid Atresia

Tricuspid atresia accounts for 1.4% of congenital heart lesions.[159] In one report, three siblings in a family had tricuspid atresia, which is consistent with autosomal recessive inheritance.[160] Other reports describe tricuspid valve hypoplasia and right ventricular hypoplasia in siblings, also suggestive of autosomal recessive inheritance.[161–163]

Ebstein Anomaly

Ebstein anomaly constitutes about 1% of CHDs,[164] and is characterized by varying degrees of tricuspid dysplasia and "atrialization" of the right ventricle. Multiple familial cases with autosomal dominant and recessive patterns of inheritance have been reported.[165, 166]

Pulmonary Atresia With Intact Ventricular Septum

Pulmonary atresia with intact ventricular septum is a rare lesion accounting for 0.7 to 3% of CHDs.[167] One report described two affected siblings, which is suggestive of autosomal recessive inheritance.[168] Another report described two affected first cousins, which is suggestive of autosomal dominant inheritance with incomplete penetrance.[169]

Pulmonary Stenosis and Noonan Syndrome

Short stature, mental retardation, abnormal facies, and other skeletal abnormalities characterize Noonan syndrome, which occurs with an incidence of approximately 1 in 1000 to 2000.[170,171] Cardiac anomalies occur frequently, including a dysplastic pulmonary valve, pulmonary stenosis without dysplasia, left ventricular hypertrophy, and atrial and ventricular septal defects. In a study of 118 patients with Noonan syndrome, 83 (70%) had associated heart defects.[172] Familial cases of Noonan syndrome suggestive of autosomal dominant inheritance have been described, and Noonan syndrome has been linked to chromosome 12q.[173] One case of Noonan syndrome with DiGeorge syndrome and another case of Noonan syndrome with velocardiofacial syndrome have also been described; both patients had a 22q11 deletion.[174]

Table 11
Right-Sided Defects

Defect	Locus	Transmission
Tricuspid atresia	—	AR
Ebstein anomaly	—	AD
Pulmonary atresia/intact ventricular septum	—	AR/AD
Pulmonary valve dysplasia	—	
(Noonan syndrome)	12q	AD

AD, autosomal dominant; AR, Autosomal recessive.

Additional Congenital Heart Defects Associated With Specific Chromosomal Loci

A large number of congenital heart defects have been associated with chromosomal abnormalities and are frequently associated with specific syndromes.[175–187] A partial list has been provided in Table 11.

Summary

Familial occurrence has been reported for most human congenital heart lesions. Linkage analyses of families with multiple affected members and studies of patients with CHD and associated chromosomal defects will lead to the identification of additional genes associated with CHD. Rigorous complementary studies can then be performed in a genetically manipulatable system, such as the mouse, in order to establish a causal role for candidate genes and specific mutations found in human subjects. Identification of these genes, their role in normal cardiac development, and how their aberrant expression can cause CHD will lead to the development of novel molecular approaches for the diagnosis, management, and prevention of human CHD.

References

1. Whittemore R, Hobbins J, Allen Engle J. Pregnancy and its outcome in women with

and without surgical treatment of congenital heart disease. *Am J Cardiol*. 1982;50:641–651.

2. Corone P, Bonaiti C, Feingold J, et al. Familial congenital heart disease: How are the various types related? *Am J Cardiol* 1983;51:942–945.

3. Rose V, Morley Gold R, Lindsay G, et al. A possible increase in the incidence of congenital heart defects among the offspring of affected parents. *J Am Coll Cardiol* 1985;6:376–382.

4. Allen LD, Crawford DC, Chita SK, et al. Familial recurrence of congenital heart disease in a prospective series of mothers referred for fetal echocardiography. *Am J Cardiol* 1986;58:334–337.

5. Boughman JA, Berg KA, Astemborski JA, et al. Familial risks of congenital heart defect assessed in a population-based epidemiologic study. *Am J Med Genet* 1987;26:839–849.

6. Nora JJ, Nora AH. Update on counseling the family with a first-degree relative with a congenital heart defect. *Am J Med Genet* 1988;29:137–142.

7. Ferencz C, Boughman JA, Neill CA, et al. Congenital cardiovascular malformations: Questions on inheritance. *J Am Coll Cardiol* 1989;14:756–763.

8. Berg KA, Astemborski JA, Boughman JA, et al. Congenital cardiovascular malformations in twins and triplets from a population-based study. *Am J Dis Child* 1989;143:1461–1463.

9. Correa Villaseñor A, McCarter R, Downing J, et al. White-black differences in cardiovascular malformations in infancy and socioeconomic factors. *Am J Epidemiol* 1991;134:393–402.

10. Chien KR. Molecular advances in cardiovascular biology. *Science* 1993;260:916–917.

11. Anderson PAW. Cardiovascular molecular genetics. *Curr Opinion Cardiol* 1994;9:78–90.

12. Bouvagnet P, Sauer U, Debrus S, et al. Deciphering the molecular genetics of congenital heart disease. *Herz* 1994;19:119–125.

13. Payne RM, Johnson MC, Grant JW, et al. Toward a molecular understanding of congenital heart disease. *Circulation* 1995;91:494–504.

14. Johnson MC, Payne RM, Grant JW, et al. The genetic basis of pediatric heart diseases. *Ann Med* 1995;27:289–300.

15. Spevak P. Myocardial disease. In: Moller JH, William NA, eds. *Fetal, Neonatal, and Infant Cardiac Disease*. East Norwalk, Conn: Appleton & Lange; 1990:809–828.

16. Kelly DP, Strauss AW. Inherited cardiomyopathies. *N Engl J Med* 1994;330:913–919.

17. Marian AJ, Roberts R. Molecular basis of hypertrophic and dilated cardiomyopathy. *Tex Heart Inst J* 1994;21:6–15.

18. Marian AJ, Roberts R. Molecular genetics of hypertrophic cardiomyopathy. *Annu Rev Med* 1995;46:213–222.

19. Schwartz K, Carrier L, Guichency P, et al. Molecular basis of familial cardiomyopathies. *Circulation* 1995;91:532–539.

20. Thierfelder L, Watkins H, MacRae C, et al. α–Tropomyosin and cardiac troponin T mutations cause familial hypertrophic cardiomyopathy: A disease of the sarcomere. *Cell* 1994;77:701–712.

21. Watkins H, McKenna WJ, Thierfelder L, et al. Mutations in the genes for cardiac troponin T and α-tropomyosin in hypertrophic cardiomyopathy. *N Engl J Med* 1995;332:1058–1064.

22. Moolman JC, Corfield VA, Posen B, et al. Sudden death due to troponin-t mutations. *J Am Coll Cardiol* 1997;29:549–555.

23. Watkins H, Conner D, Thierfelder L, et al. Mutations in the cardiac myosin binding protein-C gene on chromosome 11 cause familial hypertrophic cardiomyopathy. *Nat Genet* 1995;11:434–437.

24. Poetter K, Jiang H, Hussanzadch S, et al. Mutations in either the essential or regulatory light chains of myosin are associated with a rare myopathy in human heart and skeletal muscle. *Nat Genet* 1996;13:63–69.

25. Kimura A, Harada H, Park JE, et al. Mutations in the cardiac troponin I gene associated with hypertrophic cardiomyopathy. *Nat Genet Aug* 1997;16:379–382.

26. McMinn TR, Ross J. Hereditary dilated cardiomyopathy. *Clin Cardiol* 1995;18:7–15.

27. Oldfors A, Eriksson BO, Kyllerman M, et al. Dilated cardiomyopathy and the dystrophin gene: An illustrated review. *Br Heart J* 1994;72:344–348.

28. Muntoni F, Cau M, Ganau A, et al. Deletion of the muscle-promoter region associated with X-linked dilated cardiomyopathy. *N Engl J Med* 1993;329:921–925.

29. Fadic R, Sunada Y, Wactawik AJ, et al. Brief report; deficiency of a dystrophin-associated glycoprotein (adhalin) in a pa-

tient with muscular dystrophy and cardiomyopathy *N Engl J Med* 1996;334:362–366.

30. Duggan DJ, Gorospe JR, Zanin M, et al. Mutations in the sarcoglycan genes in patients with myopathy. *N Engl J Med* 1997; 336:618–624.

31. Bione S, D'Adamo P, Maestrini E, et al. A novel x-linked gene, G4.5, is responsible for Barth syndrome. *Nat Genet* 1996;12: 385–389.

32. Bowles KR, Gajarski R, Porter P, et al. Gene mapping of familial autosomal dominant dilated cardiomyopathy to chromosome 10q21–23. *J Clin Invest* 1996;98: 1355–1360.

33. Kass SC, MacRae HL, Graber EA, et al. A genetic defect that causes conduction system disease and dilated cardiomyopathy maps to 1p1–1q1. *Nat Genet* 1994;7:546–551.

34. Olson TM, Keating MT. Mapping a cardiomyopathy locus to chromosome 3p22–p25. *J Clin Invest* 1996;97:528–532.

35. Durand JB, Bachinski LL, Bieling LC, et al. Localization of a gene responsible for familial dilated cardiomyopathy to chromosome 1q32. *Circulation* 1995;92:3387–3389.

36. Krajinovic MB, Pinamonti G, Sinagra G, et al. Linkage of familial dilated cardiomyopathy to chromosome 9. *Am J Hum Genet* 1995;57:846–852.

37. Schultz KR, Gajarski RJ, Pignatelli R, et al. Genetic heterogeneity in familial dilated cardiomyopathy. *Biochem Mol Med* 1995;56:87–93.

38. Basso C, Thiene G, Corrado D, et al. Arrhythmogenic right ventricular cardiomyopathy. Dysplasia, dystrophy, or myocarditis? *Circulation* 1996;94:983–991.

39. Cancani B, Nava A, Toso V, et al. A causal spontaneous mutation as possible cause of the familial form of arrhythmogenic right ventricular cardiomyopathy (arrhythmogenic right ventricular dysplasia). *Clin Cardiol* 1992;15:217–219.

40. Laurent M, Descaves C, Biron Y, et al. Familial form of arrhythmogenic right ventricular dysplasia. *Am Heart J* 1987; 113:827–829.

41. Nava A, Thiene G, Canciania B, et al. Familial occurrence of right ventricular dysplasia: A study involving nine families. *J Am Coll Cardiol* 1988;12:1222–1228.

42. Nava A, Canciani A, Thiene G, et al. Analyse du mode de transmission de la dyspl-

sie ventriculaire droite. *Ach Mal Coeur* 1990;83:923–928.

43. Rampazzo A, Nava A, Daniele GA, et al. The gene for arrhythmogenic right ventricular cardiomyopathy maps to chromosome 14q23–q24. *Hum Mol Genet* 1994;3: 959–962.

44. Rampazzo A, Nava A, Erne P, et al. A new locus for arrhythmogenic right ventricular cardiomyopathy (ARVD2) maps to chromosome 1q42–q43. *Hum Mol Genet* 1995; 4:2151–2154.

45. Uhl HSM. A previously undescribed congenital malformation of the heart: almost total absence of the myocardium of the right ventricle. *Bull Johns Hopkins Hosp* 1952;91:671–676.

46. Fischer DR, Zuberbuhler JR. Familial Uhl's anomaly. *Am J Cardiol* 1984;54:940.

47. Schwartz M, Cox G, Lin AE, et al. Clinical approach to genetic cardiomyopathy in children. *Circulation* 1996;94:2021–2038.

48. Wallace DC, Lott MT, Schoffner JM, et al. Diseases resulting from mitochondrial DNA point mutation. *J Inher Metab Dis* 1992;15:472–479.

49. Ozawa T. Mitochondrial cardiomyopathy. *Herz* 1994;19:105–118.

50. Keating MT. The long QT syndrome. A review of recent molecular genetic and physiologic discoveries. *Medicine* 1996;75: 1–5.

51. Weintraub RG, Gow RM, Wilkinson JL. The congenital long QT syndromes in childhood. *J Am Coll Cardiol* 1990;16: 674–680.

52. Grace AA, Chien KR. Congenital long QT syndromes. Toward molecular dissection of arrhythmia substrates. *Circulation* 1995;92:2786–2789.

53. Towbin JA. Clinical implications of basic research: New revelations about the long-QT syndrome. *N Engl J Med* 1995; 333:384–385.

54. Roden DM, Lazzara R, Rosen M, et al. Multiple mechanisms in the long-QT syndrome. Current knowledge, gaps, and future directions. *Circulation* 1996;94: 1996–2011.

55. Vincent GM, Timothy KW, Leppert M, et al. The spectrum of symptoms and QT intervals in carriers of the gene for the long-QT syndrome. *N Engl J Med.* 1992; 327:846–852.

56. Rosen M. Long QT syndrome patients with gene mutations. *Circulation* 1995;92: 3373–3375.

57. Curran ME, Sanguinetti MC, Keating MT. Molecular basis of inherited cardiac arrhythmias. In: Chien KR, ed. *Molecular Basis of Cardiovascular Disease.* Philadelphia, Pa: WB Saunders.

58. Roy ML, Dumaine R, Brown AM. HERG, a primary human ventricular target of the nonsedating antihistamine terfenadine. *Circulation* 1996;94:817–823.

59. Jiang C, Atkinson D, Towbin JA, et al. Two long QT syndrome loci map to chromosomes 3 and 7 with evidence for further heterogeneity. *Nat Genet* 1994;8:141–147.

60. Wang Q, Shen J, Li Z, et al. Cardiac sodium channel mutations in patients with long QT syndrome, an inherited cardiac arrhythmia. *Hum Mol Genet* 1995;4:1603–1607.

61. Wang Q, Curran ME, Splawski I, et al. Positional cloning of a novel potassium channel gene: KVLQT1 mutations cause cardiac arrhythmias. *Nat Genet* 1996;12:17–23.

62. Sanguinetti MC, Curran ME, Zou A, et al. Coassembly of K_vLQT1 and minK (IsK) proteins to form cardiac I_{Ks} potassium channel. *Nature* 1996;384:80–83.

63. Splawski I, Timothy WK, Vincent GM, et al. Molecular basis of the long-QT syndrome associated with deafness. *N Engl J Med* 1997;336:1562–1567.

64. Moss AJ, Zareba W, Benhorin J, et al. ECG t-wave patterns in genetically distinct forms of the hereditary long QT syndrome. *Circulation* 1995;92:2929–2934.

65. Schwartz PJ, Priori SG, Locati EH, et al. Long QT syndrome patients with mutations of the SCN5A and HERG genes have differential responses to Na$^+$ channel blockade and to increases in heart rate. *Circulation* 1995;92:3381–3386.

66. Compton SJ, Lux RL, Ramsey MR, et al. Genetically defined therapy of inherited long-QT syndrome: Correction of abnormal repolarization by potassium. *Circulation* 1996;94:1018–1022.

67. Beyer F, Paul T, Luhmer I, et al. Familiäres idiopathisches Vorhofflimmern mit Bradyarrhythmic. *Z Kardiol* 1993;82:674–677.

68. Brugada R, Tapscott T, Czernuscewicz GZ, et al. Identification of a genetic locus for familial atrial fibrillation. *N Engl J Med* 1997;336:905–911.

69. Brink PA, Ferreira A, Moolman JC, et al. Gene for progressive familial heart block Type I maps to chromosome 19q13. *Circulation* 1995;91:1633–1640.

70. MacRae CA, Ghaisas N, Kass S, et al. Familial hypertrophic cardiomyopathy with Wolff-Parkinson-White syndrome maps to a locus on chromosome 7q3. *J Clin Invest* 1995;96:1216–1220.

71. Tsipouras P, Del Mastro R, Sarfarazi M, et al. Genetic linkage of the Marfan syndrome, ectopia lentis, and congenital contractural arachnodactyly to the fibrillin genes on chromosomes 15 and 5. *N Engl J Med* 1992;326:905–909.

72. Keating MT. Genetic approaches to cardiovascular disease. Supravalvular aortic stenosis, Williams syndrome, and long-QT syndrome. *Circulation* 1995;92:142–147.

73. Basson CT, Cowley GS, Solomon SD, et al. The clinical and genetic spectrum of the Holt-Oram syndrome (heart-hand syndrome). *N Engl J Med* 1994;330:885–891.

74. Li QY, Newbury-Ecob RA, Terrett JA, et al. Holt-Oram syndrome is caused by mutations in TBX5, a member of the Brachyury (T) gene family. *Nature Genet* 1997;15:21–29.

75. Basson CT, Bachinsky DR, Lin RC, et al. Mutations in human TBX5 [corrected] cause limb and cardiac malformation in Holt-Oram syndrome [published erratum appears in *Nat Genet* 1997;15:411]. *Nature Genet* 1997;15:30–35.

76. Basson CT, Solomon SD, Weissman B, et al. Genetic heterogeneity of heart-hand syndromes. *Circulation* 1995;91:1326–1329.

77. Schott JJ, Benson DW, Basson CT, et al. Congenital heart disease caused by mutations in the transcription factor NKX2–5. *Science* 1998;281:108–111.

78. Polymeropoulos MH, Ide SE, Wright M, et al. The gene for the Ellis-van Creveld syndrome is located on chromosome 4p16. *Genomics* 1996;35:1–5.

79. Jones KL. *Smith's Recognizable Patterns of Human Malformation.* 5th ed. Philadelphia, Pa: WB Saunders; 1997:616–617.

80. Johnson MC, Strauss AW, Dowton SB, et al. Deletion within chromosome 22 is common in patients with absent pulmonary valve syndrome. *Am J Cardiol* 1995;76:66–69.

81. Melchionda S, Digilio MC, Mingarelli R, et al. Transposition of the great arteries associated with deletion of chromosome 22q11. *Am J Cardiol* 1995;75:95–98.

82. Rohn RD, Leffell MS, Leadem P, et al. Familial third-fourth pharyngeal pouch syndrome with apparent autosomal dominant transmission. *J Pediatr* 1984;105:47–51.

83. Greenberg F, Crowder WE, Paschall V, et al. Familial DiGeorge syndrome and associated partial monosomy of chromosome 22. *Hum Genet* 1984;65:317–319.

84. Goldmuntz E, Driscoll D, Budarf ML, et al. Microdeletions of chromosomal region 22q11 in patients with congenital conotruncal cardiac defects. *J Med Genet* 1993;30: 807–812.

85. Webber SA, Hatchwell E, Barber J, et al. Importance of microdeletions of chromosomal region 22q11 as a cause of selected malformations of the ventricular outflow tracts and aortic arch: A three-year prospective study. *J Pediatr* 1996;129:26–32.

86. Burn J, takao A, Wilson D, et al. Conotruncal anomaly face syndrome is associated with a deletion within chromosome 22q11. *J Med Genet* 1993;30:822–824.

87. Amati F, Mari A, Digilio MC, et al. 22q11 deletions in isolated and sydromic patients with tetralogy of fallot. *Hum Genet* 1995;95:479–482.

88. Wulfsberg EA, Zinta EJ, Moore JW. The inheritance of conotruncal malformations: A review and report of two siblings with tetralogy of Fallot with pulmonary atresia. *Clin Genet* 1991;40:12–16.

89. Pacileo G, Musewe NN, Calabro R. Tetralogy of fallot in three siblings: A familial study and review of the literature. *Eur J Pediatr* 1992;151:726–727.

90. Pankau R, Funda J, Wessel A. Interrupted aortic arch type B1 in a brother and sister: Suggestion of a recessive gene. *Am J Med Genet* 1990;36:175–177.

91. Wilson DI, Burn J, Scambler P, et al. DiGeorge syndrome: Part of catch 22. *J Med Genet* 1993;30:852–856.

92. Driscoll DA, Salvin J, Sellinger B, et al. Prevalence of 22q11 microdeletions in DiGeorge and velocardiofacial syndromes: Implications for genetic counseling and prenatal diagnosis. *J Med Genet* 1993;30: 813–817.

93. Mulder MP, Wilke M, Langeveld A, et al. Positional mapping of loci in the DiGeorge critical region at chromosome 22q11 using a new marker (D22S183). *Hum Genet* 1995;96:133–141.

94. Halford S, Wadey R, Roberts C, et al. Isolation of a putative transcriptional regulator from the region of 22q11 deleted in DiGeorge syndrome, Shprintzen syndrome and familial congenital heart disease. *Hum Mol Genet* 1993;2:2099–2107.

95. Budarf ML, Collins J, Gong W, et al. Cloning a balanced translocation associated with DiGeorge syndrome and identification of a disrupted candidate gene. *Nat Genet* 1995;10:269–278.

96. Lamour V, Lécluse Y, Desmaze C, et al. A human homolog of the *S.cerevisiae HIR1 and HIR2* transcriptional repressors cloned from the DiGeorge syndrome critical region. *Hum Mol Genet* 1995;4:791–799.

97. Halford S, Wilson DI, Daw S, et al. Isolation of a gene expressed during early embryogenesis from the region of 22q11 commonly deleted in DiGeorge syndrome. *Hum Mol Genet* 1993;2:1577–1582.

98. Aubry M, Demczuk S, Desmaze C, et al. Isolation of a zinc finger gene consistently deleted in DiGeorge syndrome. *Hum Mol Genet* 1993;2:1583–1587.

99. Kurahashi H, Akagi K, Inazawa J, et al. Isolation and characterization of a novel gene deleted in DiGeorge syndrome. *Hum Mol Genet* 1995;4:541–549.

100. Demczuk S, Aledo R, Zucman J, et al. Cloning of a balanced translocation breakpoint in the DiGeorge syndrome critical region and isolation of a novel potential adhesion receptor gene in its vicinity. *Hum Mol Genet* 1995;4:551–558.

101. Heisterkamp N, Mulder MP, Langeveld A, et al. Localization of the human mitochondrial citrate transporter protein gene to chromosome 22q11 in the DiGeorge syndrome critical region. *Genomics* 1995;29:451–456.

102. Lindsay EA, Rizzu P, Antonacci R, et al. A transcription map in the catch 22 critical region: Identification, mapping and ordering of four novel transcripts expressed in heart. *Genomics* 1996;32:104–112.

103. Demczuk S, Aledo R, Zucman J, et al. Cloning of a balanced translocation breakpoint in the DiGeorge syndrome critical region and isolation of a novel potential adhesion receptor gene in its vicinity. *Hum Mol Genet* 1995;4:551–558.

104. Stoffel M, Karayiorgou M, Espinosa R III. The human mitochondrial citrate transporter gene (SLC20A3) maps to chromosome band 22q11 within a region implicated in DiGeorge syndrome, velo-cardio-facial syndrome and schizophrenia. *Hum Genet* 1996;98:113–115.

105. Rizzu P, Lindsay EA, Taylor C, et al. Cloning and comparative mapping of a gene from the commonly deleted region of DiGeorge and velocardiofacial syn-

dromes conserved in *C. elegans*. *Mamm Genome* 1996;7:639–643.

106. Aubry M, Demczuk S, Desmaza C, et al. Isolation of a zinc finger gene consistently deleted in DiGeorge syndrome. *Hum Mol Genet* 1993;2:1583–1587.

107. Yamagishi H, Garg V, Matsuoka R, et al. A molecular pathway revealing a genetic basis for human cardiac and craniofacial defects. *Science* 1999;283:1158–1161.

108. Jones KL. *Smith's Recognizable Patterns of Human Malformation*. 5th ed. Philadelphia, Pa: WB Saunders; 1997:8–16.

109. Kunze JK, Münster IM. *Genetics and Malformations in Art*. Berlin: Grosse Verlag; 1986.

110. Wisniewski KE, Wisniewski HM, Wen GY. Occurrence of neuropathological changes and dementia of Alzheimer's disease in Down's syndrome. *Ann Neurol* 1985;17:278–282.

111. Mazzoni DS, Ackley RS, Nash DJ. Abnormal pinna type and hearing loss correlations in Down's syndrome. *J Intellectual Dis Res* 1994;38:549–560.

112. Korenberg JR, Bradley C, Disteche CM. Down syndrome: Molecular mapping of the congenital heart disease and duodenal stenosis. *Am J Hum Genet* 1992;50:294–302.

113. Fong CT, Brodeur GM. Down's syndrome and leukemia: Epidemiology, genetics, cytogenetics, and mechanisms of leukemogenesis. *Cancer Genet Cytogenet* 1987;28:55–76.

114. Spicer RL. Cardiovascular diseases in Down syndrome. *Pediatr Clin North Am* 1984;31:1331–1343.

115. Ferencz C, et al. Congenital cardiovascular malformations associated with chromosome abnormalities. *J Pediatr* 1989;114:79–86.

116. Lejeune J, Gautier M, Turpin R. Les chromosomes humain somatiques de neuf enfants mongoliens. *C R Acad Sci Paris*. 1959;248:1721–1722.

117. Rahmani Z, Blouin JL, Creau-Goldberg N, et al. Critical role of the *D21S55* region on chromosome 21 in the pathogenesis of Down syndrome. *Proc Natl Acad Sci U S A* 1989;86:5958–5962.

118. Korenberg JR. Toward a molecular understanding of Down syndrome. In: Epstein CJ, ed. *The Phenotypic Mapping of Down Syndrome*. New York: Wiley-Liss; 1993: 87–115.

119. Marino B, deZorzi A. Congenital heart disease in trisomy 21 mosaicism. *J Peds* 1993;122:500–501.

120. Wilson L, Curtis A, Korenberg JR, et al. A large, dominant pedigree of atrioventricular septal defect (AVSD): Exclusion from the down syndrome critical region on chromosome 21. *Am J Hum Genet* 1993;43:1262–1268.

121. Cousineau AJ, Lauer RM, Pierpont ME, et al. Linkage analysis of autosomal dominant atrioventricular canal defects: Exclusion of chromosome 21. *Hum Genet* 1994;93:103–108.

122. Moller JH. Malposition of the heart. In: Moller JH, Neal WA, eds. *Fetal, Neonatal, and Infant Cardiac Disease*. East Norwalk, Conn: Appleton & Lange; 1990: 755–774.

123. Yokoyama T, Copeland NG, Jenkins NA, et al. Reversal of left-right asymmetry: A situs inversus mutation. *Science* 1993;260: 679–682.

124. Wilson GN, Stout JP, Schneider NR, et al. Balanced translocation 12/13 and situs abnormalities: Homology of early pattern formation in man and lower organisms. *Am J Med Genet* 1991;38:601–607.

125. Danos MC, Yost HJ. Linkage of cardiac left-right asymmetry and dorsal-anterior development in xenopus. *Development* 1995;121:1467–1474.

126. Yokoyama T, Copeland NG, Jenkins NA, et al. Reversal of left-right asymmetry: A situs inversus mutation. *Science* 1993; 260:679–682.

127. Burn J. Disturbance of morphological laterality in humans. In: Biological asymmetry and handedness. Chichester: Wiley Chichester (CIBA Foundation Symposium 162); 1991:282–299.

128. Carmi R, Boughman JA, Rosenbaum KR. Human situs determination is probably controlled by several different genes. *Am J Med Genet* 1992;44:246–247.

129. Narayan D, Krishnan SN, Upender M, et al. Unusual inheritance of primary ciliary dyskinesia (Kartagener's syndrome). *Am J Med Genet* 1994;31:493–496.

130. Alonso S, Pierpont ME, Radtke W, et al. Heterotaxia syndrome and autosomal dominant inheritance. *Am J Med Genet* 1995;56:12–15.

131. Britz-Cunningham SH, Shah MM, Zuppan CW, et al Mutations of the *connexin43* gap-junction gene in patients with heart malformations and defects of

laterality. *N Engl J Med* 1995;332:1323–1329.

132. Casey B, Devoto M, Jones KL, et al. Mapping a gene for familial situs abnormalities to human chromosome Xq24–q27.1. *Nat Genet* 1993;5:403–407.

133. Krabill KA, Lucas RV Jr. Total anomalous pulmonary venous connection. In: Moller JH, William NA, eds. *Fetal, Neonatal, and Infant Cardiac Disease.* East Norwalk, Conn: Appleton & Lange; 1990; 571–586.

134. Bleyl S, Nelson L, Odelberg SJ, et al. A gene for familial total anomalous pulmonary venous return maps to chromosome 4p13–q12. *Am J Hum Genet* 1995;56: 408–415.

135. Neill, Ferencz, Sabiston, Sheldon. *Bull Johns Hopkins Hosp* 1960;107:1–21.

136. Gustafson RA, Neal WA. Hypoplastic left ventricle. In: Moller JH, Neal WA, eds. *Fetal, Neonatal, and Infant Cardiac Disease.* Norwalk, Conn: Appleton & Lange; 1990:723–744.

137. Driscoll DJ, Michels VV, Gersony WM, et al. Recurrence risks for congenital heart defects in relatives of patients with aortic stenosis, pulmonary stenosis, or ventricular septal defect. *Circulation* 1993;87(2 suppl)I:114–120.

138. Brenner JI, Berg KA, Schneider DS, et al. Cardiac malformations in relatives of infants with hypoplastic left-heart syndrome. *Am J Dis Child* 1989;143:1492–1494.

139. Natovicz M, Chatten J, Clancy R, et al. Genetic disorders and major extracardiac anomalies associated with the hypoplastic left heart syndrome. *Am J Dis Child* 1988;143:1492–1494.

140. Jones KL. *Smith's Recognizable Patterns of Human Malformations.* 5th ed. Philadelphia, Pa: WB Saunders; 1997:58–59.

141. Pivnick EK, Velagaleti GVN, Wilroy RS, et al. Jacobsen syndrome: Report of a patient with severe eye anomalies, growth hormone deficiency, and hypothyroidism associated with deletion 11(q23q25) and review of 52 cases. *J Med Genet* 1996;33:772–778.

142. Penny LA, Dell'Aquila M, Jones MC, et al. Clinical and molecular characterization of patients with distal 11q deletions. *Am J Hum Genet* 1995;56:676–683.

143. Ono J, Hasegawa T, Sugama S, et al. Partial deletion of the long arm of chromosome 11: Ten Japanese children. *Clin Genet* 1996;50:474–478.

144. Jones C, Penny L, Mattina T, et al. Association of a chromosome deletion syndrome with a fragile site within the proto-oncogene CBL2. *Nature* 1995;376: 145–148.

145. Onat A, Onat T, Domanic N. Discrete subaortic stenosis as part of a short stature syndrome. *Hum Genet* 1984;65:331–335.

146. Abdallah H, Toomey K, O'Riordan AC, et al. Familial occurrence of discrete subaortic membrane. *Pediatr Cardiol* 1994; 15:198–200.

147. Moller JH, William NA. *Fetal, Neonatal, and Infant Cardiac Disease.* East Norwalk, Conn: Appleton & Lange; 1990.

148. Clementi M, Notari L, Borghi A, et al. Familial congenital bicuspid aortic valve: A disorder of uncertain inheritance. *Am J Med Genet* 1996;62:336–338.

149. Zoethout HE, Carter REB, Carter CO. A family study of aortic stenosis. *J Med Genet* 1964;1:2–9.

150. Tentolouris C, Kontozoglou T, Toutouzas P. Familial calcification of aorta and calcific aortic valve disease associated with immunologic abnormalities. *Am Heart J* 1993;126:904–909.

151. Beekman RH, Rocchini AP. Coarctation of the aorta and interruption of the aortic arch. In: Moller JH, William NA, eds. *Fetal, Neonatal, and Infant Cardiac Disease.* East Norwalk, Conn: Appleton & Lange; 1990:497–521.

152. Jones KL. *Smith's Recognizable Patterns of Human Malformation.* 5th ed. Philadelphia, Pa: WB Saunders; 1997:81–87.

153. Ogata T, Matuso N. Turner syndrome and female sex chromosome aberrations: Deduction of the principal factors involved in the development of clinical features. *Hum Genet* 1995;95:607–629.

154. Rappold GA. The pseudoautosomal regions of the human sex chromosomes. *Hum Genet* 1993;92:315–324.

155. Örstavik KH, Lindemann R, Solberg LÅ, et al. Congenital heart defects, hamartomas of the tongue and polysyndactyly in a sister and brother. *Clin Genet* 1992;42: 19–21.

156. Cornel G, Sharratt GP, Virmani S, et al. Familial coarctation of the aortic arch with bilateral ptosis: A new syndrome? *J Pediatr Surg* 1987;22:724–726.

157. Dallapiccola B, Giannotti A, Marino B, et al. Familial aplasia cutis congenita and coarctation of the aorta. *Am J Med Genet* 1992;43:762–763.

158. Rowe L, Carmody TJ, Askenazi J. Anomalous origin of the left circumflex coronary artery from the right aortic sinus: A familial clustering. *Catheterization Cardiovasc Diagn* 1993;29:277–278.

159. Driscoll DJ, Danielson GK. Tricuspid Atresia. In: Moller JH, William NA, eds. *Fetal, Neonatal, and Infant Cardiac Disease.* Norwalk, Conn: Appleton & Lange; 1990:689–700.

160. Davachi F, McLelan RH, Moller JH, et al. Hypoplasia of the right ventricle and tricuspid valve in siblings. *J Pediatr* 1967; 71:869–874.

161. Sackner MA, Robinson MJ, Jamison WL, et al. Isolated right ventricular hypoplasia with atrial septal defect or patent foramen ovale. *Circulation* 1961;24:1388–1402.

162. Kumar A, Victorica BE, Gessner IH, et al. Tricuspid atresia and annular hypoplasia: Report of a familial occurrence. *Pediatr Cardiol* 1994;15:201–203.

163. Medd WE, Neufeld HN, Weidman WH, et al. Isolated hypoplasia of the right ventricle and tricuspid valve in siblings. *Mayo Clin Proc* 1960.

164. Braunlin EQ. Ebstein's anomaly of the tricuspid valve. In: Moller JH, William NA, eds. *Fetal, Neonatal, and Infant Cardiac Disease.* East Norwalk, Conn: Appleton & Lange; 1990:701–708.

165. Connolly HM, Warnes CA. Ebstein's anomaly: Outcome of pregnancy. *J Am Coll Cardiol* 1994;23:1194–1198.

166. McIntosh N, Chitayat D, Bardanis M, et al. Ebstein anomaly: Report of a familial occurrence and prenatal diagnosis. *Am J Med Genet* 1992;42:307–309.

167. Freedom, RM. *Pulmonary Atresia with Intact Ventricular Septum.* Mount Kisco, NY: Futura Publishing Company; 1989.

168. Chitaya TD, McIntosh N, Fouron J. Pulmonary atresia with intact ventricular septum and hypoplastic right heart in sibs: A single gene disorder? *Am J Med Genet* 1992;43:304–306.

169. Grossfeld PD, Lucas VW, Sklansky MS, et al. Familial occurrence of pulmonary atresia with intact ventricular septum. *Am J Med Genet* 1997;72:294–296.

170. Chery M, Philippe C, Worms AM, et al. The Noonan syndrome. The Nancy experience revisited. *Genet Couns.* 1993;4:113–118.

171. Jones KL. *Smith's Recognizable Patterns of Human Malformation.* 5th ed. Philadelphia, Pa: WB Saunders; 1997:122–123.

172. Burch M, Sharland M, Shinebourne E, et al. Cardiologic abnormalities in Noonan syndrome: Phenotypic diagnosis and echocardiographic assessment of 118 patients. *J Am Coll Cardiol* 1993;22:1189–1192.

173. Jamieson CR, van der Burgt I, Brady AF, et al. Mapping a gene for Noonan syndrome to the long arm of chromosome 12. *Nat Genet* 1994;8:357–360.

174. Wilson DI, Britton SB, McKeown C, et al. Noonan's and DiGeorge syndromes with monosomy 22q11. *Arch Dis Child* 1993; 68:187–189.

175. Ferencz C, Neill CA, Boughman JA, et al. Congenital cardiovascular malformations associated with chromosome abnormalities: An epidemiologic study. *J Pediatr* 1989;114:79–86.

176. Chitayat D, Babul R, Silver MM, et al. Terminal deletion of the long arm of chromosome 3 [46,XX,del(3)(q27→qter)]. *Am J Med Genet* 1996;61:45–48.

177. Phipps ME, Latif F, Prowse A, et al. Molecular genetic analysis of the 3p-syndrome. *Hum Mol Genet* 1994;3:903–908.

178. Meng J, Fujita H, Nagahara N, et al. Two patients with chromosome 6q terminal deletions with breakpoints at q24.3 and q25.3. *Am J Med Genet* 1992;43:747–750.

179. Tsukahara M, Murano I, Aoki Y, et al. Interstitial deletion of 8p: Report of two patients and review of the literature. *Clin Genet* 1995;48:41–45.

180. Wu BL, Schneider GH, Sabatino DE, et al. Distal 8p deletion (8)(p23.1): An easily missed chromosomal abnormality that may be associated with congenital heart defect and mental retardation. *Am J Med Genet* 1996;62:77–83.

181. Leichtman LG, Zackowski JL, Storto PD, et al. Non-mosaic tetrasomy 9p in a liveborn infant with multiple congenital anomalies: Case report and comparison with trisomy 9p. *Am J Med Genet* 1996; 63:434–437.

182. Takano T, Yamanouchi Y, Kawashima S, et al. 11q trisomy detected by fluorescence *in situ* hybridization. *Clin Genet* 1993;44:324–328.

183. Blancata JK, Hunt M, George J, et al. Prenatal diagnosis of tetrasomy 12p by in situ hybridization: Varying levels of mosaicism in different fetal tissues. *Prenat Diagn* 1992;12:979–983.

184. Gopal Roa VVN, Carpenter NJ, Gucsavas M, et al. Partial trisomy 13q identi-

fied by sequential fluorescence in situ hybridization. *Am J Med Genet* 1995;58:50–53.

185. Milunsky JM, Wyandt HE, Huang XL, et al. Trisomy 15 mosaicism and uniparental disomy (UPD) in a liveborn infant. *Am J Med Genet* 1996;61:269–273.

186. Whiteford ML, Coutts J, Al-Roomi L, et al. Uniparental isodisomy for chromosome 16 in a growth-retarded infant with congenital heart disease. *Prenat Diagn.* 1995;15:579–584.

187. Wilson RD, Chitayat D, McGillivray BC. Fetal ultrasound abnormalities: Correlation with fetal karyotype, autopsy findings, and postnatal outcome: Five-year prospective study. *Am J Med Genet* 1992;44:586–590.

10

Analysis of the Cardiogenic Functions of NK-2 Class Homeobox Genes Using a Cross-Species Cardiac Rescue Assay in Drosophila

Gogineni Ranganayakulu, PhD, David A. Elliott, PhD, Richard P. Harvey, PhD, and Eric N. Olson, PhD

There has been exciting progress in recent years toward identifying transcription factors that control cardiac myogenesis and morphogenesis.[1] Among these factors are the NK-2 class of homeodomain proteins, which are expressed in developing cardiac lineages in organisms ranging from *Drosophila* to mammals.[2] Here, we address how these factors function to control cardiac development and the extent to which their functions are evolutionarily conserved.

In *Drosophila*, the NK-2 homeobox gene *tinman* (*tin*) is expressed in early cardiac precursors and differentiated cardiac cells of the heart-like organ, the dorsal vessel.[3,4] Loss of function mutations of *tin* result in complete ablation of the cardiac lineage, consistent with the notion that *tin* acts to specify cardiac cell identity. In addition to this early role, *tin* has been shown to control differentiation of cardiac cells by directly activating transcription of the *D-Mef2* gene, which encodes a MADS-box transcription factor required for myoblast differentiation.[5] Tin

is also required for formation of visceral mesoderm.[3,4]

In vertebrates, there are five NK-2 class homeobox genes expressed in the developing heart (*Nkx2–3, Nkx2–5, Nkx2–6, Nkx2–7* and *Nkx2–8*) (Fig. 1A). *Nkx2–5* is the only member of this family that has been knocked out in mice and the resulting phenotype, characterized by abnormalities in looping morphogenesis and chamber formation, does not resemble the early phenotype that would be predicted based on the function of tin in *Drosophila*.[6] However, recent studies in *Xenopus* embryos using dominant-negative forms of *Nkx2–5* suggest that *Nkx2–5* is required for the specification of the cardiac lineage.[7,8]

Our interest was to use a gain of function assay to determine whether Nkx2–5 shares early cardiogenic functions with tin. To address this question, we introduced Nkx2–5 and various mutant derivatives into the *Drosophila* germline and tested for their ability to restore dorsal vessel formation in *tin* mutant background.[9] Tin and Nkx2–5 (also referred to as Csx) share extensive homology within their homeodomains and both proteins contain a conserved amino-terminal sequence of 12 amino acids, known as the TN domain, but outside of these domains,

From Clark EB, Nakazawa M, Takao A (eds.): Etiology and Morphogenesis of Congenital Heart Disease: Twenty Years of Progress in Genetics and Developmental Biology. Armonk, NY: Futura Publishing Co., Inc.; © 2000.

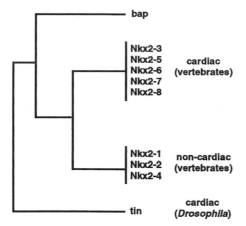

Figure 1. Simplified dendrogram of sequence relationships of NK class homeobox genes and schematic diagrams of tin and Nkx2–5 proteins.

the two proteins are unrelated[3,4,10,11] (Fig. 1B).

To express Nkx2–5 in *tin* mutant embryos, we used a binary transgenic system in which promoters for the *twist* and *D-Mef2* genes, which are expressed in mesodermal precursors of the dorsal vessel, were used to drive expression of the yeast transcriptional activator GAL4. Flies harboring these transgenes were crossed to flies harboring transgenes in which the GAL4-dependent upstream activating sequence (UAS) controlled expression of tin, Nkx2–5, or various mutants or chimeric proteins containing portions of each factor.

As predicted, expression of tin in *tin* mutant embryos using this binary transgenic system resulted in rescue of heart and visceral mesoderm formation. In contrast, Nkx2–5 was unable to rescue heart formation, though it could substitute for tin to support visceral mesoderm formation. Moreover, in wild type embryos, Nkx2–5 acted as a dominant negative repressor of cardiogenesis in *Drosophila*, presumably by competing with tin for binding sites in essential downstream genes. Thus, despite the sequence similarity and restricted expression of tin and Nkx2–5 to cardiac lineages in *Drosophila* and vertebrates,

respectively, Nkx2–5 does not possess early cardiac specification functions in the *Drosophila* embryo.

To define the domains of tin that enable it to activate cardiogenesis in *Drosophila*, we expressed several mutant forms of tin and Nkx2–5 in *Drosophila*. Deletion of the homeodomain of tin resulted in a complete loss in cardiogenic activity and replacement of the homeodomain of tin with that of Nkx2–5 restored that activity. These results demonstrate that tin must bind its target genes to activate cardiogenesis and that the homeodomain of Nkx2–5 can bind the same target genes in vivo. However, that Nkx2–5 cannot activate cardiogenesis suggests that DNA binding is not sufficient for heart formation in *Drosophila* and that domains outside the homeodomain must confer the unique cardiogenic properties of tin.

In an effort to identify potential regions outside the homeodomain of tin that are involved in cardiac specification, we created a series of tin:Nkx2–5 chimeric proteins, which were tested in the binary transgenic rescue assay. These experiments led to the identification of a novel 52-amino acid domain at the extreme amino-terminus of tin that could confer cardiogenic activity to Nkx2–5 in this assay (Fig. 1B). This novel cardiac-inducing domain does not include the transcription activation domain of tin, which lies adjacent to this domain.

These findings provide several new insights into the molecular mechanisms of mesodermal specification by NK-2 homeobox genes, as well as evolutionary conservation of these developmental pathways. The finding that both tin and Nkx2–5 can rescue visceral mesoderm formation in the *tin* mutant background demonstrates that Nkx2–5 can bind and activate the same downstream target genes as tin in the visceral mesodermal lineage. The functions of tin and Nkx2–5 in visceral mesoderm development, therefore, appear to be conserved and suggest a close evolutionary relationship between these two proteins. These results also raise the possibility that the distinct cardiogenic programs in flies and vertebrates were built upon a common and perhaps more ancient program for specification of visceral muscle.

The inability of Nkx2–5 to substitute for tin to control formation of the dorsal vessel in *Drosophila* might suggest that the mechanisms for heart formation in flies and vertebrates have diverged. However, the finding that the homeodomains of tin and Nkx2–5 are interchangeable and that Nkx2–5 can specify heart when fused to a 52-amino acid segment from the amino-terminus of tin, indicates that these factors can recognize the same downstream target genes and suggests that their ability to activate those genes is dependent on regions of the proteins outside the DNA binding domain. We propose that the cardiogenic domain at the amino-terminus of tin interacts with other important accessory factors and that these interactions are not sufficiently conserved to support heart formation by Nkx2–5. In this regard, factors that modify the selectivity of other homeodomain proteins have been identified.

Our results are in agreement with other recent studies demonstrating that different cardiac NK-2 homeobox genes rescue only visceral mesoderm formation in *tin* mutants (Fig. 2).[12] The ability of zebrafish Nkx2–5 to rescue the function of pharyngeal muscles in nematodes,[13] also reflects a common ancestral role for NK-2 homeobox genes in muscle development.

Finally, it is apparent that Nkx2–5 has acquired functions in cardiac development that do not exist in *Drosophila*. Whereas the initial molecular events involved in establishment of cellular cardiogenic activity may be at least partially evolutionarily conserved, the *Drosophila* heart does not undergo the complex morphogenetic events of looping and chamber formation that occur during vertebrate cardiogenesis. The demonstrated importance of Nkx2–5 in these processes indicates that it has acquired new functions during vertebrate evolution.

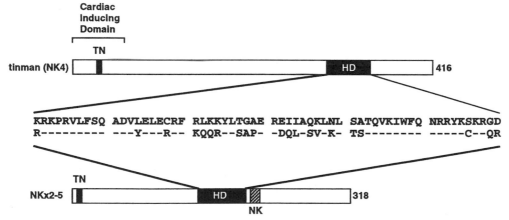

Figure 2. Genetic pathways for cardiac and visceral mesoderm formation in the *Drosophila* embryo. The transcription factor dorsal activates expression of the bHLH transcription factor twist, which is required for mesoderm formation. Twist activates expression of *tinman*, which is required for visceral and dorsal mesoderm formation. The growth factors Dpp and wingless are also required for induction of cardiogenesis. Our results suggest that the early role of *tinman* in visceral mesoderm formation can be replaced by Nkx2–5, whereas Nkx2–5 cannot substitute for *tinman* in the cardiac lineage. We postulate that *tinman* interacts with a cofactor required for cardiac induction.

References

1. Olson EN, Srivastava D. Molecular pathways controlling heart development. *Science* 1996;272:671–676.
2. Harvey RP. Nk-2 homeobox genes and heart development. *Dev Biol* 1996;178:203–216.
3. Azpiazu N, Frasch M. *tinman and bagpipe*: Two homeobox genes that determine cell fates in the dorsal mesoderm of *Drosophila*. *Genes Dev* 1993;7:1325–1340.
4. Bodmer R. The gene *tinman* is required for specification of the heart and visceral muscles in *Drosophila*. *Development* 1993;118:719–729.
5. Gajewski K, Kim Y, Lee YM, et al. D-Mef2 is a target for *tinman* activation during *Drosophila* heart development. *EMBO J* 1997;16:515–522.
6. Lyons I, Parson LM, Hartley L, et al. Myogenic and morphogenetic defects in the heart tubes of murine embryos lacking the homeobox gene *Nkx2-5*. *Genes Dev* 1995;9:1654–1666.
7. Fu Y, Yan W, Mohun TJ, et al. Vertebrate tinman homologues XNkx2-3 and XNkx2-5 are required for heart formation in a functionally redundant manner. *Development* 1998;125:4439–4449.
8. Grow MW, Krieg PA. Tinman function is essential for vertebrate heart development: Elimination of cardiac differentiation by dominant inhibitory mutants of the *tinman*-related genes, *XNkx2-3* and *XNkx2-5*. *Dev Biol* 1998;204:187–196.
9. Ranganayakulu G, Elliott D, Harvey R, et al. Divergent roles for Nk-2 class homeobox genes in cardiogenesis in flies and mice. *Development* 1998;125:3037–3048.
10. Lints TJ, Parson LM, Hartley L, et al. *Nkx2-5*: A novel murine homeobox gene expressed in early heart progenitor cells and their myogenic descendants. *Development* 1993;119:419–431.
11. Komuro I, Izumo S. *Csx*: A murine homeobox-containing gene specifically expressed in the developing heart. *Proc Natl Acad Sci U S A* 1993;90:8145–8149.
12. Park M, Lewis C, Turbay D, et al. Differential rescue of visceral and cardiac defects in Drosophila by vertebrate tinman-related genes. *Proc Natl Acad Sci, U S A* 1998;95:9366–9371.
13. Huan C, Alexander J, Stanier DY, et al. Rescue of *Caenorhabditis elegans* pharyngeal development by a vertebrate heart specification gene. *Proc Natl Acad Sci U S A* 1998;95:5072–5075.

11

Developmental Stage-Specific Transcriptional Regulation of Human Cardiac Homeobox Gene *CSX1*

Takehiko Mizuno, MD, Ichiro Shiojima, MD, and Issei Komuro, MD

Regulation of the tissue-specific gene expression by transcription factors is a central event during the development of specific tissues. Among the recently identified transcription factors that are essential for cardiac development, *Csx/Nkx-2.5*[1,2] is a homeobox-containing gene isolated as a potential vertebrate homologue of the *Drosophila* gene *tinman*.[3–5] *Csx/Nkx-2.5* is exclusively expressed in the heart from the very early developmental stage, and targeted disruption of *Csx/Nkx-2.5* gene in mice results in embryonic lethality because of the morphological abnormalities of the heart at the looping stage,[6] indicating that *Csx/Nkx-2.5* is a cardiac-restricted transcription factor that is essential for the normal heart development and morphogenesis. Therefore, the elucidation of the regulatory mechanisms of *Csx/Nkx-2.5* gene expression will provide important information to understand the molecular mechanisms by which cardiac development is regulated.

We have previously isolated *CSX1*, a human homologue of murine *Csx/Nkx2–5*,[7] and demonstrated that 965bp 5′ flanking region of *CSX1* gene is sufficient for cardiomyocyte-specific transcriptional activities at least in vitro (unpublished data). To examine the transcriptional regulation of *CSX1* during cardiomyocyte differentiation, *CSX1* promoter activity was examined in the embryonic stem (ES) cell system, which is a well-characterized in vitro model for cardiomyocyte differentiation.[8] The promoter activity of *CSX1* was very low in undifferentiated ES cells, increased sharply in erythroblasts (EBs) at day 5 of suspension culture, and remained at the relatively high levels thereafter (Fig. 1A). Because endogenous *Csx/Nkx2–5* starts to be expressed at day 5 in EB culture,[1] the time course of *CSX1* promoter activity was consistent with the endogenous *Csx/Nkx-2.5* expression pattern. Deletion analysis of *CSX1* promoter at day 5 showed that the deletion of the region between −716 and −672 decreased the promoter activity by 60% while the deletion of the same region had little effect when assayed at day 10 (Fig. 1B), suggesting that the positive cis-element located between −716 and −672 is involved in the transcriptional regulation of *CSX1* gene only in the early stage of cardiomyocyte differentiation. We termed this positive cis-element between −716 and −672 as CDE (for *CSX Distal Element*).

Early morning specimen analysis (EMSA) with nuclear lysates prepared from ES cells and EBs at day 5 and day 10

From Clark EB, Nakazawa M, Takao A (eds.): Etiology and Morphogenesis of Congenital Heart Disease: Twenty Years of Progress in Genetics and Developmental Biology. Armonk, NY: Futura Publishing Co., Inc.; © 2000.

A.

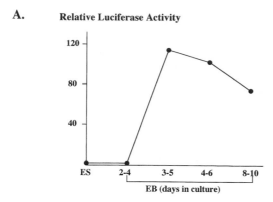

B.

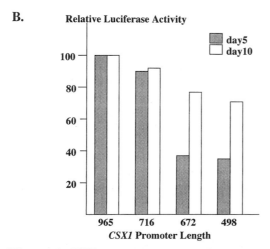

Figure 1. *CSX1* promoter activity during cardiomyocyte differentiation. **A.** Reporter plasmids containing 965bp promoter region of the *CSX1* gene were transfected to ES cells and EBs at various time points of differentiation, and promoter activities were determined. Transcriptional activities of 965bp *CSX1* promoter showed a marked increase at day 5 in culture and remained at the significantly high level thereafter. **B.** Deletion analysis of *CSX1* promoter was performed in EBs at day 5 and day 10 in suspension culture. Deletion of the promoter region between −716 and −672 reduced the promoter activity only at day 5 of EB differentiation.

revealed a day 5 EB-specific CDE-binding activity (Fig. 2A), suggesting that a developmental stage-specific DNA-binding factor regulates the expression of *CSX1* at the early stage of cardiomyocyte differentiation via CDE. Because CDE contained two 6-bp elements highly homologous to a BS.p half site, a binding sequence of Brachyury (T) that is essential for the mesoderm development (Fig. 2B),[9−11] we examined the possibility that Brachyury (T) is identical with CDE-binding factor. However, EMSA with the nuclear extracts prepared from *Xenopus* T gene (XeT)-overexpressed COS-7 cells revealed a strong BS.p-binding activity that was competed by BS.p itself but not by CDE (Fig. 2C), indicating that Brachyury (T) binds to BS.p but not to CDE. Next we examined the possibility that the CDE-binding factor binds to the E-box in CDE. The oligonucleotides mutated outside of the E-box (m2 and m5) abolished the CDE binding activity, whereas the oligonucleotides with mutated E-box (m1, m3, and m4) did not compete the wild-type probe (Fig. 2E). These results suggest that CDE-binding factor binds to the E-box motif in CDE.

Because the 965-bp 5′-flanking region of *CSX1* gene exhibited cardiomyocyte-specific transcriptional activity (unpublished data), and mediated a sharp increase in promoter activity that mimicked the endogenous *Csx/Nkx-2.5* gene expression, this region is thought to be involved in both the spatial and the temporal regulation of *CSX1* gene expression during cardiomyocyte differentiation. Deletion analysis of the *CSX1* promoter at day 5 and day 10 of EB differentiation identified CDE, a cis-regulatory element that is involved in the transcriptional regulation of *CSX1* only in the early stage of cardiomyocyte differentiation. Although the expression of *Csx/Nkx-2.5* starts from the early stage of embryonic development and persists in the adult heart in mice,[1,2] our present study suggests that the regulatory mechanisms of *Csx/Nkx-2.5* gene expression are different between the early and late stage of development. Our present results also indicate that CDE-binding factor is the E-box binding factor but not Brachyury (T). Because E-box is a consensus DNA binding sequence for the basic helix-loop-helix (bHLH) transcription factors, these results suggest that CDE-binding factor may belong to the bHLH transcription factor superfamily. At present, however, no transcription factor

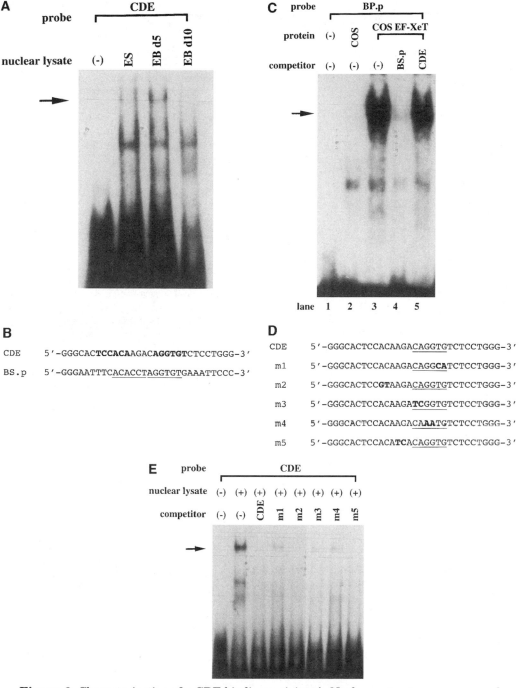

Figure 2. Characterization of a CDE-binding activity. **A.** Nuclear extracts were prepared from undifferentiated ES cells and EBs at day 5 and day 10, and EMSA was performed with CDE as a probe. One shifted band (arrow) was detected only in the extracts from EBs at day 5. **B.** Sequence comparison of CDE and BS.p. CDE contains two tandem repeat of sequences (bolded) highly homologous to the Brachyury half site (underlined). **C.** Nuclear extracts prepared from COS-7 cells transfected with the *Xenopus* T expression plasmids were analyzed by EMSA with BS.p as a probe. The binding activity of T protein to BS.p was not competed by excess amount of CDE oligonucleotides, suggesting that CDE-binding factor is distinct from Brachyury (T). **D.** Sequences of CDE and mutant oligonucleotides. The E-box is underlined and mutations introduced are bolded. **E.** Nuclear extracts prepared from day 5 EBs were analyzed by EMSA with CDE probe. Oligonucleotides containing mutations in the E-box motif do not compete for the wild type probe, suggesting that the CDE-binding factor binds to the E-box motif.

other than dHAND and eHAND has been characterized as tissue-specific bHLH proteins expressed in the developing heart. dHAND and eHAND were identified as E12-binding proteins and are expressed in the future right and left ventricle during murine cardiogenesis, respectively.[12,13] Recent studies have shown that dHAND and eHAND are involved in the left and right chamber specification of the heart and this process is, at least in part, under the control of *Csx/Nkx-2.5*.[14] Furthermore, in *dHAND* –/– embryos, expression of *Csx/Nkx-2.5* is not affected,[15] while in *Csx/Nkx-2.5* –/– embryos eHAND expression is downregulated.[14] From these results, it is unlikely that CDE-binding factor is identical with dHAND or eHAND.

Twist is also a bHLH factor that functions as a key regulator in the initial step of mesoderm formation in *Drosophila*, and is an upstream regulator of *tinman*.[16,17] However, *M-twist*, a murine homologue of *Drosophila twist*, is not expressed in the heart, and *M-twist* –/– embryos exhibit normal heart development until they die from abnormal head mesenchyme formation,[18] suggesting that *M-twist* is not the upstream regulator of *Csx/Nkx-2.5* and therefore is distinct from CDE-binding factor. Possibly *twist-tinman* genetic cascade cannot be applicable to vertebrates; *twist* seems to regulate the initial expression of *tinman* in all mesodermal cells while *Csx/Nkx-2.5* is expressed only in the precardiac mesoderm.

At present, no upstream transcription factor is known that directly regulates the expression of *Csx/Nkx-2.5*-family genes in vertebrates. The isolation and characterization of CDE-binding factor will provide novel insight for the understanding of the genetic cascade that regulates the initial step of cardiac development and differentiation.

References

1. Komuro I, Izumo S. *Csx*: A murine homeobox-containing gene specifically expressed in the developing heart. *Proc Natl Acad Sci U S A* 1993;90:8145–8149.

2. Lints TJ, Parsons LM, Hartley L, et al. *Nkx-2.5*: A novel murine homeobox gene expressed in early heart progenitor cells and their myogenic descendants. *Development* 1993;119:419–431.

3. Bodmer R, Jan LY, Jan YN. A new homeobox-containing gene, *msh-2*, is transiently expressed early during mesoderm formation of *Drosophila*. *Development* 1990;110:661–669.

4. Azpiazu N, Frasch M. *tinman* and *bagpipe*: Two homeo box genes that determine cell fates in the dorsal mesoderm of *Drosophila*. *Genes Dev* 1993;7:1325–1340.

5. Bodmer R. The gene *tinman* is required for specification of the heart and visceral muscles in *Drosophila*. *Development* 1993;118:719–729.

6. Lyons I, Parsons LM, Hartley L, et al. Myogenic and morphogenetic defects in the heart tubes of murine embryos lacking the homeo box gene *Nkx2-5*. *Genes Dev* 1995;9:1654–1666.

7. Shiojima I, Komuro I, Mizuno T, et al. Molecular cloning and characterization of human cardiac homeobox gene. *CSX1 Circ Res* 1996;79:920–929.

8. Robbins J, Gulick J, Sanchez A, et al. Mouse embryonic stem cells express the cardiac myosin heavy chain genes during development in vitro. *J Biol Chem.* 1990;265:11905–11909.

9. Herrmann BG, Labeit S, Poustka A, et al. Cloning of the T gene required in mesoderm formation in the mouse. *Nature* 1990;343:617–622.

10. Kispert A, Herrmann BG. The Brachyury gene encodes a novel DNA binding protein. *EMBO J* 1993;12:3211–3220.

11. Kispert A, Koschorz B, Herrmann BG. The T protein encoded by Brachyury is a tissue-specific transcription factor. *EMBO J* 1995;14:4763–4772.

12. Cserjesi P, Brown D, Lyons GE, et al. Expression of the novel basic helix-loop-helix gene eHAND in neural crest derivatives and extraembryonic membranes during mouse development. *Dev Biol* 1995;170:664–678.

13. Srivastava D, Cserjesi P, Olson EN. A subclass of bHLH proteins required for cardiac morphogenesis. *Science* 1995;270:1995–1999.

14. Biben C, Harvey RP. Homeodomain factor Nkx2-5 controls left/right asymmetric expression of bHLH gene *eHAND* during murine heart development. *Genes Dev* 1997;11:1357–1369.

15. Srivastava D, Thomas T, Lin Q, et al. Regulation of cardiac mesodermal and neural crest development by the bHLH transcription factor, dHAND. *Nat Genet* 1997;16: 154–160.

16. Thisse B, Stoetzel C, Gorostiza-Thisse C, et al. Sequence of the *twist* gene and nuclear localization of its protein in endomesodermal cells of early *Drosophila* embryos. *EMBO J* 1988;7:2175–2183.

17. Lee YM, Park T, Schulz RA, et al. Twist-mediated activation of the NK-4 homeobox gene in the visceral mesoderm of *Drosophila* requires two distinct clusters of E-box regulatory elements. *J Biol Chem* 1997; 272:17531–17541.

18. Chen ZF, Behringer RR. *M-twist* is required in head mesenchyme for cranial neural tube morphogenesis. *Genes Dev* 1995;9:686–699.

12

Functional Analysis of the Csx/Nkx2.5 Homeobox Gene in Murine Cardiac Development

*Makoto Tanaka, MD, Naohito Yamasaki, MD,
Ike W. Lee, MD, Stephanie Burns Wechsler, MD,
Joel A. Lawitts, MD, and Seigo Izumo, MD*

Introduction

Molecular mechanisms for cardiac development have been intensively studied during the last five years. Several genes critical for heart formation have been isolated and the function of each gene was analyzed in vivo by a gene targeting technique.[1,2] Among those genes, the Csx/Nkx2.5-eHAND pathway and the MEF2C-dHAND pathway have been shown to play critical roles at early stages of cardiac development.[3-8]

Csx/Nkx2.5 is a homeobox gene and a murine homolog of *tinman*,[9,10] whose disruption causes complete loss of the heart structure in *Drosophila*.[11] This gene starts to be expressed in the bilateral cardiac primordia as early as 7.5 days p.c. (post coitum), and continues to be expressed in the myocardium throughout gestation and in the adult.[9,10] The expression pattern suggested that this gene might play similar roles in cardiac development in vertebrates as *tinman* does in *Drosophila*. In this chapter, we will discuss the role of Csx/Nkx2.5 in cardiac development.

From Clark EB, Nakazawa M, Takao A (eds.): Etiology and Morphogenesis of Congenital Heart Disease: Twenty Years of Progress in Genetics and Developmental Biology. Armonk, NY: Futura Publishing Co., Inc.; © 2000.

Inactivation of Csx/Nkx2.5 Arrested Heart Formation, but Did Not Abolish the Cardiac Cell Lineage

It was reported that homozygous mice for Csx/Nkx2.5 disruption were embryonically lethal due to absence of cardiac looping.[4] However, the primitive heart tube formed normally, indicating that specification of the cardiac cell lineage occurred in these mutant mice. Because the mutant mice were generated by the insertion of a targeting construct into the homeodomain and transcripts encoding a truncated Csx/Nkx2.5 protein were abundantly expressed in embryoid bodies made from mutant ES cells homozygous for Csx/Nkx2.5,[4] a question was raised whether a complete null mutation of this gene might result in a different phenotype. Accordingly we generated and analyzed a null allele (a removal of both exons) for Csx/Nkx2.5.[8] Even in the complete null mutant mice for Csx/Nkx2.5, the cardiac cell lineage was induced normally, indicating that the function of Csx/Nkx2.5 is different from that of *tinman*. The null mutant mice showed a similar phenotype to the mutant mice with a truncation mutation, but, surprisingly, the phenotype was milder. At E9.5, the beginning of the outflow tract was located on the right side and the atrioventricular canal on the left side, indicating that cardiac looping was initiated, unlike the truncation mutant. Expression pattern of myosin light chain 2V (MLC2V) was also different. In the truncation mutant mice, expression of MLC2V was abolished except for a small cluster of cells.[4] However, in the null mutant embryos, MLC2V was homogeneously expressed, albeit at low levels in the ventricle, suggesting that the ventricular specification was more advanced in the null mutant embryos. It is possible that a truncated Csx/Nkx2.5 protein had additional negative effects, for example, "squelching" of cofactors into nonfunctional complexes.

It is now clear that Csx/Nkx2.5 is not functionally equivalent to *Drosophila tinman*. It is possible that "gene redundancy" accounts for normal formation of the heart tube in Csx/Nkx2.5 null mutant mice. There may be other NK2 homeobox genes that have overlapping functions with Csx/Nkx2.5 in the murine embryonic heart. Nkx2.6 is a potential candidate in the mouse.[1] It has been shown that in *Xenopus*, XNkx2.3 and XNkx2.5 are expressed in the early heart and have overlapping functions.[12,13] However, the mouse Nkx2.3 is not expressed in the cardiac mesoderm. In the chicken, cNkx2.8 has been shown to be expressed in the early heart,[14] but no murine homolog of cNkx2.8 has been isolated to date. Alternatively, in vertebrates, other classes of transcription factors, such as MEF2 or GATA, may specify the cardiac cell lineage in concert with Csx/Nkx2.5.

Csx/Nkx2.5 Mutation Affects Expression of Several Downstream Genes in the Embryonic Heart

In order to examine molecular mechanisms whereby Csx/Nkx2.5 regulates heart formation, we searched potential downstream target genes of Csx/Nkx2.5[8] (Table 1). Among myofilament genes tested, only MLC2V was down-regulated in the mutant

heart as described above. Interestingly, expression of atrial natriuretic factor (ANF) and brain natriuretic peptide (BNP) in the ventricle was abolished in homozygous mutant embryos, while expression of these genes in the atrium was maintained. These results indicated that ANF and BNP expression in the ventricle is dependent on Csx/Nkx2.5 and that expression of these genes in the atrium and in the ventricle is differentially regulated.

As for transcription factors, expression of N-myc, eHAND and MEF2C was down-regulated in the mutant heart, whereas TEF-1, dHAND, and GATA4 were normally expressed. N-myc is required for normal expansion of the compact layer at mid-gestation stages.[15] Csx/Nkx2.5 may regulate this process through N-myc. Homozygous mutant embryos for eHAND arrested by E7.5 because of yolk sac abnormalities.[6,7] However, tetraploid-rescued eHAND mutants showed a similar cardiac phenotype to Csx/Nkx2.5 mutant embryos,[7] suggesting that eHAND may play critical roles in the molecular pathway downstream of Csx/Nkx2.5. *Drosophila* has one copy of MEF2 (D-mef2), and D-mef2 is a direct target of *tinman*.[16] In the mouse, MEF2C seems partly regulated by Csx/Nkx2.5.

Table 1
Summary of Changes in Gene Expression
in Csx/Nkx2.5 −/− Mice

Myofilament genes		Secreted factors, receptors and others	
α-cardiac actin	→		
αMHC	→		
β MHC	→	ANF	↓
MLC2v	↓	BNP	↓
Transcription factors		TGFβ1	→
		BMP4	→
N-myc	↓	erbB4	→
TEF1	→	N-cadherin	→
eHAND	↓	fibronectin	→
dHAND	→		
MEF2C	↓		
GATA4	→		
Msx1	→		
Msx2	*		
Csx/Nkx2.5	↑		

Expression of 21 potential downstream target genes were examined. Æ, no changes; ∅, down-regulation; ≠, upregulation; *, changes in gene expression pattern.

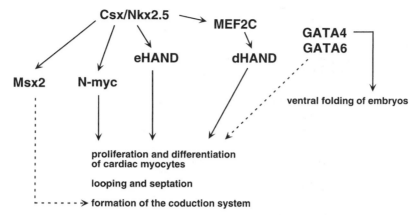

Figure 1. Transcriptional cascade controlling cardiac development. Csx/Nkx2.5 controls cardiac development by regulating several downstream transcription factors.

Expression of the Msx2 homeobox gene was also disturbed in the mutant heart. Msx2 is normally expressed in the myocardium at the atrioventricular junction and at later stages at the crest of the interventricular septum and coalescing trabeculae, suggesting that Msx2 may play a role in the formation of the conduction system.[17] In the mutant heart, Msx2 was expressed in the entire ventricle, indicating that Csx/Nkx2.5 may negatively regulate Msx2 expression in the ventricle. Csx/Nkx2.5 may suppress ectopic formation of the conduction system through down-regulation of Msx2 expression.

These results indicated that Csx/Nkx2.5 controls heart formation by regulating, either directly or indirectly, several downstream target genes, in particular, transcription factors (Fig. 1). Identification of more downstream target genes will further elucidate mechanisms by which Csx/Nkx2.5 regulates cardiac development.

Csx/Nkx2.5-Expressing Cardiac Myocytes Are Required for Cardiac Development in a Dose-Sensitive Manner

To examine the fate of Csx/Nkx2.5 deficient cells in the heart, we did a chimera study using Csx/Nkx2.5-deficient ES cell lines ("double knock-out" ES cell lines).[8] Examination of chimeric embryos revealed that embryos with more than 30% contribution of Csx/Nkx2.5-deficient cells in the heart showed the same phenotype as homozygous mutant embryos. Interestingly, chimeric embryos with 20% to 30% contribution of Csx/Nkx2.5-deficient cells in the heart exhibited a milder phenotype. These chimeric embryos showed moderate growth retardation and less pericardial effusion, and histologically there was some degree of trabeculation in the chimeric heart. Interestingly, Csx/Nkx2.5-deficient cells could differentiate into trabecular cells in the presence of wild-type cardiac myocytes, in contrast with the germline null embryos that do not form trabeculae. These results indicated that there might be some autocrine or paracrine factors downstream of Csx/Nkx2.5 that could either positively or negatively regulate differentiation of cardiac myocytes. This hypothesis is intriguing, because gene targeting studies of the neuregulin pathway[18] and the RXRα pathway[19] have shown that paracrine factors play critical roles in cardiac development at around E12.5.

Regulation of Csx/Nkx2.5 Expression During Development

We next examined regulation of Csx/Nkx2.5 during development using transgenic embryos carrying a LacZ reporter gene. We analyzed a total of 23 kb of 5'and 3' flanking sequence of Csx/Nkx2.5 and found that cis-acting elements of Csx/Nkx2.5 were surprisingly complex and modular[20] (Fig. 2). There were three different transcription start sites and two untranslated exons in addition to the two coding exons. Primer extension assay revealed that the transcript III initiating upstream of the first ATG was the major start site. Whole-mount β-gal staining of transgenic embryos showed that 3.3 kb of 5' flanking sequence contained cis-acting elements driving extracardiac expression of Csx/Nkx2.5, such as in the pharyngeal floor, thyroid gland, and stomach. This region also possessed regulatory elements to drive Csx/Nkx2.5 expression in the outflow tract and a basal part of the right ventricle. At E15.5, this regulatory element could also drive LacZ expression in the spleen. At this stage, cardiac expression of this enhancer was restricted to the outflow region of the right ventricle. In the adult, this enhancer element was inactive.

Additional cardiac enhancers were mapped to 5' flanking sequence between −14 and −6 kb. This region was able to direct transgene expression in most of the right and left ventricles except for the compact layer of the lateral walls. This region was also enough to direct the transgene expression in the cardiac crescent at E7.5. In the adult, LacZ expression was restricted to the luminal surface of the right ventricle.

We also found that 6 kb of 3' flanking sequence could drive LacZ expression throughout the right ventricle. Interestingly, there was a potent negative cis-acting element between −6 and −4 kb that could eliminate cardiac and extracardiac transgene expression by the downstream enhancers. The upstream regulatory elements could override this repressor element.

These results indicated that complex and modular cis-acting elements regulate expression of Csx/Nkx2.5 at different time points of development. There have been three other reports describing regulatory elements of Csx/Nkx2.5. Olson and colleagues focused on the upstream cardiac enhancer and narrowed it down to an approximately 500-bp fragment, which contains two GATA binding sites. A mutation of one of these sites eliminated LacZ expression in transgenic embryos, suggesting that this enhancer was GATA dependent.[21] Schwartz and collaborators showed that one of the upstream exons (exon 1b in Fig. 2) could be alternatively spliced into the coding exons in four different ways. They also identified another RV enhancer between the inhibitory domain and exon 1b.[22] Yutzey and colleagues studied the proximal 3 kb of 5' regulatory elements. In this region, they identified a 505-bp regulatory element driving LacZ expression in the cardiac

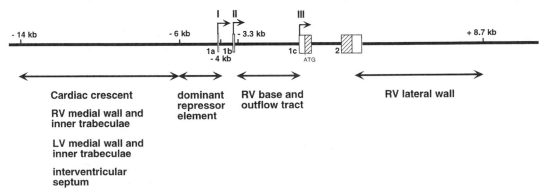

Figure 2. Transcription start sites and cis-regulatory elements of the Csx/Nkx2.5 gene. The Csx/Nkx2.5 gene consists of two untranslated exons and two coding exons. There are three transcription start sites (I, II, III). Four enhancers were studied.

crescent, the outflow tract and extracardiac tissues. Disruption of paired GATA binding sites in this element eliminated the transgene expression.[23] However, their results were different from those of the other groups in that the proximal 3 kb could direct LacZ expression in the cardiac crescent. The other three groups, including our group, showed that the proximal 3-kb element was not sufficient and the distal cardiac enhancer is required for transgene expression in the cardiac crescent.[20–22]

Conclusion

We studied functions of Csx/Nkx2.5 and regulation of the Csx/Nkx2.5 gene expression using gene targeting and transgenic technique. In human, heterozygous mutations of Csx/Nkx2.5 were reported to cause familial atrial septal defect (ASD) and atrioventricular (AV) conduction delays.[24] This human study not only showed that mutations of Csx/Nkx2.5 were linked to congenital heart disease, but also suggested that Csx/Nkx2.5 is required for later stages of heart formation and maintenance of AV nodal functions. The functions of Csx/Nkx2.5 are more divergent than *tinman* and the spatiotemporal regulation of the Csx/Nkx2.5 gene expression is more complex than we initially anticipated. Analysis of the molecular pathways upstream and downstream of Csx/Nkx2.5 will certainly contribute to a better understanding of molecular mechanisms of cardiac development.

References

1. Tanaka M, Kasahara H, Bartunkova S, et al. Vertebrate homologs of tinman and bagpipe: roles of the homeobox genes in cardiovascular development. *Dev Genet* 1998;22:239–249.
2. Olson EN, Srivastava D. Molecular pathways controlling heart development. *Science* 1996;272:671–676.
3. Lin Q, Schwarz J, Bucana C, et al. Control of mouse cardiac morphogenesis and myo-genesis by transcription factor MEF2C. *Science* 1997;276:1404–1407.
4. Lyons I, Parsons LM, Hartley L, et al. Myogenic and morphogenetic defects in the heart tubes of murine embryos lacking the homeo box gene Nkx2–5. *Genes Dev* 1995;9:1654–1666.
5. Srivastava D, Thomas T, Lin Q, et al. Regulation of cardiac mesodermal and neural crest development by the bHLH transcription factor, dHAND. *Nat Genet* 1997;16:154–160.
6. Firulli A, McFadden D, Lin Q, et al. Heart and extra-embryonic mesodermal defects in mouse embryos lacking the bHLH transcription factor Hand1. *Nat Genet* 1998;18:266–270.
7. Riley P, Anson-Cartwright L, Cross J. The Hand1 bHLH transcription factor is essential for placentation and cardiac morphogenesis. *Nat Genet* 1998;18:271–275.
8. Tanaka M, Chen Z, Bartunkova S, et al. The cardiac homeobox gene Csx/Nkx2.5 lies genetically upstream of multiple genes essential for heart development. *Development* 1999;126:1269–1280.
9. Komuro I, Izumo S. Csx: a murine homeobox-containing gene specifically expressed in the developing heart. *Proc Natl Acad Sci USA* 1993;90:8145–8149.
10. Lints TJ, Parsons LM, Hartley L, et al. Nkx-2.5: a novel murine homeobox gene expressed in early heart progenitor cells and their myogenic descendants. *Development* 1993;119:419–431.
11. Bodmer R. The gene tinman is required for specification of the heart and visceral muscles in Drosophila. *Development* 1993;118:719–729.
12. Fu Y, Yan W, Mohun TJ, et al. Vertebrate tinman homologues XNkx2–3 and XNkx2–5 are required for heart formation in a functionally redundant manner. *Development* 1998;125:4439–4449.
13. Grow MW, Krieg PA. Tinman function is essential for vertebrate heart development: elimination of cardiac differentiation by dominant inhibitory mutants of the tinman-related genes, XNkx2–3 and XNkx2–5. *Dev Biol* 1998;204:187–196.
14. Reecy JM, Yamada M, Cummings K, et al. Chicken Nkx-2.8: a novel homeobox gene expressed in early heart progenitor cells and pharyngeal pouch-2 and -3 endoderm. *Dev Biol* 1997;188:295–311.
15. Moens CB, Stanton BR, Parada LF, et al. Defects in heart and lung development in

compound heterozygotes for two different targeted mutations at the N-myc locus. *Development* 1993;119:485–499.

16. Gajewski K, Kim Y, Lee YM, et al. D-mef2 is a target for Tinman activation during Drosophila heart development. *Embo J* 1997;16:515–522.

17. Chan-Thomas PS, Thompson RP, Robert B, et al. Expression of homeobox genes Msx-1 (Hox-7) and Msx-2 (Hox-8) during cardiac development in the chick. *Dev Dyn* 1993;197:203–216.

18. Meyer D, Birchmeier C. Multiple essential functions of neuregulin in development. *Nature* 1995;378:386–390.

19. Chen J, Kubalak SW, Chien KR. Ventricular muscle-restricted targeting of the RXRalpha gene reveals a non-cell-autonomous requirement in cardiac chamber morphogenesis. *Development* 1998;125:1943–1949.

20. Tanaka M, Wechsler SB, Lee IW, et al. Complex modular cis-acting elements regulate expression of the cardiac specifying homeobox gene Csx/Nkx2.5. *Development* 1999;126:1439–1450.

21. Lien CL, Wu C, Mercer B, et al. Control of early cardiac-specific transcription of Nkx2–5 by a GATA-dependent enhancer. *Development* 1999;126:75–84.

22. Reecy JM, Li X, Yamada M, et al. Identification of upstream regulatory regions in the heart-expressed homeobox gene Nkx2–5. *Development* 1999;126:839–849.

23. Searcy RD, Vincent EB, Liberatore CM, et al. A GATA-dependent nkx-2.5 regulatory element activates early cardiac gene expression in transgenic mice. *Development* 1998;125:4461–4470.

24. Schott JJ, Benson DW, Basson CT, et al. Congenital heart disease caused by mutations in the transcription factor NKX2–5. *Science* 1998;281:108–111.

13

Identification of Upstream Regulatory Regions in the Murine *Tinman* Homologue, *Nkx2-5*

James M. Reecy, MD, Xuyang Li, BZ, MS,
Miho Yamada, MD, Francesco J. Demayo, PhD,
and Robert J. Schwartz, PhD

The *Nkx2-5* gene contains two coding exons.[1] However, the presence of an additional 5' exon was suggested by the DNA sequence of a single *Nkx2-5* cDNA clone isolated from an adult mouse heart library.[2] Sequence analysis of 5' RACE fragments and comparison with *Nkx2-5* genomic sequences confirmed the presence of a novel exon of at least 89-bp (exon 1a; Fig. 1A) alternatively spliced into the TN-domain of exon 1. Four novel *Nkx2-5* transcripts that involve the alternative splicing of exon 1a were detected by RT-PCR analysis (see Fig. 1B). Exon 1a was spliced into exon 1 at three separate sites (1) 5' UTR, (2) within the TN-domain, and (3) toward the 3' end and into exon 2. However, the translated proteins from these *Nkx2-5* splice variants were ineffectual in transfection assays (Fig. 1C). Although these possibilities for novel *Nkx2-5* proteins are intriguing, our RNase protection analysis (data not shown) suggests that their mRNAs are very low in abundance in the hearts of midgestation embryos and adults. It is possible that they result from cryptic transcriptional initiation within or close to an enhancer. However, we cannot discount the possibility that at other times in development, in other tissues, or under certain physiological or pathological conditions, these transcripts could play an important role.

We tested the ability of *Nkx2-5/LacZ* transgenes to recapitulate the endogenous *Nkx2-5* expression pattern in F_0 transgenic embryos (Fig. 2A). At 13.5 d.p.c., a transgene construct that contained 10.7 kbp of DNA 5' of the *Nkx2-5* initiator methionine (−10765D) was highly expressed in the atrioventricular canal, interventricular septum, and the trabecula of the right ventricle and outflow tract of the heart, spleen primordia, pyloric region of the stomach, thyroid diverticulum, and ventral endoderm of the pharynx (Fig. 1B–D). In contrast, endogenous *Nkx2-5* was normally expressed throughout the heart myocardium, as well as in the tongue. In addition, the −10765D transgene directed *LacZ* expression at the earliest time points of cardiac development in bilaterally symmetrical progenitor pools in anterior lateral plate mesoderm and in the linear heart tube (Fig. 2E, F). It also directed expression in the spleen, pharynx, thyroid, and stomach.

From Clark EB, Nakazawa M, Takao A (eds.): Etiology and Morphogenesis of Congenital Heart Disease: Twenty Years of Progress in Genetics and Developmental Biology. Armonk, NY: Futura Publishing Co., Inc.; © 2000.

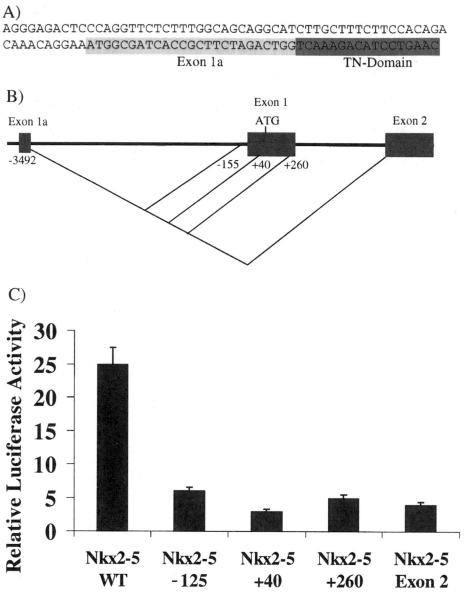

Figure 1. Identification and characterization of a novel 5′ exon. **A.** Total RNA (0.5 μg) isolated from adult mouse tissues was analyzed by 5′ RACE. **B.** Pictorial of exon 1a alternative splicing as determined by sequencing of RT-PCR products. **C.** Transcriptional ability of *Nkx2-5* splice variants. Luciferase activities (average of two independent experiments) were measured in extracts from CV1 cells transfected with *Nkx2-5* expression constructs (−155, +40, +260, Exon 2; 400 ng) in combination with A20-TATA-Luc reporter construct (1 μg) and corrected for protein content. The bars represent the average of two independent transfections and the error bars represent the standard error of corrected luciferase activity relative to the pCG vector within an experiment.

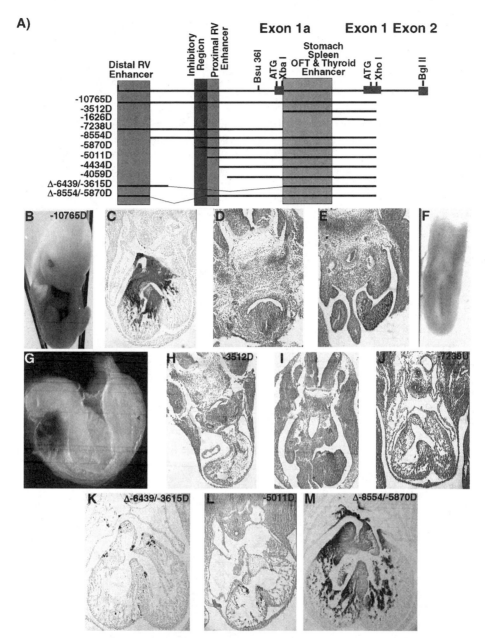

Figure 2. A. Schematic representation of the *Nkx2-5* promoter constructs analyzed in F$_0$ embryos. (i) Restriction map of the *Nkx2-5* gene showing the three *Nkx2-5* exons (Red) and the 5′ flanking sequences tested for promoter activity. (ii) The *LacZ* gene was fused in-frame into the coding region of exon 1 and 1a. In the construct name, D and U (downstream or exon 1 and upstream or exon 1a) denotes which exon the *LacZ* cDNA was fused in-frame into. Base pair positions are numbered relative to the start methionine in exon 1, except −7238U, which is numbered relative to the start methionine in exon 1a. ATG refers to the *Nkx2-5* translation start sites. No β-gal activity was detected in −1626D, −8554D, or −5870D transgenic mice. **B–M.** The *LacZ* expression pattern induced by the transgenes used in this study. **B–G.** −10765D transgene expression pattern. **H, I.** −3512D transgene expression pattern. **J.** −7238U transgene expression pattern. **K.** Δ−6439/−3615DU transgene expression pattern. **L.** −5011D transgene expression pattern. **M.** Δ−8554/−5870D transgene expression pattern.

To determine where the *Nkx2-5* regulatory domains were located, we first constructed two *LacZ* transgenes, −3512D and −7238U, which contained *LacZ* fused in-frame to exons 1 or 1a, respectively (Fig. 2A). In −3512D transgenic embryos, *LacZ* expression was detected in the outflow tract of the heart, pharynx, thyroid, spleen primordium, and stomach (Fig. 2G, H). In contrast, the −7238U transgene was expressed exclusively in the atrioventricular canal, interventricular septum, and outflow tract of the heart (Fig. 2I). In −1626D transgenic mice, no β-gal activity was detected (data not shown). Thus, there appear to be two promoters capable of guiding *Nkx2-5* expression, as well as, enhancers that direct expression to the right ventricle and outflow tract of the heart and several extra-cardiac sites.

To further delineate the cardiac element(s), we generated a series of deletion mutants that lacked 5′ flanking sequences (−8554D, −5870D, −5011D, −4434D, and −4059D). *LacZ* expression was lost in the atrioventricular canal, interventricular septum and right ventricle when sequences 5′ of −8554 were deleted (Fig. 2J). However, the cis-acting element located 5′ of −8554 was incapable of directing high-level expression in the right ventricle when analyzed in conjunction with the proximal *Nkx2-5* promoter (Fig. 2K). Thus, an essential enhancer would appear to be located between −10765 and −8554. Although no expression in heart was seen with −5870D, *LacZ* expression was again detected, albeit sparsely, throughout the right ventricle when sequences 5′ of −5011 were deleted (Fig. 2L). In this case, however, ectopic expression was detected. Furthermore, it appears that this proximal right-ventricular enhancer works in conjunction with the distal enhancer (−10765 to −8554) to override the negative cis-acting element located between −5870 and −5011 to direct high level transgene expression in the atrioventricular canal, interventricular septum, and right ventricular trabecula (Fig. 2M). Thus, multiple cardiac elements are modified in a complex way by

an inhibitory domain located between −5870 and −5011. Deletion of this inhibitory domain also leads to ectopic *Nkx2-5* expression, suggesting that it may work in collaboration with the cardiac elements to ensure spatial specificity.

Nkx2-5 is expressed uniformly throughout the heart myocardium. One theoretical way to accomplish this would be to have a single element that controls *Nkx2-5* expression in this tissue layer. However, the lack of evidence for a master gene regulatory mechanism for cardiac myogenesis,[3] and the results of our transgenic analysis, favor a model in which distinct but interactive positive and negative cis-acting elements control regional expression of *Nkx2-5* in the heart. This model is consistent with the compartmental-specific expression of a growing number of transgenes and endogenous genes in the developing heart.[4−6] Based on genetic and evolutionary considerations, it has been suggested that the heart is a modular organ, with individual modules that represent unique and separate innovations that were added to the heart in a stepwise manner during evolution. This model accounts for the null phenotypes of several heart-expressed genes, in which individual modules were deleted with little effect on overall patterning.[7,8]

In the developing Drosophila embryo, Lee et al.[9] and Yin et al.[10] have recently reported the identification of four cis-acting elements that regulate *tinman* expression. Each of these elements was differentially utilized throughout development in a cell type-specific and temporal-specific manner. In addition, they responded to different signaling molecules. By analogy, the control of *Nkx2-5* transcription may also be highly modular, with individual elements able to respond to different developmental cues. For example, bone morphogenic proteins (BMPs) appear to have an early role in signaling the formation of heart mesoderm in vertebrate embryos.[11,12] We can expect that sequences within the *Nkx2-5* locus will include those capable of directing transgene expression in the lateral plate mesoderm under BMP control. Recently, Xu et al.[13] reported that *Tinman* was required in combination with the *Dpp* signaling pathway to induce *Tinman* transcription, which suggests that *Nkx2-5* such as tinman may function in a feedback loop to regulate their own transcription. Further analysis of the regulatory elements highlighted in this study may help to identify such factors.

Acknowledgements: We would like to thank Katherine Yutzey, Robin Searcy, Ching-Ling Lien, and Eric Olson for communication of results prior to publication and Thierry Lints and Linda Parsons for isolation and sequencing of Nkx2-5 cDNA clones. This work was supported by a grant from the National Institutes of Health (NIH PO1 HL49953) to R.J.S.

References

1. Lyons I, Parsons LM, Hartley L, et al. Myogenic and morphogenetic defects in the heart tubes of murine embryos lacking the homeo box gene Nkx2–5. *Genes Dev* 1995;9:1654–1666.
2. Lints TJ, Parsons LM, Hartley L, et al. Nkx-2.5: A novel murine homeobox gene expressed in early heart progenitor cells and their myogenic descendants. *Development* 1993;119:419–431.
3. Evans S, Yan W, Murillo MP, et al. *Tinman,* a *Drosophila* homeobox gene required for heart and visceral mesoderm specification, may be represented by a family of genes in vertebrates: *XNkx-2.3,* a second homologue of *tinman. Development* 1995;121:3889–3899.
4. Ross RS, Navankasattusas S, Harvey RP, et al. An HF-1a/HF-1b/MEF-2 combinatorial element confers cardiac ventricular specificity and establishes an anterior-posterior gradient of expression. *Development* 1996;122:1799–1809.
5. Franco D, Kelly R, Lameres WH, et al. Regionalized transcriptional domains of myosin light chain 3f transgenes in the embryonic mouse heart: Morphogenetic implications. *Dev Biol* 1997;188:17–33.
6. He CZ, Burch JB. The chicken GATA-6 locus contains multiple control regions that confer distinct patterns of heart region-specific expression in transgenic mouse embryos. *J Biol Chem* 1997;272:28550–28556.
7. Fishman MC, Chien KR. Fashioning the vertebrate heart: Earliest embryonic decisions. *Development* 1997;124:2099–2117.
8. Fishman MC, Olson EN. Parsing the heart: Genetic modules for organ assembly. *Cell* 1997;91:153–156.
9. Lee YM, Park T, Schulz RA, et al. Twist-mediated activation of the NK-4 homeobox gene in the visceral mesoderm of *Drosophila* requires two distinct clusters of E-box regulatory elements. *J Biol Chem* 1997; 272:17531–17541.
10. Yin Z, Xu XI, Frasch M. Regulation of the twist target gene *tinman* by modular cis-regulatory elements during early mesoderm development. *Development* 1997;124:4971–4982.
11. Schultheiss TM, Burch JB, Lassar AB. A role for bone morphogenetic proteins in the induction of cardiac myogenesis. *Genes Dev* 1997;11:451–462.
12. Andree B, Duprez D, Vorbusch B, et al. BMP-2 induces ectopic expression of cardiac lineage markers and interferes with somite formation in chicken embryos. *Mech Dev* 1998;70:119–131.
13. Xu X, Yin Y, Hudson JB, et al. Smad proteins act in combination with synergistic and antagonistic regulators to target Dpp responses to the *Drosophila* mesoderm. *Genes Dev* 1998;12:2354–2370.

14

Role of FGF1 in Specification of Mesoderm to Cardiac Muscle Lineage

*Masako Okada, MD, Chiaki Hidai, MD,
Hirotaka Nagashima, MD, Hiromi Ikeda, MD,
Rumiko Matsuoka, MD, Hiroshi Kasanuki, MD,
and Masatoshi Kawana, MD*

Recent studies have indicated that the primitive streak is an important region for cardiac differentiation in chick and mouse embryos.[1,2] The cardiac primordium becomes directed at the primitive streak stage in the early gastrula and then undergoes terminal differentiation in the anterolateral mesoderm.[3] Some cytokines take part in the commitment and differentiation of cardiac myocytes and bone morphogenic protein 4 (BMP4) is an essential factor for cardiogenesis.[4] However, the upstream signaling has not been determined. Using an in vitro system, we demonstrated that fibroblast growth factor 1 (FGF1) from the endoderm adjacent to the primitive streak induces premature cells to differentiate in the cardiac lineage in the early stage of development.

P19 cell, a mouse embryonal carcinoma cell line, differentiates into cardiac and skeletal myocytes, and neurocytes at low, medium, and high concentrations of retinoic acid (RA), respectively.[5] We employed developmental markers for gastrulation, cardiac muscle and skeletal muscle to analyze P19 differentiation (Table 1).[6-13] Semiquantitative reverse transcription PCR (RT-PCR) analysis showed that Brachyury[14,15] and Wnt8[6,16] were markedly expressed on days 2 to 3 of induction (data not shown). The expression of GATA4[17,18] showed a marked increase in cultures with 10^{-12} M RA on day 3. From these data, days 2 and 3 in our in vitro system were considered to correspond to the early primitive streak stage of embryo. When P19 cells were cultured with 10^{-12} M RA, the cells started to beat on day 7. GATA4 was upregulated from day 3, and the expression of cardiac alpha myosin heavy chain (αMHC) was induced on day 6. *MyoD* did not show any remarkable change, and myosin light chain (MLC1), a marker of skeletal muscle differentiation, was not induced (data not shown). When the cells were incubated with 10^{-8} M RA, they exhibited the morphology of skeletal myoblasts. The expression of MyoD increased markedly and MLC1 gene was induced. However, the expression of αMHC was not detected (data not shown).

Next we designated cultures with 10^{-12} M RA and 10^{-8} M RA as cardiac and skeletal muscle-inducing conditions, respectively, and compared expression patterns of several cytokines between the two conditions. Transcription of FGF1 and FGF2 showed interesting differences in the expression pattern (Fig. 1). Expres-

From Clark EB, Nakazawa M, Takao A (eds.): Etiology and Morphogenesis of Congenital Heart Disease: Twenty Years of Progress in Genetics and Developmental Biology. Armonk, NY: Futura Publishing Co., Inc.; © 2000.

Table 1
Developmental Markers in P-19 Differentiation.

Gene	cDNA Length (bp)	Annealing Temp (°C)	5' Primer (5' to 3')	3' Primer (5' to 3')	Reference
Wnt8	418	66	AAGTCAGCCAGCTGCAGCCAA	GGTGGAATTGTCCTGAGCAT	6
αMHC	384	62	GCTGTGGTCCACATTCTTCAGG	CTTGAGGTTGTACAGCACAGCC	7
GATA4	483	68	TGCCGCTTCGCTTCGAAGGG	GCTCTGAGCACGAGGCAGAC	8
FGF1	437	60	GAAACAAGATGGCTTTCTGGC	TGAAGGGGAGATCACAACC	9
FGF2	344	60	TTCTGTCCAGGTCCCGTTTTGG	AAGCGGCTCTACTGCAAGAACG	9
FGFR1	882	64	TGGGAGCATCAACCACACCTACC	GCCCGAAGCAGCCCTCGCCAAG	10
TGFβ1	260	64	CTTTAGGAAGGACCTGGGTT	CAGGAGCGCACAATCATGTT	11
BMP4	566	50	TGTGAGGTGTTTCCATCACG	TTATTCTTCTTCCTGGACCG	12
ms16	103	68	AGGAGCGATTTGCTGGTGTGGA	GCTACCAGGCCTTTGAGATGGA	13

sion of both FGFs peaked on day 3 of induction. FGF1 expression was dominant in the cardiac muscle-inducing condition and FGF2 was dominant in the skeletal muscle-inducing condition in the early few days of differentiation.

To investigate whether FGF1 contributes to cardiac differentiation, we conducted administration of FGF1 under the skeletal muscle-inducing condition. Cells induced to differentiate into skeletal muscle were treated with 1ng/ml FGF1 from day 2 to 3. The cells did not develop spontaneous beating. However, RT-PCR showed that αMHC gene was induced, and GATA4 was upregulated by FGF1 (Fig. 2A). The expression of MLC1 was suppressed. Longer treatment with FGF1 did not have any additional effect on dif-

ferentiation. These data indicate that FGF1 supports cardiac differentiation in the early stage of development.

To study the signal transduction of FGF1, Fibrinoblast growth factor, RT-PCR was performed for developmental markers (Fig. 2A). The expression levels of Brachyury and Wnt8 did not change. Interestingly, upregulation of FGFR1, BMP4, and GATA4 genes was observed.[3] Therefore, the target stage of FGF1 is thought to be just after mesoderm induction, that is, the early primitive streak stage corresponding to day 2 to 3 of our system.

To investigate whether FGFR1 participates in FGF1 signal transduction, blocking experiments were conducted. Anti-FGFR1 antibody blocked the induction of

FGF1   FGF2

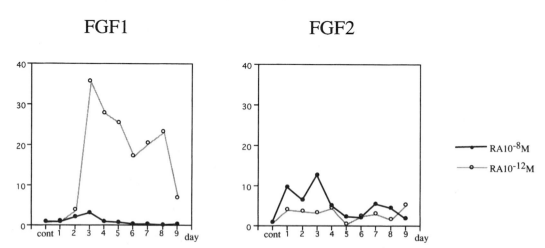

Figure 1. Expression pattern of FGF1 and FGF2 following induction with 10^{-8} M RA (**A**) and 10^{-12} M RA (**B**). The level of induction in pre-induced P19 cells was equated to 1.

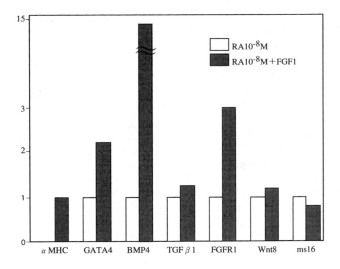

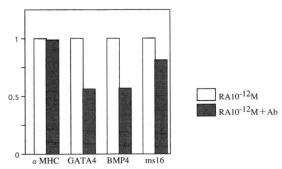

Figure 2. Effects of exogenous FGF1 on induction with 10^{-8} M RA (**A**) and anti-FGFR1 antibody on induction with 10^{-12} M RA (**B**). Expression of developmental marker genes following FGF1 administration from day 2 to 3 is shown. RNA was harvested on day 4 and day 9. Analysis of αMHC was performed on day 9, and of other markers on day 4. Mouse S16 ribosomal protein gene (ms16) was used as a standard for RT-PCR. The value of expression in 10^{-8} M RA (**A**) and 10^{-12} M RA (**B**) was equated to 1. This, however, was not possible for αMHC, because the mRNA of αMHC was not detectable in 10^{-8} M RA (**A**). As an alternative, the value of αMHC induced by FGF1 was equated to 1.

αMHC by exogenous FGF1 (data not shown). Anti-FGFR1 antibody added to the cardiac muscle-inducing condition did not attenuate the expression of αMHC, but suppressed BMP4 and GATA4 expression (Fig. 2B). These data indicate that FGF1 signaling through FGFR1 induces BMP4 expression and contributes to cardiomyocyte differentiation.

The distribution of developmental molecules has been intensively studied with in situ hybridization and immunohistochemical methods. FGFR1 is known to be expressed at the primitive streak.[19] BMP4 is localized in the posterior part of the primitive streak during gastrulation.[4] To investigate the relationship among these molecules spatially, FGF1 localization in the early embryo was examined immunohistochemically in rat embryo 8 days post-coitum (dpc), corresponding to the early primitive streak stage (data not shown). The embryos generally displayed pale staining, but the primitive endoderm of the mid-posterior primitive streak region in the base of egg cylinder was strongly stained. It is considered that FGF1, FGFR1, and BMP4 co-localize at the posterior primitive streak of this stage.

Taken together, our results suggest that FGF1 from the primitive endoderm positively regulates BMP4 expression and supports cardiac differentiation. Further in vivo studies should be conducted to elucidate the mechanism of cardiomyocyte differentiation.

Materials and Methods

P19 Cell Culture and in Vitro Differentiation

The cells were cultured and induced to differentiate according to McBurney et al.[5] Human recombinant FGF1 (R&D Systems, Mineapolis, MN) and mouse anti-bovine FGFR1 monoclonal antibody (Chemicon, Temecula, CA) were added at the concentrations and duration indicated in the text and figures.

Expression Analysis

Transcripts were detected by RT-PCR (Table 1) and analyzed with BAS2000 system (Fujinon, Inc., Wayne, NJ) after Southern blotting.[8] The relative levels of expression were quantitatively determined as indicated in the figures.

Immunohistochemistry

Rat embryos 8.5 dpc were dissected and fixed with freshly prepared 4% paraformaldehyde. Immunohistochemical studies were performed with ABC method using rabbit polyclonal anti-bovine FGF1 antibody (Upstate Biotechnology, Lake Placid, NY) diluted to 2 mg/mL and a secondary biotinylated antibody (goat anti-rabbit IgG;

Dako, Carpenteria, CA) (1:200). Control sections were incubated with normal rabbit IgG (100 mg/mL).

References

1. Schoenwolf GC, Garcia-Martinez V. Primitive-streak origin and state of commitment of cells of the cardiovascular system in avian and mammalian embryos. *Cell Mol Biol Res* 1995;41:233–240.
2. Tam PPL, Parameswaran M, Kinder SJ, et al. The allocation of epiblast cells to the embryonic heart and other mesodermal lineages: The role of ingression and tissue movement during gastrulation. *Development* 1997;124:1631–1642.
3. Schultheiss TM, Burch JBE, Lassar AB. A role for bone morphogenetic proteins in the induction of cardiac myogenesis. *Genes Dev* 1997;11:451–462.
4. Winnier G, Blessing M, Labosky PA, et al. Bone morphogenic protein-4 is required for mesoderm formation and patterning in the mouse. *Genes Dev* 1995;9:2105–2116.
5. McBurney MW. Isolation of male embryonal carcinoma cells and their chromosome replication patterns. *Dev Biol* 1982;89:503–508.
6. Bouillet P, Oulad-Abdelghani M, Ward SJ, et al. A new mouse member of the Wnt gene family, mWnt-8, is expressed during early embryogenesis and is ectopically induced by retinoic acid. *Mech Dev* 1996;58:141–152.
7. Quinn-Laquer BK, Kennedy JE, Wei SJ, et al. Characterization of allelic differences in the mouse cardiac a-myosin heavy chain coding sequence. *Genomics* 1992;13:176–188.
8. Grepin C, Robitaille L, Antakly T, et al. Inhibition of transcription factor GATA-4 expression blocks in vitro cardiac muscle differentiation. *Mol Cell Biol* 1995;15:4095–4102.
9. Hebert JM, Basilico C, Goldfarb M, et al. Isolation of cDNA encoding four mouse FGF family members and characterization of their expression patterns during embryogenesis. *Dev Biol* 1990;138:454–463.
10. Kouhara H, Kasayama H, Saito H, et al. Expression cDNA cloning of fibroblast growth factor (FGF) receptor in mouse breast cancer cells; a variant from in FGF-responsive transformed cells. *Biochem Biophys Res Commun.* 1991;176:31–37.

11. Derynck R, Jarrett JA, Chen EY, et al. The murine transforming growth factor-beta precursor. *J Biol Chem* 1986;261: 4377–4379.
12. Johansson BM, Wiles MW. Evidence for Involvement of Activin A and Bone Morphogenic Protein 4 in mammalian mesoderm and hematopoietic development. *Mol Cell Biol* 1995;15:141–151.
13. Leonard MW, Lim K-C, Engel JD. Expression of the chicken GATA factor family during early erythroid development and differentiation. *Development* 1993;119:519–531.
14. Smith JC, Price BM, Green JBA, et al. Expression of a *Xenopus* Homolog of Brachyury (T) is an immediate-early response to mesoderm induction. *Cell* 1991; 67:79–87.
15. Vidricaire G, Jardine K, McBurney MW. Expression of Brachyury gene mesoderm development in differentiating embryonal carcinoma cell cultures. *Development* 1994;120:115–122.
16. Christian JL, McMahon JA, McMahon AP, et al. Xwnt-8, a *Xenopus* wnt-1/int-1 related gene responsive to mesoderm-inducing growth factors, may play a role in ventral mesodermal patterning during embryogenesis. *Development* 1991;111:1045–1055.
17. Kelley C, Blumberg H, Zon LI, et al. GATA-4 is a novel transcription factor expressed in endocardium of the developing heart. *Development* 1993;118:817–827.
18. Grepin C, Nemer G, Nemer M. Enhanced cardiogenesis in embryonic stem cells overexpressing in the GATA-4 transcription factor. *Development* 1997;124:2387–2395.
19. Yamaguchi TP, Conlon RA, Rossant J. Expression of the fibroblast growth factor receptor FGFR-1/flg during gastrulation and segmentation in the mouse embryo. *Dev Biol* 1992;152:75–88.

15

Increased Expression of Cardiotrophin-1 in Dilated Cardiac Myocytes

Mariko Tatsuguchi, MD, Setsuko Noda, PhD,
Yoshiyuki Furutani, BS, Susumu Minamisawa, MD, PhD,
Eriko Hiratsuka, BSc, Keiko Komatsu, BSc,
Hiroshi Kasanuki, MD, and Rumiko Matsuoka, MD

Recently, in the cardiomyopathic Syrian hamster (BIO14.6), a deletion has been found in the first exon of δ-sarcoglycan,[1, 2] which leads to a physiological and functional disorder [3] that causes cardiac hypertrophy from 20 weeks, and cardiac dilatation from 40 weeks of age.

A novel cytokine, cardiotrophin-1 (CT-1), which displays structural similarities to the interleukin (IL)-6 related cytokines,[4,5] and which activates several features of cardiomyocyte hypertrophy,[4,6,7] in vitro, including sarcomeric organization and embryonic gene expression,[8] was discovered. Chien et al.[4–6] indicated that CT-1 caused myofibrils to orient along the longitudinal cell axis, and extend to the cell periphery. Also, the morphological changes in cardiac myocytes induced by CT-1 were similar to those found when the myocytes were subjected to chronic volume overload.

On the other hand, it has also been reported that IL-1 alpha contributes to cardiomyocyte hypertrophy in transgenic mice.[9] The type of cardiac hypertrophy induced by IL-1 alpha is different than that due to CT-1 as IL-1 alpha induces concentric left ventricular hypertrophy. Ventricular hypertrophy, indicating different regulatory mechanisms of cytokines, plays a role in hypertrophy or heart failure.

In this study, we examined the expression of CT-1 in the left ventricle (LV) of the BIO14.6 in the hypertrophic and dilated phases and in the LV of the congenic normal Syrian hamsters (CN) by light and electron microscopic immunohistochemistry. We also investigated the relative amount of CT-1 and IL-1 alpha protein in the LV of the BIO14.6 and in the LV of the CN by dot blot analysis.

In the light microscopic study, staining with CT-1 antisera was more diffuse and dense in the 41w-BIO14.6 LV than in the 23w-BIO14.6, 23w-CN, and 41w-CN (Fig. 1).

To observe the detailed localization of CT-1, we performed an electron microscopic study. The Z bands containing intercalated disks in the cardiac myocytes were stained predominantly in the 41w-BIO14.6 LV. Also the T system, and sarcoplasmic reticulum were stained (Fig. 2). There was no significant staining of CT-1 in the non-

From Clark EB, Nakazawa M, Takao A (eds.): Etiology and Morphogenesis of Congenital Heart Disease: Twenty Years of Progress in Genetics and Developmental Biology. Armonk, NY: Futura Publishing Co., Inc.; © 2000.

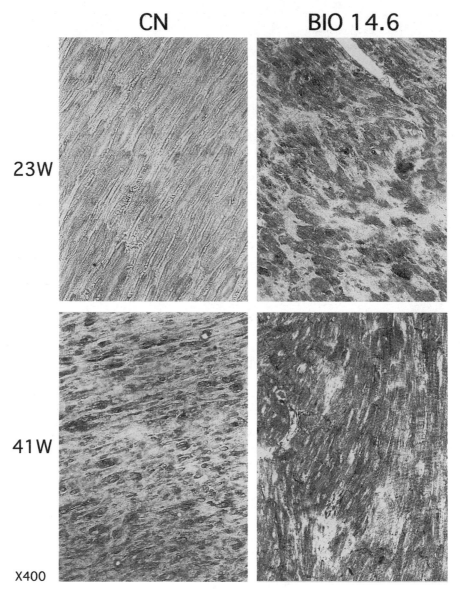

Figure 1. Immunohistochemical localization of CT-1 staining in BIO14.6 and CN under a light microscope. The CT-1 antisera stained strongest in the left ventricle of the 41w-BIO14.6.

cardiac myocytes. Further study is necessary on noncardiac myocytes.

Dot blot analysis revealed that the expression of CT-1 protein was strongest in the 41w-BIO14.6. On the other hand, there was no significant difference in the expression of IL-1 alpha in the 23w-BIO14.6, 23w-CN, 41w-BIO14.6, and 41w-CN.

Several recent studies have shown that the plasma levels of IL-6 or its family are increased in patients with congestive heart failure or an animal model of cardiac hypertrophy.[10–13] As CT-1 is a member of the IL-6 family, this theory may support our conclusion that CT-1 may be expressed in the dilated phase of cardiac

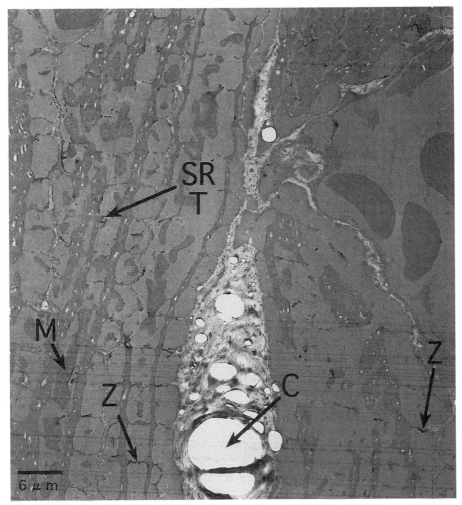

Figure 2. Immunoelectron microscopic localization of CT-1 in the left ventricle of the BIO14.6 in the dilated phase. M, mitochondria; Z, Z bands; T, T system; C, capillary; SR, sarcoplasmic reticulum. Z bands containing intercalated disks are predominantly stained.

myocytes in the BIO14.6 and there it may be related to the dilatation of cardiac myocytes in the BIO14.6.

Materials and Methods

Hypertrophic phase (23w) and dilated phase (41w) BIO14.6 and CN were kindly donated by Professor Nishimura (Nagoya University, Japan). They were inbred at Tokyo Women's Medical Univer-

sity for this study. The animals were allowed free access to food and water.

Immunohistochemistry

Immunohistochemistry was performed in the left ventricular tissue of BIO14.6 in the hypertrophic and dilated phases and that of CN, utilizing mouse CT-1 antisera. The sections were first washed with xylene for 15 minutes and then hydrated with a series of 100% to 65% ethanol. After blocking with 1.5% of goat serum/phosphate-buffered PBS for 10 minutes, the sections were incubated with the anti-CT-1 serum at room temperature for 1 hour, washed with PBS three times, and incubated with horseradish peroxidase-conjugated goat anti-rabbit IgG (Amersham, Bucks, United Kingdom). After washing with PBS three times, the peroxidase was revealed by diaminobenzidine (DAB). The sections were finally co-stained with methyl green. A set of control slides were prepared in parallel, using the preimmune serum.

Immunoelectron Microscopic Study

For the electron-microscopic examination, the above-mentioned immuno-stained sections were osmicated in 2% OsO_4 in 100 mM sodium phosphate buffer (pH7.2) for 1 hour, dehydrated in a series of graded ethanols (70% to 100%), and embedded in Quetol 812. Ultra-thin sections were prepared on an LKB 2088 ultrasome and examined with a JEM-120EM electron microscope without uranyl acetate staining.

Dot Blot Analysis

One hundred micrograms of proteins in 0.5l tissue solution extracted from the hamsters' left ventricles were blotted in cellulose nitrate (Schleider and Schuell, Dassel, Germany). Nonspecific binding was reduced by incubating a nitrate sheet for 1 hour in PBS containing 4% skim milk. Anti-CT-1-serum and polyclonal rabbit anti-mouse IL-1 alpha Ab (Genzyme, Cambridge, Mass) were allowed to react for 1 h at room temperature. They were then incubated with donkey anti-rabbit Ig antiserum (Amersham, Life Science), and colored with DAB-Ni-Co.

Acknowledgments: We would like to thank Kenneth R Chien for his generosity in supplying the mouse CT-1 antisera.

References

1. Nigro V, Piluso G, Belsito A, et al. Identification of a novel sarcoglycan gene at 5q33 encoding sarcolemmal 35kDa glycoprotein. *Hum Mol Genet.* 1996;5:1179–1186.
2. Nigro V, Okazaki Y, Belsito A, et al. Identification of the Syrian hamster cardiomyopathy gene. *Hum Mol Genet* 1997;6:601–607.
3. Sakamoto A, Ono K, Abe M, et al. Both hypertrophic and dilated cardiomyopathies are caused by mutation on the same gene, -sarcoglycan, in hamster. *Proc Natl Acad Sci U S A* 1997;94:13873–13878.
4. Wollert K, Chien KR. Cardiotrophin-1 and the role of gp130-dependent signaling pathways in cardiac growth and development. *J Mol Med* 1997;75:492–501.
5. Pennica D, Wood WI, Chien KR. Cardiotrophin-1: A multifunctional cytokine that signals via LIF receptor-gp130-dependent pathways. *Cytokine Growth Factor Rev* 1996;7:81–91.
6. Pennica D, King KL, Shaw KJ, et al. Expression cloning of cardiotrophin-1, a cytokine that induces cardiac myocyte hypertrophy. *Proc Natl Acad Sci U S A* 1995;92:1142–1146.
7. Wollert K, Taga T, Maito M, et al. Cardiotrophin-1 activates a distinct form of cardiac muscle cell hypertrophy. Assembly of sarcomeric units in series VIA gp 130/leukemia inhibiting factor receptor-dependent pathways. *J Biol Chem* 1996; 271:9535–9545.
8. Sheng Z, Pennica D, Wood WI, et al. Cardiotrophin-1 displays early expression in the murine heart tube and promotes cardiac myocyte survival. *Development* 1996;122:419–428.
9. Isoda K, et al. Overexpression of human interleukin-1 alpha gene is coupled with both cardiomyocyte hypertrophy and left ventricular dysfunction in transgenic mice. *Circulation* 1997;96(suppl.):116.
10. Testa M, Yeh M, Lee P, et al. Circulating levels of cytokines and their endogenous modulators in patients with mild to severe congestive heart failure due to coronary artery disease or hypertension. *J Am Coll Cardiol* 1996;28:964–971.

11. Blum A, Miller H. Role of cytokines in heart failure. *Am Heart J* 1998;135:181–186.

12. Tsutamoto T, Hisanaga T, Wada A, et al. Interleukin-6 spillover in the peripheral circulation increases with the severity of heart failure, and the high plasma level of interleukin-6 is an important prognostic predictor in patients with congestive heart failure. *J Am Coll Cardiol* 1998;31:391–398.

13. Ishikawa M, Saito Y, Miyamoto Y, et al. cDNA cloning of cardiotrophin-1 (CT-1): Augmented expression of CT-1 gene in ventricle of genetically hypertensive rats. *Biochem Biophys Res Commun* 1996;219:377–381.

Section III

16

Overview: Formation of the Primary Heart Tube

Roger R. Markwald, PhD, Takashi Nakaoka, MD, and Corey H. Mjaatvedt, PhD

Segmental Basis of Heart Tube Formation

The progenitor of the vertebrate tubular heart is a pair of heart forming fields established within the lateral plate mesoderm following gastrulation.[1] What distinguishes the heart forming fields from other mesodermal cells is that they express genes homologous to the *Drosophila tinman* gene,[2] like *nkx2.5*[3] or *nkx 2.8*.[4] The latter, together with downstream transcriptions factors, e.g., MEF 2c[5] or GATA 4[6] regulate cardiac specific gene expression. In turn, secreted morphogens may act to regulate *tinman* homologs or other cardiogenic transcription factors. Two such categories of morphogens would include bone morphogenic proteins[7] and *wnt* proteins.[8] Bone morphogenetic proteins 2 and 4, which are secreted by adjacent endoderm and ectoderm,[9] have been shown to induce undifferentiated mesoderm to enter a cardiogenic lineage.[10] Eisenberg et al.[11] have shown that *wnt 11* is expressed in the posterior region of the heart fields in the area where it is proposed that undifferentiated mesoderm is being recruited into the heart fields.[12] When transfected into an undifferenti-

ated mesodermal cell line, *wnt 11* can induce a cardiomyocyte phenotype.[11] In vivo, sarcomeric myosin is first expressed

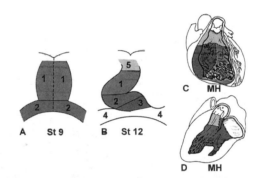

Figure 1. Formation and integration of the segments of the chick primary heart tube are shown as they develop *over time* from the fused heart forming fields. Their "birthdates" are given below in parentheses. A: Segment 1 immediately upon fusion of the heart fields (stage 9−); the so-called straight tube heart is composed almost entirely of this single segment. Segment 2 (stage 10) appears concomitantly with the onset of looping, which places segment 1 in the anterior (outlet) limb and segment 2 in the posterior (inflow) limb of the U-shaped heart. B: Segment 3 (stage 12) and future segment 4 (stage 13/14) will complete the anterior limb. Segment 5 develops progressively (stages 12–22) at the distal end of segment 1 to complete the anterior limb. The fate of each segment is described in the text. An important point is that each anatomical ventricular chamber of the mature heart is formed *over time* by the integration of 3 embryonic segments C: (1 + 3 + 5 for the right ventricle; D: 2 + 3 + 5 for the left ventricle).

From Clark EB, Nakazawa M, Takao A (eds.): Etiology and Morphogenesis of Congenital Heart Disease: Twenty Years of Progress in Genetics and Developmental Biology. Armonk, NY: Futura Publishing Co., Inc.; © 2000.

at stage 7 in chick heart fields just prior to their fusion.[13,14] However, expression of the myosin at this time does not appear to be sarcomerically organized and appears to be iterated at sites where adherens junctions are established by N-cadherins and beta catenins.[15] Cardiac-specific actins are not expressed in the heart fields. The first muscle actin to be expressed is alpha smooth muscle actin which is present in all segments of the tubular heart prior to any specific cardiac actin.[16] A major morphogenetic event within the heart fields is the segregation of endocardial endothelial precursor cells from those committed to a myogenic lineage.[17–19] In the chick, TGF beta3 appears to be a potent signal for endocardial endothelial precursor formation and segregation with VEGF and VEGF receptors and important for integration of endocardial angio-

blasts into the definitive endocardium (Sugi, personal communication).[20]

The fate of the heart fields is to fuse ventrally beneath the foregut. Fused heart fields create a crescent-shaped structure from which a linear or straight tube heart emerges (Fig. 1).[15] Two epithelia—endocardium and myocardium—separated by an acellular matrix (cardiac jelly) form the wall of the linear heart tube.[21] One of the most important questions concerning formation of the tubular heart is whether all future chambers of the mature heart have their primordium within the straight tube heart? In other words, are the future chambers of the heart arranged along a rostral-caudal sequence as frequently shown for the straight heart tube? Based on studies in living embryos, the answer is no. The only area of the four chambered heart represented in the linear heart tube

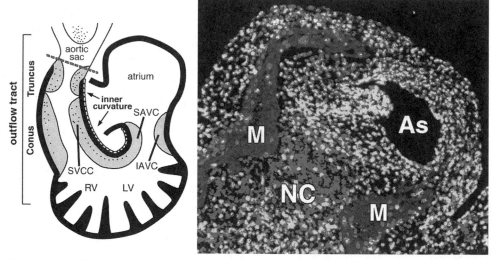

Figure 2. A. Diagram of the outflow tract of a stage 19 chick heart. Note the conus and the (still developing) truncus form the outlet segment; the latter together with the aortic sac constitute the complete outflow tract. The myocardial epithelium ends at the level of the aortic sac. The solid line indicates the site of the putative anterior heart forming field. The dots indicate the future migratory pathway of neural crest cells into the conus and truncus. SAVC, superior atrioventricular cushion; IAVC, inferior atrioventricular cushion; LV, left ventricle; RV, right ventricle; SVCC, sinistroventral conal cushion. **B.** Oblique section through the junction between the posterior aortic sac and the truncus 48 hours later in development than shown in 2a. The tissue had been labeled for 16 hours with BrdU prior to preparation for staining with anti-BrdU (yellow/white), anti-myosin or HNK (green) antibodies. Note that the cuffs of myocardium (M) or the HNK+ condensed mesenchyme (presumably neural crest) have few BrdU (+) cells compared to the mesoderm of the posterior aortic sac (the proposed anterior heart forming field). M, myocardium; NC, neural crest; AS, aortic sac.

is the future trabeculated region of the right ventricle.[22] Rather, when development is traced *over time* using in vivo markers, the heart tube appears to be put together "piece by piece" or segmentally.[23] Each segment arises at a different time-point or birthdate from the heart fields.[12,24] In the chick, four segments arise sequentially from the fused heart fields between stages 9 and 14 (Fig. 1). Looping or bending of the heart tube begins at the seam or junction between the first two segments once the second is fully "clear" of the fused heart fields. The trabeculated regions of the right and left ventricles arise from these two segments, respectively. The third segment—the atrioventricular (AV) canal—is initially the largest segment of the posterior limb of the looped heart.[25] It forms the inlet region of each ventricle. The fourth segment—the sinuatrial segment—forms the future venous pole. The fifth and final segment—the conotruncus or outlet segment—develops between stages 12 and 24 at the distal end of the original first segment (Figs. 1 and 2). The outlet segment develops at the arterial pole and, as such, appears to be the only one to not be derived directly from primordial cells located within the original fused heart fields.[12] Thus, the segments have different birthdates and, perhaps for the outlet segment, birthplaces.

Significance of Segmentation

One implication of forming segments sequentially *over time* is that there may be spatial and temporal "windows" that may be developmentally regulated. If there are genes that regulate the formation and differentiation of segments, they could explain why some segments form cushion tissues and others myocardial invaginations (e.g., ventricular trabeculae or the primary atrial septum). Although the myocardial and endocardial epithelium blend imperceptibly between segments, there are several examples of genes that are expressed segmentally or intersegmentally. For example, *d-*

HAND and *e-HAND* are expressed in the future trabeculated regions of the right and left ventricles, respectively.[26,27] *Mouse tolloid-like-1 (mt1–1)*[28] is expressed in the spina vestibuli of the atrium and the interventricular primary septum. Conversely, in one or both cushion forming segments (AV canal and outlet), the endocardium uniquely expresses the type 3 TGF beta receptor[29] whereas the adjacent myocardium expresses SLIM 1,[30] *wnt 11* (Fig. 3A), *bmp4* (Fig. 3B), and the *heart defect gene (hdf)* (Fig. 3C). There are also examples where a homeobox gene can regulate segment specific patterns of myosin genes[31] or specific elements of a promoter can direct (or restrict) expression of a myosin gene to a particular segment of the heart.[32,33] Whether such promoter elements normally do this in vivo is not known but it demonstrates there is potential for even some globally expressed genes to become restricted to a specific segment. Conversely, in mammalian or chick embryos, exogenously administered retinoic acid can expand expression of genes like *hdf* or atrial versus ventricular myosins across segmental boundaries.[34] The effect of obscuring or neutralizing segmental identity is unclear, however, in those instances where retinoids modify laterality, the consequences can include abnormal looping and misalignment of internal septa.[35,36] In zebrafish, exogenously added retinoids selectively truncate the formation of the ventricle and bulbus arteriosus without affecting the sinus venosus, atrium or AV canal.[37] This further supports the hypothesis that segments are under different genetic regulation.

Another significance of segmental development as revealed by in vivo labeling is that no segment is the sole progenitor of an anatomical chamber of the mature heart[22,24]; as illustrated in Figure 1, the anatomic right and left ventricles are derived from three segments: the trabeculated region from original segments one and two respectively while the inlet and outlet (up to the level of the valves) of each are derived from the AV junction (segment 3) and the conus and truncus of the outlet segment, respectively. Thus,

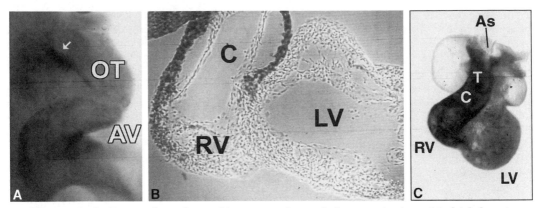

Figure 3. A. Expression of *wnt 11* message in a whole mount, stage 14 chick heart; arrow denotes the junction of the distal end of the heart tube and the aortic sac, the approximate position of the hypothetical anterior heart forming field. **B.** LacZ expression driven by the *bmp 4* promoter in a section taken from a day 10.5 heterozygous mouse heart; note that the beta galactosidase reaction product occurs as an increasing gradient beginning with the distal portion of the right ventricular segment and extending into the developing conus. This pattern of expression is consistent with the hypothesis that the distal (posterior) end of the heart tube induces the formation ("recruitment) of precursor cells for the conus and truncus from an anterior heart field. **C.** Expression of the *hdf* gene in a heterozygous, day 10, whole mouse heart; note expression parallels that of *bmp 4*, suggesting the *hdf*/versican gene may be expressed as a result of *bmp 4* signaling. OT, outflow tract; AV, atrioventricular; RV, right ventricle; C, conus; LV, left ventricle; T, truncus; AS, aortic sac.

mature ventricular chambers are anatomical but *not* embryological units. Although the variation in trabeculation can be used to confirm the identity of a ventricle (e.g, as in persistent AV canal or situs inversus), most congenital defects of the ventricle involve either the inlet segment (e.g., tricuspid atresia) or the outlet segment (double outlet right ventricle). For this and other reasons, Anderson[38] developed the *sequential segmental analysis* approach as a means of more precisely characterizing and identifying congenital heart defects. It is important to recognize that the majority of heart defects are problems in the integration or alignment of segments or the septa that form within or between segments.[12,36,39–41]

Origin of the Outlet Segment

The term outlet segment and "outflow tract" are used to describe the vascular conduit between the embryonic right ventricular segment and the aortic arches which includes the conus, truncus and aortic sac.[42,43] Only the conus and truncus have a myocardial epithelial mantle (Fig. 2A). The conus forms cushions that fuse to form the outlet septum that divides the conus into an outlet for both the left and right ventricle (the "infundibulum" and "aortic vestibule," respectively).[44] Cushions also develop within the truncus, which, if they really fuse at all, soon become "impaled" by the leading edge of the aorticopulmonary septum that divides the aortic sac into the root of the aorta and the pulmonary trunk.[44] Truncal cushions differentiate into the valve leaflets that guard the entrances to the aorta and pulmonary trunk.[18,45] The transcription factors, *NFAT-C* and *SOX-4* are expressed in the endocardium of the truncal cushions and appear required for differentiation of the subjacent mesenchyme into valvular tissues.[46,47]

Despite its enormous relevance to congenital heart disease, little is known about the origin of the precursors for the conotruncus or how they are integrated or recruited into a conotruncal segment. Two logical possibilities come to mind. The precursors could form by an extension (outward growth) of myocardial cells from the existing right ventricle (or bulbus cordis)[48] or they could be derived de novo from mesoderm located at or rostral to the distal rim or the heart tube. The concept of a rostral or anterior heart forming field for the conotruncus has never been described to our knowledge but was clearly inferred by the experimental findings of de la Cruz.[49] Based on in vivo labeling studies (reviewed in Reference 12), no in vivo marker placed into the heart fields or into the distal most segment of the heart tube (i.e., the future trabeculated right ventricular segment) ever traced to the conus or truncus. Rather, the conotruncal segment was labeled only when markers are placed into mesodermal cells located rostal or anterior to the distal end of the heart tube at stages 9 or 12 and incubation continued until stage 17 (end of conus formation) or stage 22–24 (end of truncal formation).[49] The conclusion from these studies was that the conus and truncus are added as new structures to the distal of the tubular heart. A similar interpretation was recently made by Fisher and Watanabe[50] who used adenoviral/lacZ vectors to infect, in situ, all myocardial cells at stage 14; when incubation was then continued until stage 24, part of the conus and all the truncus were unlabelled, i.e., they did not express beta galactosidase, a finding consistent with the hypothesis of an anterior heart field. Had they been "blue" (lacZ+) like the rest of the tubular heart, it would have suggested an origin from the myocardium at the distal rim of the tubular heart that existed at the time of infection.

If a rostral/anterior heart field exists, it would have to be at or near the junction of the truncal end of the tubular heart and the posterior wall of the aortic sac (Fig. 2A). This junction is shown at stage 24 following 16-hour labeling period with BrdU (Fig. 2B). The boundary is not a sharp one as "cuffs" of myocardial cells extend beyond the distal end of the heart tube into the aortic sac. The condensed core of mesenchyme within the truncal cushions is part of the leading edge of the aorticopulmonary septum (APS). The latter is well-known to be of neural crest origin.[51] As shown in Figure 2B, BrdU-positive cells are abundant in the mesenchyme of the posterior wall of the aortic sac but not in the cuffs of myocardial cells or the APS. The BrdU-positive cells appear to be mesenchymal tissue which is most likely a derivative of the splanchnic mesoderm or dorsal mesocardium that persists at the arterial pole after the onset of looping. Thus, the posterior wall of the aortic sac (and any associated dorsal mesocardium) is a candidate site for an anterior heart forming field. As described elsewhere in this book (see Chapter 17), this hypothesis was tested by microinjecting the vital dye, *mitotracker* directly into the mesodermal tissue located immediately rostral to the distal rim of the heart tube at stage 16 and incubation continued to stage 22. Unlike results obtained by labeling the entire heart tube at stage 14, the distal conus and all the truncus were the only labeled structures, a finding consistent with the existence of an anterior heart field located at the level of the posterior aortic sac.

Also, in preliminary experiments, we have isolated the candidate anterior heart field (posterior wall of the aortic sac) and co-cultured it with myocardial tissue explanted from the distal end of the heart tube versus a region of right ventricle not directly associated with the candidate anterior heart field. When aortic sac/dorsal mesocardium is explanted on collagen gels, mesodermal cells migrate from the explant and form an epithelial monolayer of myosin-negative cells. However, after 48 hours in co-culture, mesodermal cells in close association with the distal myocardial rim of the heart tube begin to express myosin markers, become contractile and, by 3 days, establish links (i.e., they integrate) with the original myocardial explant (Fig. 4). Conversely, mesodermal cells in contact with myocardial explants

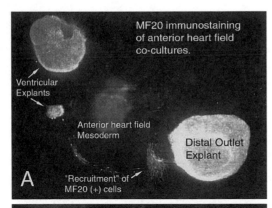

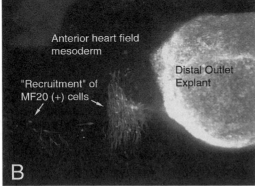

Figure 4. Co-culture assay to test the hypothesis that the distal end of the heart tube can recruit undifferentiated mesodermal cells from the anterior heart field (posterior aortic sac) to enter a myocardial (MF20+) lineage. **A.** An explant containing the candidate anterior heart forming field was dissected from tissue surrounding the aortic sac and placed on the surface of a 3-dimensional collagen gel. After 24-hour incubation, other explants were isolated from the left ventricle (*bmp 4* negative) or the distal rim of the outlet (*bmp 4* positive) from stage 19 hearts and positioned to directly contact the periphery of the mesoderm that had grown out of the explant taken from the posterior wall of the aortic sac. Co-cultures were incubated for 48 hours, fixed, and immunostained for cardiac sarcomeric myosin (MF20 antibody). Distal outlet explants appeared to recruit MF20 positive (+) cells from the anterior heart field mesoderm near the outlet explant. Few or no MF 20 (+) cells were observed near the ventricular explants. **B.** Higher magnification of the site of potential recruitment of elongated MF20 positive cells from the anterior heart field mesoderm.

from the left ventricle do not show any signs of entering a myocardial lineage. Based on these observations, we have proposed a conceptual working hypothesis that the outlet segment is derived from an anterior heart field located at the arterial pole and that an inductive interaction may occur between the putative anterior heart field and the distal end (i.e., the "growing rim/tip") of the looped heart tube. This interaction is envisioned as enhancing the recruitment of undifferentiated (but probably committed) mesoderm into the future myocardial cells of the conus and truncus. If the hypothesis is correct, the future right ventricle would initiate at stage 12–14 the recruitment of mesodermal from the anterior heart field into conal cells. In turn, between stages 14–24, the most recently recruited conal or truncal cells would then sustain the recruitment process until the outlet segment was completed.

Molecular Morphogenesis of the Outlet Segment?

One interpretation of the co-culture data shown in Figure 4 is, if myocardial cells secrete inductive signals that recruit aortic sac mesoderm into a myocardial lineage, they might be acting at relatively short range. A similar possibility was suggested by other preliminary co-culture experiments using QCE-6 cells and myocardial explants (Fig. 5). QCE-6 cells are undifferentiated mesodermal cell line which has been developed as a model for heart field mesoderm.[52] They are highly responsive to cues in their microenvironment, which can induce them to enter a myocardial lineage.[53] When an aggregate of myocardial tissue was co-cultured with undifferentiated QCE-6 cells, the only QCE-6 cells to express myocardial markers were those that had become integrated into the ventricular explant (Fig. 5). Again, this suggests that putative inductive interaction may be limited to a very short range.

Coculture of HH stage 16 OFT and β-Gal-labeled QCE6 cells

β-Gal

MF20

β-Gal + MF20

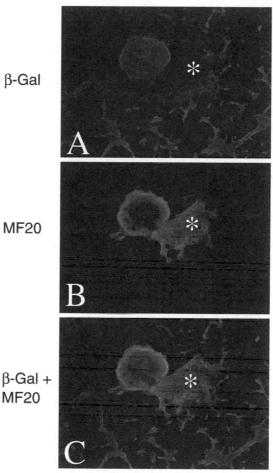

Figure 5. Co-culture of stage 16 outlets and lacZ-labeled QCE-6 cells. **A.** LacZ (beta galactosidase) expression showing the distribution of the lacZ transfected QCE-6 cells co-cultured with a distal outlet heart explant. **B.** Distribution of MF20 (+) cells in the co-culture visualized by indirect immunofluorescence. **C.** Co-localization of the MF20 (+) and QCE-6 (lacZ) positive cells within the co-culture. A co-localization of signals was observed within an aggregate of QCE-6 cells that had formed adjacent to an OFT explant, suggesting a short range interaction occurs between the outflow explant and QCE-6 cells acts to "recruit" the latter into a MF20 (+) lineage. QCE-6 cells alone did not express MF20 markers under the culture conditions. (*) denotes the site of the OFT explant in all figures.

The same two classes of morphogens that act at short range to recruit cells into the classic heart forming fields are also expressed in the region proposed as the candidate anterior heart. These are *wnt 11* and *bmp 4* (Fig. 3A). Because *wnt 11* is expressed only within the candidate anterior heart forming field, it is more likely to play an intrinsic role in the recruitment of mesoderm into a myocardial lineage than *bmp 2* or *4*. The expression pattern of the latter suggests an extrinsic role (Fig. 3B). Specifically, in a transgenic mouse expressing a lacZ reporter driven by the *bmp 4* promoter, the *bmp 4* gene at day 10 is expressed in an increasing gradient beginning with the the distal portion of the right ventricle and continuing through the developing outlet segment (Fig. 3B). We suggest that this pattern of *bmp 4* expression would appear to correlate closely with the pattern predicted by the hypothesis of an outlet segment that is added progressively *over time* to the distal end of the heart tube. Unfortunately, the knockout of either *bmp 2* or *bmp 4* is an early day 9 lethal[54,55] that precludes using this mouse model in its present form to test the role of this morphogen in the formation of the outlet segment. We are currently placing the *bmp 4* knockout mouse onto different genetic backgrounds to attempt to prolong development. In another approach, we have constructed an adenoviral vector expressing *bmp 4*. Microinjection of the virus at high titers ($>10^6$) into the growing outlet segment at day 16 indicate that constitutively expressing *bmp 4* significantly increases the length of the truncal region at the expense of the aortic sac which appears to become actually a part of the heart tube itself rather that remaining as the pharyngeal vascular basket that feeds the aortic arches (Fig. 6).

This raises the question as to why the aortic sac normally does not become "myocardialized." As shown in Figure 2B, cuffs of myocardial cells enter the aortic sac but their extension does not proceed more rostrally. From the work of Ya et al.,[44] the fate of the cuffs within the aortic sac may be to transdifferentiate or revert back into a mesenchymal-like phenotype. This raises the question whether the rostral extension of the distal end of the heart tube toward the aortic sac and aortic arches is ultimately stopped because the stability of newly recruited cardiomyocytes is dependent upon some signal that is normally absent in the aortic sac.

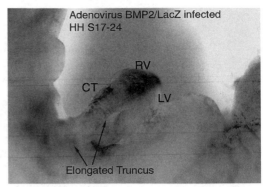

Figure 6. Microinjection of an adenoviral vector constructed to express *bmp 2* and lacZ into the growing outlet segment of a stage 17 chick heart and incubated for an additional 3 days (stage 24). Results indicate an abnormally elongated truncus segment that appears to have completely "incorporated" (myocardialized) the aortic sac. These results are consistent with the hypothesis that bone morphogenetic proteins may play a role in formation of the outlet segment. CT, conotruncus; RV, right ventricle; LV, left ventricle.

A candidate for such a signal is *hdf* gene. The *hdf* mouse was created through an insertion of a transgene containing a lacZ reporter into chromosome 13.[56] The transgene was found to have disrupted the CSPg2 gene, also known as versican.[57] In heterozygous embryos, the expression pattern of the *hdf* gene closely parallels *bmp 4* in the mouse and, like the latter, does not extend rostrally into the aortic sac beyond the level of the candidate anterior heart field (Fig. 3C). In homozygous mutant embryos, the extracellular space that normally separates endocardium from myocardium was deficient or absent and the right ventricular and conotruncal segments were highly truncated. Exon 6 of versican normally encodes the hyaluronate binding region of versican.[57] Interestingly, the knockout of the *hyaluronate synthesis 2 gene* which encodes an enzyme required for hyaluronate synthesis also produces a phenotype very similar to *hdf* (John McDonald, personal communication). These findings indicate that "downstream" extracellular molecular complexes like versican/hyaluronate can affect morphogenesis of an entire embryonic cardiac segment. It is possible that versican/hyaluronate might directly promote recruitment of mesoderm into a myocardial lineage, however, this is unlikely since a looped heart tube forms in homozygous *hdf* mutants. Given its reciprocal relationship to the myocardial cuffs and the consequence of its knockout, a reasonable role for this gene is to regulate the integration of conotruncal precursor cells into concentric epithelia and/or to sustain their myocardial epithelial phenotype.

Cushion Formation Versus Trabeculation

Each segment of the heart participates in forming septal tissues that collectively integrate *over time* to divide the primary heart tube into four chambers. In the AV and outlet segments, the septal tissues are mesenchymal swellings called cushions which fuse to form mesenchymal septal structures from which the valve leaflets arise.[40,41,58] In the ventricles, clonal expansions of myocardial cells project into the lumen to form trabeculae.[59] Historically, the coalescence of trabeculae at the interventricular junction has been the mechanism proposed for the formation of the primary ventricular muscular septum.[60] However, in vivo labeling studies point to a specific site of origin for the ventricular septum from cells derived from the original ventral fusion line of the heart fields,[61] a finding supported by the expression of the mammalian *tolloid-like 1* gene.[28] In the sinuatrium, infoldings of the myocardium form the muscular portion of the primary atrial septum. Formation of the septum is dependent upon an association with extracardiac mesenchymal tissue derived, in part, from the spina vestibuli (right pulmonary ridge),[40,62,63] a structure that also expresses *tolloid-like-1*.[28] The mesenchyme of the fused AV cushions serves to knit together and stabilize the primary atrial and ventricular muscular septa.[40,58] In the outlet segment, the fusion of the conal cushions forms

a septum, which, when brought into alignment with the primary ventricular septum, creates a separate outlet for each ventricle. Thus, the formation of cushions is critical for cardiac morphogenesis.

A central tenet of cushion tissue formation is that the myocardium of the AV and outlet segments induces a competent endocardium to transform into mesenchyme.[64,65] Myocardial cells of these segments secrete multicomponent complexes we have called adherons, which promote some but not all endothelial cells to transform into mesenchyme (reviewed in References 57, 66, 67). Endothelial cells competent to transform express a marker, JB3, which may reflect their origin from the heart fields.[18,66] Overall, some 40+ genes or proteins have been identified that affect endothelial transformation or whose expression is modified during transformation and migration. These include ES 130,[68] hLAMP,[69] transferrin,[70] serine proteases,[71] growth factors, particularly of the TGF beta family,[72–74] receptors to TGF beta growth factors,[29,30] and cell and extracellular adhesion molecules.[75–79] Thus, multiple levels of myocardial-endocardial interaction appear to be required to initiate, sustain or amplify the formation of cushion tissue or to "fine tune" its final form or shape.

However, to date, no consensus myocardial signal has been confirmed as the one "master" upstream signal that starts the whole process. That such a signal exists was reaffirmed in a recent, high stringency, temporal refinement of the culture assay for myocardial-endocardial interaction.[80,81] Using early activation markers, these studies indicated that myocardial induction actually began during the formation of the actual AV or outlet segments (much earlier than previously thought). Thus, the search for the myocardial inducer logically should include consideration of those proteins that are segmentally expressed during morphogenesis of the segment itself. To our knowledge, *bmp 4* (and probably *bmp 2* also) is the only TGF gene family member to be uniquely expressed by myocardial cells during formation of the AV and outlet segments and whose expression continues until the onset of endocardial transformation to cushion mesenchyme. Although their temporal and spatial expression makes *bmp 2/4* "perfect" candidates for being the upstream myocardial signal that initiates cushion formation, neither has been experimentally tested. Unfortunately, the early lethality of *bmp2/4* knockouts precludes determining any link to cushion formation. In a paper by Nakajima et al. in this volume, the *bmp 2* protein-induced cushion cell formation in culture, particularly when combined with TGF beta3. These findings suggest that the regulatory mechanisms that establish the AV and conotruncal segments (e.g., *bmp 2/4*) may also be linked downstream to the activation of endocardial transformation to mesenchyme.

Similar links between segmental morphogenesis and trabeculation may occur in the ventricles. Results from gene knockouts indicate that it is highly unlikely that myocardial cells invade the cardiac jelly to form trabeculae only if endocardial endothelial cells do not first fill the extracellular space with cushion tissues. Rather, specific endocardial-myocardial interactions appear to drive trabeculation as shown by the profound disruption of trabeculae formation in mice null for either Tie 2 or angiopoitin 1. Tie 2 is a receptor tyrosine kinase on endocardial cells whose ligand, angiopoitin 1, is secreted by the myocardium.[82] In this instance, it is proposed that signaling from the myocardium through secretion of angiopoitin 1 is received by the endocardium via the Tie 2 receptor, which in turn feeds back to affect myocardial development, in some yet unknown manner.[82]

Transforming the Primary Heart Tube Into a Four Chambered Organ

In this overview, we have described development of the primary heart tube up to the onset of cushion formation and trabeculation (approximately stage 20 in the chick and day 9 in the mouse). For the primitive tubular heart to become a four-chambered organ, several major morphogenetic events must follow: (1) the formation of an epicardium from which is derived the coronary vasculature as well as a population of epicardial derived cells (EPDCs) that invade the tubular heart[83]; (2) the invasion of neural crest cells into the aortic sac (as the aorticopulmonary septum) and into the conus and truncus where their role remains to be determined[84–86]; (3) remodeling of the inner curvature to complete looping and to align segments and septa[12]; (4) formation of the central and peripheral myocardial conduction system.[87] However, each of these defining morphogenetic processes must be preceded by first successfully establishing a rostrocaudal sequence of segments with differing birthdates and, probably, birthplaces.

Acknowledgments: Support for this work was provided by grants HL19136 and HL33756 from the National Heart, Lung, and Blood Institute. We also express our appreciation to Dr. John McDonald for allowing us to cite his unpublished observations. The assistance of the Molecular Morphology Core under the direction of Dr. Thomas Trusk and Mr. Spruill is most gratefully appreciated.

References

1. Rosenquist GC, DeHaan RL. Carnegie Inst Washington, *Contrib Embryol* 1966; 38:111–121.
2. Bodmer R. The gene tinman is required for specification of the heart and visceral muscles in Drosophila. *Development* 1993; 118(3):719–729.
3. Lints TJ, Parson LM, Hartley, et al. Nkx-2.5: a novel murine homeobox gene expressed in early heart progenitor cells and their myogenic descendants. *Development* 1993;119:419–431.
4. Brand T, Andree B, Schneider A, et al. Chicken NKx2-8, a novel homeobox gene expressed during early heart and foregut. *Mech Dev* 1997;64:53–59.
5. Lin Q, Schwartz, JA, Olsen EN. Control of mouse cardiac morphogenesis and myogenesis by transcription factor MEF2C. *Science* 1997;276:1404–1407.
6. Molkentin JD, Kalvakolanu DV, Markham BE. Transcription factor GATA-4 regulates cardiac muscle-specific expression of the

alpha-myosin heavy-chain gene. *Mol Cell Biol* 1994;14:4947–4957.

7. Wall NA, Hogan B. TGF-beta related genes in development. *Curr Opinion Genet Dev* 1994;4:517–522.

8. Nusse R, Varmus HE. Wnt genes. *Cell* 1992;69:1073–1087.

9. Ladd, AN, Yatskievych TA, Antin PB. Regulation of avian cardiac myogenesis by activin/TGFbeta and bone morphogenetic proteins. *Dev Biol* 1998;204:407–419.

10. Lough J, Barron M, Brogley M, et al. Combined BMP-2 and FGF-4, but neither factor alone, induces cardiogenesis in nonprecardiac embryonic mesoderm. *Dev Biol* 1996;178:198–202.

11. Eisenberg CA, Gourdie RG, Eisenberg LM. Wnt-11 is expressed in early avian mesoderm and required for the differentiation of the quail mesoderm cell line QCE-6. *Development* 1997;124:525–536.

12. Markwald RR, Trusk T, Moreno-Rodriguez. In: de la Cruz MV, Markwald RR, eds. Formation and septation of the tubular heart: integrating the dynamics of morphology with emerging molecular concepts. *Living Morphogenesis of the Heart*. Boston, Mass: Birkhauser (Springer–Verlag); 1998:43–84.

13. Han Y, Dennis JE, Cohen-Gould L, et al. Expression of sarcomeric myosin in the presumptive myocardium of chicken embryos occurs within six hours of myocyte commitment. *Dev Dynam* 1992;193:257–265.

14. Montgomery MO, Litvin J, Gonzalez-Sanchez A, et al. Staging of commitment and differentiation of avian cardiac myocytes. *Dev Biol* 1994;164:63–71.

15. Linask KK, Lash JW. In: de la Cruz MV, Markwald RR, eds. Morphoregulatory mechanisms underlying early heart development: pre-cardiac stages to the looping, tubular heart. *Living Morphogenesis of the Heart*. Boston, Mass: Birkhauser (Springer Verlag); 1998:1–41.

16. Ruzicka DL, Schwartz RJ. Sequential activation of alpha-actin genes during avian cardiogenesis: vascular smooth muscle alpha-actin gene transcipts mark the onset of cardiomyocyte differentiation. *J Cell Biol* 1988;107(6 Pt 2):2575–2586.

17. Linask KK, Lash JW. Early heart development: dynamics of endocardial cell sorting suggests a common origin with cardiomyocytes. *Dev Dynam* 1993;195:62–69.

18. Wunsch A, Markwald RR, Little CD. Cardiac endothelial heterogeneity defines valvular development as demonstrated by the diverse expression of JB3, an antigen of the endocardial cushion tissue. *Dev Biol* 1994;165:585–601.

19. Sugi Y, Markwald RR. Formation and early morphogenesis of endocardial endothelial precursor cells and the role of endoderm. *Dev Biol* 1996;175:66–83.

20. Dumont DJ, Jussila L, Taipale J, et al. Cardiovascular failure in mouse embryos deficient in VEGF receptor-3. *Science* 1999;282:946–949.

21. Viragh S, Szabo E, Challice CE. Formation of the primitive myo- and endocardial tubes in the chicken embryo. *J Mol Cell Cardiol* 1989;21:123–137.

22. de la Cruz MV, Sanchez Gomez C, Cayre R. *Cardiol Young* 1991;1:123–128.

23. de la Cruz MV, Sanchez-Gomez C. In: de la Cruz MV, Markwald RR, eds. Straight Tube Heart: Primative Cardiac Cavities Vs. Primitive Cardiac Segments. *Living Morphogenesis of the Heart*. Boston, Mass: Birkhauser (Springer Verlag); 1998:85–99.

24. de La Cruz MV, Sanchez-Gomez C, Palomino MA. *J Anat* 1989;165:121–131.

25. Gittenberger-de Groot AC, Bartelings MM, Poelmann RE. In: Clark EB, Markwald RR, Takao, A, eds. Overview: Cardiac Morphogenesis. *Developmental Mechanisms of Heart Disease*. Armonk, NY: Futura Publishing Company; 1995:157–168.

26. Olsen EN, Srivastava D. Molecular pathways controlling heart development. *Science* 1996;272:671–676.

27. Srivastava D, Thomas T, Lin Q, et al. *Nature* 1997;16:154–160.

28. Clark TG, Conway SJ, Scott IC, et al. The mammalian Tolloid-like 1 gene, T111, is necessary for normal septation and positioning of the heart, *Development* 1999; 126:2631-2642.

29. Brown CB, Boyer AS, Runyan RB, et al. Requirement of type III TGF-beta receptor for endocardial cell transformation in the heart. *Science* 1999, 26;283(5410):2080–2082.

30. Brown S, Biben C, Ooms LM, et al. The cardiac expression of striated muscle LIM protein 1 (SLIM1) is restricted to the outflow tract of the developing heart. *J Mol Cell Cardiol* 1999;31:837–843.

31. Bao Z-Z, Bruneau BG, Seidman JG, et al. Regulation of chamber-specific gene expression in the developing heart by Irx4. *Science* 1999;283:1161–1164.

32. Ross RS, Navankasattusas S, Harvey RP, et al. An HF-1a/HF-1b/MEF-2 combinatorial element confers cardiac ventricular specificity and established an anterior-

posterior gradient of expression. *Development* 1996;122:1799–1809.

33. Franco D, Kelly R, Buckingham M, et al. Regionalized transcriptional domains of myosin light chain 3f transgenes in the embryonic mouse heart: morphogenetic implications. *Dev Biol* 1997;187:17–33.

34. Yutzey KE, Rhee JT, Bader DM. Expression of the atrial-specific myosin heavy chain AMHC1 and the establishment of antero-posterior polarity in the developing chicken heart. *Development* 1994;120:871–883.

35. Smith SM, Dickman ED, Thompson RP, et al. Retinoic acid directs cardiac laterality and the expression of early markers of precardiac asymmetry. *Dev Biol* 1997;182:162–171.

36. Bouman HGA, Broekhuizen MLA, Baasten MJ, et al. Spectrum of looping disturbances in stage 34 chicken hearts after retinoic acid treatment. *Anat Rec* 1995;243:101–108.

37. Stanier DYR, Fishman MC. GAP-43 as a plasticity protein in neuronal form and repair. *Dev Biol* 1992;153:91–101.

38. Shinbourne EA, Macartney FJ, Anderson RH. Editorial: Connexions, relation, discordance, and distorsions. *Br Heart J* 1976;38:327–340.

39. Lamers WH, Wessels A, Verbeek FJ, et al. New findings concerning ventricular septation in the human heart. Implications for maldevelopment. *Circulation* 1992;86:1194–1205.

40. Webb S, Brown NA, Anderson RH. Formation of the atrioventricular septal structures in the normal mouse. *Circ Res* 1998;82:645–656.

41. Mjaatvedt CH, Yamamura H, Ramsdell A, et al. In: Harvey RP, Rosenthal N, eds. *Heart Development*. New York: Academic Press; 1999:159–177.

42. Thompson RP, Fitzharris TP. Morphogenesis of the truncus arteriosus of the chick embryo heart: tissue reorganization during septation. *Am J Anat* 1979;156:251–264.

43. Pexieder T. In: Clark EB, Markwald RR, Takao A, eds. Conotruncus and Its Septation at the Advent of the Modecular Biology Era. *Developmental Mechanisms of Heart Development*. Armonk, NY: Futura Publishing; 1995:227–247.

44. Ya J, Van den Hoff MJB, de Boer PAJ, et al. Heart defects in connexin43-deficient mice. *Circ Res* 1998;82:464–472.

45. Noden DM, Poelmann RE, Gittenberger-de Groot AC. *Trends Cardiovasc Med* 1995;5:69–75.

46. Ranger A, Grusby M, Hodge M, et al. The transcription factor NF-ATc is essential for cardiac valve formation. *Nature* 1998;392:186–190.

47. Schilham MW, Oosterwegel MA, Moerer P. Defects in cardiac outflow tract formation and pro-B-lymphocyte expansion in mice lacking Sox-4. *Nature* 1996;380:711–714.

48. Castro-Quezada A, Nidal-Ginard B, de la Cruz MV. Experimental study of the formation of the bulboventricular loop in the chick. *J Embryol Exp Morphol* 1972;27:623–637.

49. de la Cruz MV, Sanchez-Gomez C, Arteaga MM, et al. Experimental study of the development of the truncus and the conus in the chick embryo. *J Anat* 1977;123:661–686.

50. Fisher SA, Watanabe M. Expression of exogenous protein and analysis of morphogenesis in the developing chicken heart using an adenoviral vector. *Cardiovasc Res* 1996;31:E86–E95.

51. Kirby ML. Cellular and molecular contributions of the cardiac neural crest to cardiovascular development. *Trends Cardiovasc Med* 1993;3:18–23.

52. Eisenberg C, Bader D. Prenatal sonographic diagnosis of dacryocystocele: a case and review of the literature. *Dev Biol* 1995;167:469–481.

53. Eisenberg CA, Markwald RR. Mixed cultures of avian blastoderm cells and the quail mesoderm cell line QCE-6 provide evidence for the pluripotentiality of early mesoderm. *Dev Biol* 1997;191:167–181.

54. Winnier G, Blessing M, Labosky PA, et al. Bone morphogenetic protein-4 is required for mesoderm formation and patterning in the mouse. *Genes Dev* 1995;9:2105–2116.

55. Zhang H, Bradley A. Mice deficient for BMP2 are nonviable and have defects in amnion/chorion and cardiac development. *Development* 1996;122:2977–2986.

56. Yamamura H, Zhang M, Mjaatvedt CH, et al. A heart segmental defect in the anterior-posterior axis of a transgenic mutant mouse. *Dev Biol* 1997;186:58–72.

57. Mjaatvedt CH, Yamaura H, Capehart AA, et al. The Cspg2 gene, disrupted in the hdf mutant, is required for right cardiac chamber and endocardial cushion formation. *Dev Biol* 1998;202:56–66.

58. de la Cruz MV, Moreno-Rodriguez R, Markwald RR. In: de la Cruz MV, Markwald RR, eds. Embryological development of the apical trabeculated region of both ventricals: the contribution of the primitive intraventricular septum in the ventricular septation. *Living Morphogenesis*

of the Heart. Boston, Mass: Birkhauser (Springer-Verlag); 1998:l131–1156.

59. Mikawa T, Borisov A, Brown AMC, et al. Clonal analysis of cardiac morphogenesis in the chicken embryo using a replication-defective retrovirus. III: Polyclonal origin of adjacent ventricular myocytes. *Dev Dynam* 1992;195:133–141.

60. Ben-Shachar G, Arcilla RA, Lucas RV, et al. Ventricular trabeculations in the chick embryo heart and their contribution to ventricular and muscular septal development. *Circ Res* 1985;57:759–766.

61. de la Cruz MV, Castillo MM, Villavicencio L, et al. Primitive interventricular septum, its primordium, and its contribution in the definitive interventricular septum: in vivo labelling study in the chick embryo heart. *Anat Rec* 1997;247:512–520.

62. Tasaka H, Krug EL, Markwald RR. Origin of the pulmonary venous orifice in the mouse and its relation to the morphogenesis of the sinus venosus, extracardiac mesenchyme (spina vestibuli), and atrium. *Anat Rec* 1996;246:107–113.

63. Webb S, Anderson RH, Lamers WH, et al. Mechanisms of deficient cardiac septation in the mouse with trisomy 16. *Circ Res* 1999;84:897–905.

64. Bernanke DH, Markwald RR. Migratory behavior of cardiac cushion tissue cells in a collagen-lattice culture system. *Dev Biol* 1982;91:235–245.

65. Runyan RB, Markwald RR. Invasion of mesenchyme into three-dimensional collagen gels: a regional and temporal analysis of interaction in embryonic heart tissue. *Dev Biol* 1983;95:108–114.

66. Eisenberg LM, Markwald RR. Molecular regulation of atrioventricular valvuloseptal morphogenesis. *Circ Res* 1995;77:1–6.

67. Markwald R, Eisenberg C, Eisenberg L, et al. Epithelial-mesenchymal transformations in early avian heart development. *Acta Anat* 1996;156:173–186.

68. Krug EL, Rezaee M, Isokawa K, et al. Transformation of cardiac endothelium into cushion mesenchyme is dependent on ES/130: temporal, spatial, and functional studies in the early chick embryo. *Cell Mol Biol Res* 1995;41:263–277.

69. Sinning AR, Hewitt CC. Identification of a 283-kDa protein component of the particulate matrix associated with cardiac mesenchyme formation. *Acta Anat* 1996;155:219–230.

70. Isokawa K, Rezaee M, Wunsch A, et al. Identification of transferrin as one of multiple EDTA-extractable extracellular proteins involved in early chick heart morphogenesis. *J Cell Biochem* 1994;54:207–218.

71. McGuire PG, Alexander SM. Inhibition of urokinase synthesis and cell surface binding alters the motile behavior of embryonic endocardial-derived mesenchymal cells in vitro. *Development Camb* 1993;118:931–939.

72. Potts JD, Dagle JM, Walder JA, et al. Epithelial-mesenchymal transformation of embryonic cardiac endothelial cells is inhibited by a modified antisense oligodeoxynucleotide to transforming growth factor beta 3. *Proc Natl Acad Sci U S A* 1991; 88:1516–1520.

73. Runyan RB, Potts JD, Weeks DL. TGF-beta-3-mediated tissue interaction during embryonic heart development. *Mol Reprod Dev* 1992;32:152–159.

74. Nakajima Y, Yamagishi T, Nakamura H, et al. *Dev Biol* 1997;194:58–72.

75. Bernanke DH, Markwald RR. Effects of two glycosaminoglycans on seeding of cardiac cushion tissue cells into a collagen-lattice culture system. *Anat Rec* 1984;210: 25–31.

76. Crossin KL, Hoffman S. Expression of adhesion molecules during the formation and differentiation of the avian endocardial cushion tissue. *Dev Biol* 1991;145: 277–286.

77. Little CD, Rongish BJ. The extracellular matrix during heart development. *Experentia* 1995;51:873–882.

78. Bouchey D, Argraves WS, Little CD. Fibulin-1, vitronectin, and fibronectin expression during avian cardiac valve and septa development. *Anat Rec* 1996;244:540–551.

79. Markwald RR, Trusk T, Gittenberger-de Groot AC, et al. In: Kavlock R, Datson G, eds. *Handbook of Experimental Pharmacology,* 124/I. Berlin: Springer–Verlag; 1997:11–40.

80. Ramsdell A, Markwald R. Induction of endocardial cushion tissue in the avian heart is regulated, in part, by TGFbeta-3-mediated autocrine signaling. *Dev Biol* 1997; 187:64–74.

81. Ramsdell AF, Moreno-Rodriguez RA, Weinecke MM, et al. Identification of an autocrine signaling pathway that amplifies induction of endocardial cushion tissue in the avian heart. *Acta Anat* 1998; 162:1–15.

82. Suri C, Jones PF, Patan S, et al. Requisite role of angiopoietin-1, a ligand for the TIE2 receptor, during embryonic angiogenesis *Cell* 1996;87:1172–1180.

83. Gittenberger-deGroot AC, Vranken Peeters MP, Mentink MM, et al. Epicardium-derived cells contribute a novel population to the myocardial wall and the atrioventricular cushions. *Circ Res* 1998;82:1043–1052.

84. Poelmann RE, Mikawa T, Gittenberger-deGroot AC. Neural crest cells in outflow tract septation of the embryonic chicken heart: differentiation and apoptosis. *Dev Dynamics* 1998;212:373–384.

85. Waldo K, Miyagawa-Tomita S, Kumiski D, et al. Cardiac neural crest cells provide new insight into septation of the cardiac outflow tract: aortic sac to ventricular septal closure. *Dev Biol* 1998; 196:129–144.

86. Waldo K, Zdanowicz M, Burch J, et al. A novel role for cardiac neural crest in heart development. *J Clin Invest* 1999;103:1499–1507.

87. Gourdie RG, Kubalak S, Mikawa T. Conducting the embryonic heart: orchestrating development of specialized cardiac tissues. *Trends Cardiovasc Med* 1999;9:18–26.

17

Segmental Heart Development of the *hdf*/Versican Gene

Roger R. Markwald, PhD, Hideshi Yamamura, MD,
Maria Victoria de la Cruz, MD, Wanda Litchenberg, PhD,
Rob Gourdie, PhD, Robert Thompson, PhD,
Simon Conway, PhD, and Corey Mjaatvedt, PhD

Based on the results of a series of tissue marking experiments on living embryos, we have determined that between stages 9– and 14[1] most segments of the primary heart tube are established through a progressive and irreversible recruitment of lateral mesoderm derived from the classically recognized heart forming fields. In a novel tissue marking assay, five or six 10 μm Sepharose beads were implanted along the rostral-caudal axis of the classically defined heart forming fields at specific developmental time points and then followed as development was allowed to proceed. Results showed that most of the beads implanted at one specific time point (e.g., stage 4 vs. stage 5) in the heart field would be found at later stages clustered into a single phenotypically defined segment. For example, if the heart field is marked at stage 6+, the beads would track to the atrioventricular segment of the looped heart (Fig. 1A, B). These results of the microbead marking experiments were then confirmed in other experiments using a recombinant B-galactosidase-expressing retrovirus[2] to label individual cells of the heart forming

fields. Collectively, these data indicated that cardiac cells are recruited from the heart forming fields into the posterior end of the forming heart tube by a progressive mechanism that forms the linear series of four segments. These segments are (1) the future trabeculated regions of the right ventricle; (2) the trabeculated left ventricle; (3) the atrioventricular (AV) canal; and (4) the sinuatrium. The first indication of heart looping is initiated only after the formation of the first two segments at their boundary interface. However, none of the tissue or cell marking experiments that labeled the classically defined heart forming fields ever mapped the region of mesoderm that gives rise to the conotruncus.[3] The origin of this segment is of particular interest since the conotruncus displays a high incidence of congenital heart defects. In vivo markers have indicated that precursors for this region of the outflow tract are derived between stages 12–22 from undifferentiated mesoderm possibly associated with the dorsal mesocardium that persists between the future trabeculated right ventricular (RV) and the aortic sac. In multiple experiments, a bead placed in the mesoderm anterior to the heart at stage 9 (Fig. 1C) was tracked to the conus/truncus segment of a stage 12 heart (Fig. 1C', shaded region). Similarly, a bead placed at the base of the

From Clark EB, Nakazawa M, Takao A (eds.): Etiology and Morphogenesis of Congenital Heart Disease: Twenty Years of Progress in Genetics and Developmental Biology. Armonk, NY: Futura Publishing Co., Inc.; © 2000.

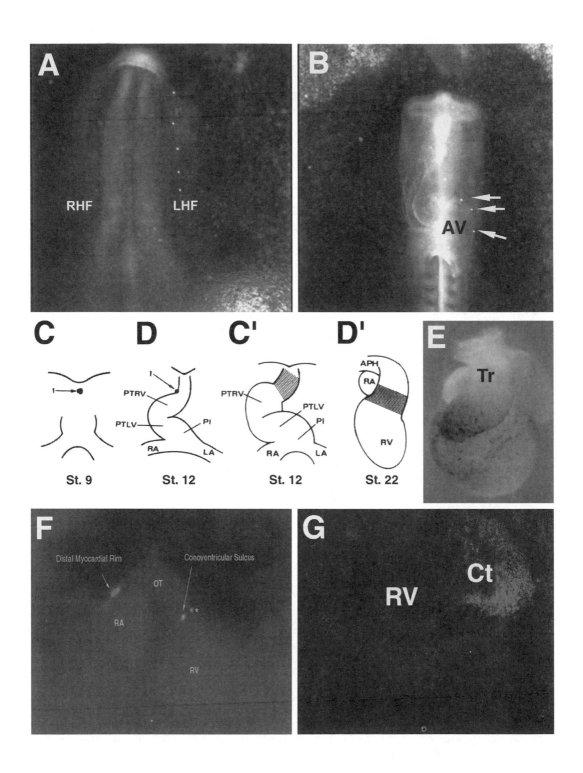

forming conus just anterior to the primitive trabeculated RV at stage 12 (Fig. 1D) was found to remain, with further development to stage 22, in the definitive conus region (Fig. 1D', shaded area), and was never found in the newly formed truncus. Other marking experiments using a lacZ expressing adenovirus (Fig. 1E) and microinjections of a fluorescent dye (mitotracker) have confirmed the observations made in the bead implant experiments and support the hypothesis that the conotruncus arises from a mesocardial mesoderm anterior to the traditionally defined heart forming fields. We have proposed that this mesocardial mesoderm is an "anterior heart forming field."

An unexpected finding of the tissue marking experiments was that microbeads implanted over either the right or left heart fields only, would consistently trace to only one AV cushion segment. For example, when the left heart field was initially marked, beads were subsequently traced to only the inferior AV cushion. Conversely, beads labeling the right heart field always were found in the superior AV cushion (Fig. 1A, B). This appears to be the first experimental evidence suggesting that the left and right heart fields may give rise to separate heart structures.

The establishment of these segmental boundaries within the single heart tube has led us to hypothesize that there are specific morphoregulatory genes that determine and regulate the phenotype of a specific segment. The segmental expression of two genes, *hdf* and dHAND indicates a regulatory role in establishment of the conus/truncus. We have characterized the heart defect (*hdf*) mouse which fails to form a conus/truncus. The *hdf* mouse arose from the insertion of a transgene containing a lacZ reporter into a single site on mouse chromosome 13.[4] In homozygous mutants (*hdf* –/–), the right ventricular portion of the anterior limb was found to be poorly developed or absent and the future conus region represented only by a narrow ring of variably condensed, mesodermal tissue (the hypothetical anterior heart field; Fig. 2A). Histological analysis at days 9.5–11 p.c., showed *hdf* driven lacZ to be distally expressed into the elongated, tapered region of the anterior limb (future conus/truncus) that formed during this period between its future RV portion and the aortic sac (Fig. 2B). Chromosome mapping studies initially identified Cspg2 (versican) as a candidate *hdf* gene and the identity of the *hdf* gene as Cspg2 was confirmed by independent lines of evidence.[5] These findings suggest that versican is required for morphogenesis of the

---

Figure 1. A. Placement of 10 um beads along the anterior-posterior axis of a stage 6+ chick embryo that were tracked through continued development until stage 12 (shown in **B**) most of the beads are found in the AV and ventricle segment of the heart tube, but were never found in the conotruncus segment. **C.** In vivo fate mapping of the CT segment using bead implants at stage 9 (**C**) in the "anterior heart forming field." At stage 12 (**C'**) beads were found only within the shaded region shown which is within the boundaries of the conotruncus segment. **D.** Beads placed at the distal tip of the ventricle at the conus/ventricular boundary at stage 12 (**D**) were found only in the conus (shaded region **D'**) at stage 22 and not found in the newly formed truncus. **E.** Hearts infected with adenovirus expressing lacZ at stage 17 and then harvested 48 hours later show labeling throughout the heart segments except the newly formed truncus. **F.** Labeling site on a stage 15 heart tube at the distal myocardial tip next to the body wall using a red fluorescent dye (mitotracker). **G.** Labeled heart shown in F) after 24-hour incubation shows labeling in the forming conotruncus. RHF, right heart field; LHF, left heart field; AV, atrioventricular segment; PTRV, primitive trabeculated right ventricle; PTLV, primitive trabeculated left ventricle; PI, primitive inlet; RA, right atrium; LA, left atrium; Tr, truncus; OT, outflow tract; RV, right ventricle; Ct, conotruncus. See color appendix.

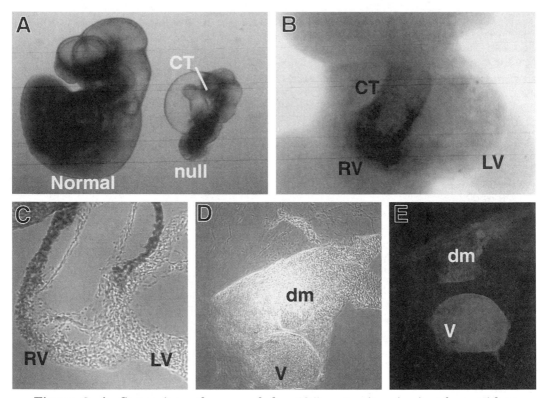

Figure 2. A. Comparison of a normal day 10.5 post coitus (p.c.) embryo with a homozygous *hdf* embryo (Cspg2/versican null). The Cspg2 null embryo displays impaired conotruncal (CT) formation. **B.** LacZ expression in a day 10.5 p.c. *hdf* hemizygous heart shows a segmental expression pattern associated with the conotruncus and RV development. **C.** Transgenic lacZ expression in a heterozygous BMP4/LacZ knock-in heart shows a segmentally restricted pattern associated with conotruncus development. **D.** Phase-contrast image of an explanted piece of the dorsal mesocardium (dm) dissected from a stage 12 embryo and co-cultured on a collagen gel with the distal tip of a stage 12 ventricular (V) explant. Within 24 hours of co-culture the dm began to beat spontaneously and express the MF20 muscle marker. CT, conotruncus; RV, right ventricle; LV, left ventricle. See color appendix.

conus/truncus segment if not the entire anterior limb of the looped heart but may not be needed to bring mesodermal cells into a heart lineage.

The lacZ expression patterns and phenotype of the *hdf*/versican homozygous mice suggests that the myocardium at the distal end of the tube may induce anterior heart field cells to enter the cardiocyte lineage by a signaling mechanism involving Bmp/Nkx and *hdf*/versican. Bone morphogenetic protein 4 is both expressed in a manner consistent with the formation of the conotruncus and may function in anterior heart field recruit-

ment (Fig. 2C). As a first step in testing this hypothesis, we dissected, from stage 12+ embryos, anterior heart field explants from the dorsal mesocardium and cultured them with an explant of the distal heart tube (Fig. 2E). In the presence of a distal heart tube explant, the anterior heart field cells began spontaneous contractions within 24 hours of incubation. Immunohistochemical analysis with the antibody MF20 confirmed the presence of cardiac muscle in the anterior heart field explants (Fig. 2F) and is consistent with the hypothesis that the conotruncus arises from a mesocardial mesoderm anterior to classically defined heart forming fields.

Acknowledgement: *Supported by NIH grants HL52813 and HL33756.*

References

1. V Hamburger, HL Hamilton. *Dev Dyn* 1951;195:231–272.
2. Mikawa T, Cohen-Gould L, Fischman DA. Clonal analysis of cardiac morphogenesis in the chicken embryo using a replication-defective retrovirus. III: Polyclonal origin of adjacent ventricular myocytes. *Dev Dyn* 1992;195:133–141.
3. Mjaatvedt CH, Yamamura H, Ramsdell A. In: Harvey RP, Rosenthal N, eds. *Heart Development*. Vol. 1. New York: Academic Press; 1998:159–174.
4. Yamamura H, Zhang M, Markwald R, et al. A heart segmental defect in the anterior-posterior axis of a transgenic mutant mouse. *Dev Biol* 1997;186:58–72.
5. Mjaatvedt CH, Yamamura H, Capehart T, et al. The Cspg2 gene, disrupted in the hdf mutant, is required for right cardiac chamber and endocardial cushion formation. *Dev Biol* 1998;202:56–66.

18

A Role Of *rae28*, A Member of the *Polycomb* Group of Genes, in Cardiac Morphogenesis

Yoshihiro Takihara, MD, Manabu Shirai, PhD, Daihachiro Tomotsune, PhD, and Kazunori Shimada, MD

Although congenital heart disease is one of the most common malformations observed in humans,[1] the molecular mechanisms underlying the disease still remain unsolved. The CATCH22 syndrome has recently attracted attention for gaining an insight into the genetic defects.[2] The main developmental defects of the syndrome involve cardiac anomalies, abnormal facies, thymic hypoplasia, cleft palate, and hypocalcemia (hypoparathyroidism). It is related to a wide spectrum of clinical manifestations, including DiGeorge,[3] conotruncal anomaly face,[4] and velocardiofacial syndromes.[5] These disorders are a major source of birth defects with an incidence greater than 1 in 5,000,[6] and are believed to result from systemic neural crest defects, because all the affected organs are derivatives of the third and fourth pharyngeal arches.[7,8] Although recently microdeletions in chromosomes 22q11.2[2] and 10p13–14[9] have been found in patients with the syndrome, the causative genes have remained unidentified and the underlying genetic defects are presumed to be heterogeneous.

We generated a mouse model for the CATCH22 syndrome by disrupting the *rae28* gene and demonstrated that a defect in a single genetic locus can cause all the developmental defects observed in the CATCH22 syndrome.[10] The *rae28* gene, also designated as a *mph1* gene,[11] is a mouse homologue of the *Drosophila polyhomeotic* (*ph*) gene,[12,13] which is a member of the *Polycomb* group of (*Pc*-G) genes.[14–16]

The *rae28*[−/−] homozygous mice displayed skeletal posterior transformations and multiple developmental defects in the facies (Fig. 1a), eyes (Fig. 1a,b), hard palate (Fig. 1b), parathyroid glands (Fig. 1c), thymus (Fig. 1d), and heart (Fig. 1e–h).[9] In the frontal histological section of the *rae28*[−/−] homozygote (Fig. 1b), the right optic cup was completely absent but a hypoplastic optic cup was present on the left. The majority of *rae28*[−/−] homozygous newborns featured a bilateral cleft of the secondary palate (Fig. 1b). All homozygotes showed hypoplasia of the parathyroid glands and thymus, and the positions of the parathyroid glands were markedly altered (Fig. 1c, d). Serial histological sections of the hearts revealed anomalies in all *rae28*[−/−] homozygotes (Fig. 1e–h). Pulmonary stenosis (PS), including infundibular stenosis and pulmonary valve stenosis, a ventricular septal defect (VSD), and aortic stenosis (AS) were present in the majority of the homozygotes. The representative homozygotes showed tetralogy

From Clark EB, Nakazawa M, Takao A (eds.): Etiology and Morphogenesis of Congenital Heart Disease: Twenty Years of Progress in Genetics and Developmental Biology. Armonk, NY: Futura Publishing Co., Inc.; © 2000.

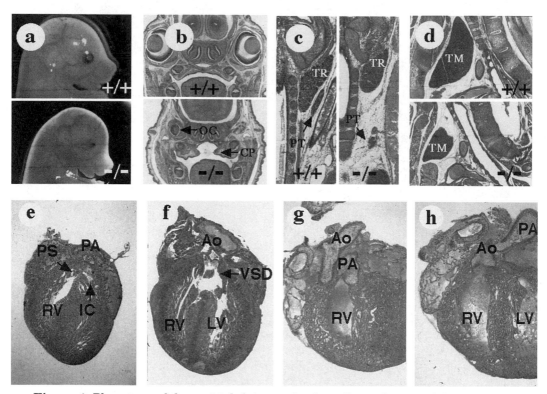

Figure 1. Phenotype of the *rae28*-deficient animals. **a.** Lateral views of the 15.5 d.p.c. embryos. The eyes were smaller in the homozygous embryos than those in the wild-type embryos. **b.** Frontal histological sections through heads of the 17.5 d.p.c. embryos. The right optic cup is completely absent and the left is hypoplastic, as indicated by OC with an arrow, in the homozygous embryo. Cleft palate is indicated by CP with an arrow. **c, d.** Frontal and parasagittal histological sections through cervical and thoracic regions of the 17.5 d.p.c. embryos. TR, thyroid; PT, parathyroid gland; TM, thymus. +/+, wild-type mice; –/–, homozygotes. **e–h.** Cardiac anomalies in homozygous newborns. Serial histological sections of the hearts were observed and representative cardiac findings in homozygous newborns are shown. **e, f.** Histological sections through the right and left outflow tracts are shown in the homozygous newborns with TOF. Stenosis in the right ventricular infundibulum is indicated by PS with an arrow. Note hypoplasia of the pulmonary trunk and dilatation of the right ventricle (RV). A large ventricular septal defect is indicated by VSD with an arrow. The findings shown in **e** and **f** are compatible with TOF. **g, h.** Histological sections through the outflow tracts in a homozygous newborn with DORV. Note that both the aorta and the pulmonary artery originate from the right ventricle. PA, pulmonary artery; Ao, aorta; RV, right ventricle; LV, left ventricle; IC, infundibular chamber; PS, pulmonary stenosis; VSD, ventricular septal defect. See color appendix.

of Fallot (TOF).[1] In the histological section through the right outflow tracts of the homozygous newborn, stenosis in the right ventricular infundibulum and hypoplasia of the pulmonary trunk were evident (Fig. 1e). The infundibular chamber appeared between the infundibular stenotic region and pulmonary valve. Enlargement of the right ventricle was confirmed in serial histological sections (data not shown). In addition, the aorta straddled a large ventricular septal defect and originated from both ventricles, as shown in the histological section through the left outflow tract (Fig. 1f). All these findings were compatible with TOF. Furthermore, we found homozygous embryos with a double-outlet right ventricle (DORV).[1] In histological sections through the outflow tracts in the newborn (Fig. 1g, h), both the aorta and the pulmonary artery were found to originate from the right ventricle. Subaortic stenosis in the right outflow tract and atresia in the left outflow tract were present. Both ventricles were severely dilated and the thickness of the myocardium was reduced. No cardiac anomalies were, on the other hand, observed in the wild-type and heterozygous mice (data not shown).

Because in *Drosophila* the *Pc*-G genes are known to be involved in the maintenance of homeotic gene expression,[17,18] we examined the expression pattern of *Hox* genes in the mutant embryos at various stages by means of the in situ hybridization method. The anterior expression boundaries of the *Hox* genes, including the *Hoxa-3, a-4, a-5, b-3, b-4,* and *d-4* genes, were shifted in the rostral direction in the paraxial mesoderm of the 12.5 day post-coitum (d.p.c.) *rae28*$^{-/-}$ homozygous embryos (Table 1),[9] that may be responsible for the skeletal posterior transformations in the mutants. We further examined the expression of the *Hox genes* in the head brachial regions of the 10.5 d.p.c. embryos and detected altered expression of the *Hoxb-3* and *b-4* genes in the head brachial regions of the *rae2*$^{-/-}$ homozygous embryos.[9] In the rhombomere of the 10.5 d.p.c. *rae28*$^{-/-}$ homozygous embryos, the anterior expression boundary of the *Hoxb-3* gene was shifted from the fifth to the fourth and that of *Hoxb-4* from the seventh to the sixth (Table 1). The anterior expression boundary of the *Hoxb-3* gene in the pharyngeal arches was also shifted from the third to the second (data not shown). The abnormal expression of the *Hoxb-3* gene in the pharyngeal arches correlated well with the anterior shifts of the corresponding *Hox* gene expression boundary in the rhombomeres, because the neural crest cells in the fourth rhombomere are known to migrate into the second pharyngeal arch.[8] Because these neural crest cells are known to be involved in the formation of

Table 1

Hox Genes Affected in the *rae28*-Deficient Embryos

Hox genes	Rhombomers	Paraxial mesoderm
Hox a-2	0/2	nd
Hox a-3	0/4	2/3
Hox a-4	0/1	2/2
Hox a-5	0/2	3/3
Hox a-9		0/2
Hoxa-10		0/3
Hoxa-11		0/2
Hox b-1	0/5	nd
Hox b-3	5/5	5/5
Hox b-4	4/4	2/2
Hox b-5		0/4
Hox b-6		0/3
Hox c-6		0/5
Hox c-8		0/3
Hox d-3	0/3	0/2
Hox d-4	0/2	3/3
Hox d-9		0/2

Summary of altered expression of *Hox* genes in *rae28*-deficient embryos. The index is as follows; the number of embryos with ectopic *Hox* expression in the rhombomeres and paraxial mesoderm/the number of embryos examined by section *in situ* hybridization.

the face, palate, parathyroid, thymus, and cardiac outflow tracts, ectopic expression of these *Hoxb-3* and *b-4* genes were presumed to cause the systemic neural crest defects observed in the *rae28*-deficient mice. Furthermore, we recently found that expression of the genes involved in cardiogenesis and looping was also impaired in homozygous embryos (Shirai, M., Takihara, Y., and Shimada, K., in preparation). Thus, the *rae28* gene may play a crucial role not only in neural crest development but also in cardiac morphogenesis.

In *Drosophila*, the *Pc*-G genes are required for the spatially restricted expression of homeotic genes along the anteroposterior (A-P) axis and for segment specification.[17,18] The Pc-G proteins form multimeric protein complexes and maintain long-range repression of homeotic genes, presumably through alterations in the higher-order chromatin structure.[17,18] The *rae28* gene encodes a protein sharing several characteristic motifs and highly homologous regions with the *Drosophila ph* protein; a single zinc finger, a glutamine-rich region and two highly homologous regions, the H-1 region consisting of 28 amino acid residues and the H-2/SPM/SET domain consisting of 66 amino acid residues.[11,12,19] The H-2/SPM/SET domain is conserved among *Drosophila* ph, Sex comb on midleg, lethal(3)-malignant brain tumour and RAE28 proteins.[19] We and others showed that the RAE28 protein forms homodimers and heterodimers with the Bmi1 and Mel18 proteins and constitutes a multimeric Polycomb protein complex with the addition of the M33 protein through these conserved domain regions.[11,20,21] Because mice deficient in the *bmi1*, *mel18* and *M33* genes show neither the systemic neural crest defects nor the cardiac anomalies,[22–24] *Pc*-G multimeric complexes may include heterogenous members with functional specificity.[20] Further study of the *Pc*-G genes therefore appears to be crucial for clarification of the genetic network regulating cardiac morphogenesis.

Methods

Generation of *rae28*-deficient Mice

The mouse *rae28* genomic DNA was cloned from a 129/Sv mouse liver genomic library. A 12 kb *Sal*I-*Kpn*I fragment containing the *rae28* gene was subcloned into pBluescript (Stratagene, La Jolla, Calif). The promoterless neomycin-resistance (*neo*^{r}) gene was inserted in-frame in the *Sal*I site of exon 4, and a 5.3-kb *Sal*I-*Eco*RI fragment was deleted. The D3 ES cells were electroporated with the construct linearized with *Sal*I and *Kpn*I, plated and selected with G418 (300 μg/ml). After 11 to 14 days, G418-resistant (G418^r) colonies were screened for homologous recombination. Chimeric mice, generated by the injection of positive ES clones into C57BL/6 blastocysts, were mated to C57BL/6 females to generate outbred offspring. Heterozygous mice were backcrossed to C57BL/6 for consecutive generations. The genotypes were determined by Southern blotting and polymerase chain reaction.[10]

Phenotypic Analysis

Embryos and newborns were generated from heterozygous intercrosses, and anatomical and histological examinations were performed. The embryos were fixed in 9% formaldehyde, 5% acetic acid, and 0.9% picric acid (Bouin's solution) for at least 24 hours, dehydrated in a graded series of ethanol and embedded in paraffin. Histological sections (2–10 μm) were obtained on a standard paraffin microtome and stained with hematoxylin and eosin.[10]

In Situ Hybridization

Wild-type and mutant embryos were obtained and genotyped as described above. Embryos were fixed in phosphate-buffered saline (PBS) containing 4% paraformaldehyde (PFA) and embedded in paraffin. Histological sections (5 μm) were mounted on slides coated with 3-aminopropyltriethoxysilane (Sigma), treated with xylene for 3 min three times, and hydrated in a series of ethanol (100%, 90%, 70%, 50% ethanol and PBS containing 0.1% Tween-20 [PBT]). After treatment with 10 μg/ml proteinase K (Sigma Chemicals, St. Louis, Mo) for 10 min, sections were fixed again for 10 min in PBS containing 4% PFA, treated with 0.2 N HCl, and acetylated in 0.02 N HCl, 1.2% triethanolamine (Wako Pure Chemicals, Osaka, Japan), and 0.02% acetic anhydrate. Then, embryos were soaked in prewarmed prehybridization buffer (50% formamide, 5 × SSC, 50 μg/ml yeast total RNA, 1% SDS, 50 μg/ml heparin) for 1 hour at 70°C, and hybridized overnight with a digoxigenin-labeled riboprobe. A riboprobe was synthesized with digoxygenin-UTP and T3 or T7 polymerase (Boehringer Mannheim, Mannheim, Germany), using *Hox* genes as templates. After washing in Solutions I (50% formamide, 5 × SSC, 1% SDS), II (50% formamide, 2 × SSC), and III (50% formamide, 0.2 × SSC) at 70°C, and blocking, sections were incubated overnight at 4°C in the preabsorbed antibody solution. Alkaline phophatase-conjugated antidigoxigenin Fab (Boehringer Mannheim) was preabsorbed for 1 hour at 4°C with heat-inactivated mouse embryonic powder (0.6%) and sheep serum (1%). Following further washing in NTMT (100 mM NaCl, 100 mM Tris-HCl [pH 9.5], 50 mM $MgCl_2$, 0.1% Tween, 2 mM levamisol) for 10 min three times, alkaline phophatase reaction was performed in PVA/NTM solution (12.5% polyvinylalchol [Aldrich Chemicals, Milwaukee, Wisc], 100 mM NaCl, 100 mM Tris-HCl [pH 9.5], 50 mN $MgCl_2$, 2 mM levamisole) containing 300 μg/ml NBT (4-Nitro blue tetrazolium chloride [Boehringer Mannheim]) and 150 μg/ml BCIP (5-Bromo-4-chloro-3-indolylphosphate [Boehringer Mannheim]). After stopping the reaction, hybridization was observed under microscopy.[10]

Acknowledgments: We thank Drs. T. Higashi-nakagawa, Y. Katoh-Fukui, K. Nishii, Y. Shibata, K. Y.-Takihara, T. Takeuchi, and H. W. Brock for generous assistance and advice, M. Miyazaki and T. Sakaura for technical support, and Drs. D. Duboule, P. Gruss, R. Krumlauf, and O. Chisaka for providing Hox probes.

References

1. Schlant RC, Alexander RW, eds. *Hurst's the Heart: Arteries and Veins*. 8th ed, New York: McGraw-Hill; 1994.
2. Wilson DI, Burn J, Scambler P, et al. DiGeorge syndrome: Part of CATCH 22. *J Med Genet* 1993;30:852–856.
3. McKusick VA, ed. *Mendelian Inheritance in Man*. Baltimore: Johns Hopkins Univ Press; 1992:1078–1080.
4. Takao A, Ando M, Cho K, et al. Etiologic categorization of common congenital heart disease. In: Van Praagh R, Takao A, eds. *Etiology and Morphogenesis of Congenital Heart Disease*. New York: Futura; 1978: 253–269.
5. Shprintzen RJ, Goldberg RB, Lewin ML, et al. A new syndrome involving cleft palate, cardiac anomalies, typical faces, and learning disabilities: Velo-cardio-facial syndrome. *Cleft Palate J* 1978;15:56–62.
6. Glover TW. CATCHing a break on 22. *Nature Genet* 1995;10:257–258.
7. Bockman DE, Kirby ML. Dependence of thymus development on derivatives of the neural crest. *Science* 1984;233:498–500.
8. Gilbert SF, ed. Early vertebrate development: Neurulation and the ectoderm. In *Developmental Biology*. 4th ed. Sunderland, MA: Sinauer Associates Inc.; 1994: 244–294.
9. Daw SCM, Taylor C, Kraman M, et al. A common region of 10p deleted in DiGeorge and velocardiofacial syndromes. *Nature Genet* 1996;13:458–460.
10. Takihara Y, Tomotsune D, Shirai M, et al. Targeted disruption of the mouse homologue of the *Drosophila polyhomeotic* gene leads to altered anteroposterior patterning and neural crest defects. *Development* 1997;124:3673–3682.
11. Alkema MJ, Bronk M, Verhoeven E, et al. Identification of Bmi1-interacting proteins as constituents of a multimeric mammalian Polycomb complex. *Genes Dev.* 1997; 11:226–240.
12. Nomura M, Takihara Y, Shimada K. Isolation and characterization of retinoic acid-inducible cDNA clones in F9 cells: One of the early inducible clones encodes a novel protein sharing several highly homologous regions with a *Drosophila Polyhomeotic* protein. *Differentiation* 1994;57:39–50.
13. Motaleb MdA, Takihara Y, Nomura M, et al. Structural organization of the *rae28* gene, a putative murine homologue of the *Drosophila polyhomeotic* gene. *J Biochem Tokyo* 1996;120:797–802.
14. Dura J-M, Brock HW, Santamaria P. *Polyhomeotic*: A gene of *Drosophila melanogaster* required for correct expression of segmental identity. *Mol Gen Genet* 1985; 198:213–220.
15. Dura J-M, Randsholt NB, Deatrick J, et al. A complex genetic locus, *polyhomeotic*, is required for segmental specification and epidermal development in D. melanogaster. *Cell* 1987;51:829–839.
16. Deatrick J, Daly M, Randsholt NB, et al. The complex genetic locus *polyhomeotic* in *Drosophila melanogaster* potentially encodes two homologous zinc-finger proteins. *Gene* 1991;105:185–195.
17. Paro R. Propagating memory of transcriptional states. *Trends Genet* 1995;11:295–297.
18. Simon J. Locking in stable states of gene expression: transcriptional control during *Drosophila* development. *Curr Opin Cell Biol* 1995;7:376–385.
19. Bornemann D, Miller E, Simon J. The *Drosophila Polycomb* group gene *Sex comb on midleg* (*Scm*) encodes a zinc finger protein with similarity to polyhomeotic protein. *Development* 1996;122:1621–1630.

20. Hashimoto N, Brock HW, Nomura M, et al. RAE28, BMI1, and M33 are members of heterogeneous multimeric mammalian Polycomb group of complexes. *Biochem Biophys Res Commun* 1998;245:356–365.

21. Kyba M, Brock HW. The *Drosophila* Polycomb group protein Psc contacts ph and Pc through specific conserved domains. *Mol Cell Biol* 1998;18:2712–2720.

22. van der Lugt NMT, Domen J, Linders K, et al. Posterior transformation, neurological abnormalities, and severe hematopoietic defects in mice with a targeted deletion of the *bmi-1* proto-oncogene. *Genes Dev* 1994:8:757–769.

23. Akasaka T, Kanno M, Balling R, et al. A role for *mel-18*, a polycomb group-related vertebrate gene, during the anteroposterior specification of the axial skeleton. *Development* 1996;122:1513–1522.

24. Katoh-Fukui Y, Tsuchiya R, Shiroishi T, et al. Male-to-female sex reversal in *M33* mutant mice. *Nature* 1998;393:688–692.

19

Control of Mouse Cardiac Morphogenesis and Myogenesis by *jumonji*

Takashi Takeuchi, MD

The *jumonji* (*jmj*) gene and *jmj* mutant mice were obtained by a mouse gene trap strategy.[1] The *jmj* gene encodes a nuclear protein that is partially homologous to the AT-rich interaction domain (ARID) identified in the DNA binding protein dead ringer in *Drosophila,* in transcription factor Bright in mouse, and in SWI1 in yeast,[2–5] implying the possibility that the Jmj protein is a transcription factor. Homozygous *jmj* mice fail to express normal *jmj* mRNA.[1] The phenotypes of *jmj* mutant mice are dependent on the genetic background.[6] All homozygous *jmj* embryos with a C3H/He background show neural tube defects and die around E11.5. Moreover, these embryos have cardiac defects. *jmj* mutant embryos with a BALB/cA, C57BL/6J, or DBA/2J background, however, display neither neural tube defects nor apparent heart abnormalities, and mutant embryos die around E15.5 with impairment in definitive hematopoiesis.[6,7] Thus, *jmj* mutant phenotypes, can be classified into two distinct types, a C3H/He type and a BALB/c type.

Here, we performed analyses on cardiac defects in a C3H/He type in order to further our understanding of the role of *jmj* gene in the normal development of the heart.

First, we examined the expression pattern of the *jmj* gene during the heart development. Because the expression pattern of the *jmj* gene can be monitored by a reporter gene, *lacZ* introduced into *jmj* gene, we stained embryos with X-gal.[5,6] Expression of the *jmj* gene was detected weakly in the whole heart at the 6-somite stage, restricted to the bulbus cordis at the 8-somite stage when elongation of the bulbus cordis is evident, and stronger in the whole bulbus cordis at the 11-somite stage when looping is apparent. When the right ventricle becomes formed in the bulbus cordis, the expression disappears in the region of the right ventricle but still remains in the outflow tract. Histological analysis revealed that *jmj* expression in the bulbus cordis and the outflow tract is observed in the cardiac myocytes in the wall, and that *jmj* is also expressed in the myocytes of the trabeculae, but not of the compact layer, in the ventricles.

Abnormal phenotypes were observed in these two regions (bulbus cordis and trabeculae) of *jmj* homozygous embryos. The proximal region of the bulbus cordis appeared swollen after 11-somite stage and connected to the ventricle at an abnormal position, more rostral than in control embryos (Fig. 1). Histological sections showed that trabeculation was observed in swollen morphology of the bulbus cordis, as well as the left ventricle, of mutant embryos after E9.5. In situ hybridization was used to analyze the expression of *myosin light-chain 2V* (MLC2V), a ventricu-

From Clark EB, Nakazawa M, Takao A (eds.): Etiology and Morphogenesis of Congenital Heart Disease: Twenty Years of Progress in Genetics and Developmental Biology. Armonk, NY: Futura Publishing Co., Inc.; © 2000.

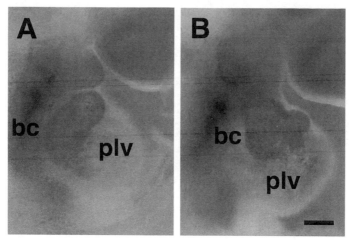

Figure 1. Abnormal morphology of the bulbus cordis of the *jmj* mutant embryo. Lateral views of hearts of heterozygous (**A**) and homozygous embryos (**B**) at E9.5. Embryos were stained with X-gal. Note that *jmj* is expressed in the bulbus cordis (bc) (**A**) and the proximal region of the bulbus cordis of mutant embryos appeared swollen (**B**). plv, primitive left ventricle. Bar, μm.

lar specific marker[8] and the expression was detected in the swollen morphology. Together with that the right ventricle develops from the proximal region of the bulbus cordis, these results suggest that impairment of morphogenesis of the right ventricle results in formation of the abnormal structure in mutant embryos.

We also found abnormal phenotypes in the trabecular myocytes (Fig. 2). Normal embryos at E10.5 evidenced developing trabeculae with many erythroid cells visible in the interspace between the endocardial layers of the left ventricle. On the other hand, the left ventricles of the mutant embryos at E10.5 were occupied by cells, mainly cardiac myocytes in the trabeculae with many bubblelike structures apparent. There were almost no spaces between the endocardial layers and very few erythroid cells could be detected. At E11.5, the same or more severe morphology was found in the left ventricles and the swollen morphologies of the mutants. We investigated cell density and the proliferation of cardiac myocytes in the trabeculae and endocardial cells by counting these cells as well as mitotic cells per field in the left ventricles. The densities of total and mitotic endocardial cells showed no significant differences be-

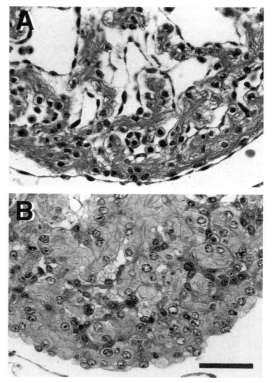

Figure 2. Abnormal morphology of the trabeculae of the *jmj* mutant embryo. Transverse sections of left ventricles of wild type (**A**) and homozygous (**B**) embryos at E11.5. Note that the ventricles of mutant embryos are occupied by trabecular myocytes. Bar, μm. See color appendix.

tween normal and mutant embryos at either E10.5 or E11.5. On the other hand, total and mitotic trabecular cardiac myocyte densities and mitotic index in the mutant embryos showed a significant increase compared with control embryos. Next, the average cell size was calculated by measuring the area occupied by cells. The average cell area of the trabecular myocytes and endocardial cells revealed no significant differences compared with controls at E10.5 and E11.5. These data suggest that hyperplasia but not hypertrophy occurs in the trabecular myocytes of mutant embryos. We examined the fine cellular ultrastructure by transmission electron microscopy. The myocytes in the trabeculae of control embryos adhere tightly to one another and often show long myofilaments. On the other hand, many spaces are apparent between the trabecular myocytes of mutant embryos while cells in which myofilaments are observed are very few. Moreover, the myofilaments appeared to be short and show a disordered orientation. Many myocytes in the mutant embryos showed abnormal vacuoles in their cytoplasm, suggesting the bubblelike structure. In situ hybridization was used to analyze myogenesis in these abnormal cells. Using probes for a-cardiac actin, myosin heavy-chain a (MHCa), myosin light-chain 2A (MLC2A), and MLC2V, comparable levels and patterns of expression were found across the myocardium of the compact layer in both mutant and normal embryos at E10.5. However, the expression of all genes examined in the trabecular cardiac myocytes was either very weak or not detectable in many cells, although some cells showed strong signals. These results show that trabecular myocytes of *jmj* mutants proliferate abnormally and lose myogenic markers.

Our present study shows that *jmj* gene has essential roles in morphogenesis of the right ventricle, and growth and differentiation of ventricular myocytes on a C3H/He background. It will be interesting to identify the genes that modify the cardiac defects in *jmj* mutant mice because these modifying genes are involved in the function of the *jmj* gene and in cardiac development.

Acknowledgements: We thank Mizuyo Nakajima, Kuniko Nakajima, and Shuzo Kondo for technical assistance. This work was partially supported by a Grant-in-Aid for Creative Basic Research from the Ministry of Education, Science, Sports, and Culture of Japan.

References

1. Takeuchi T, Yamazaki Y, Katoh-Fukui Y, et al. Gene trap capture of a novel mouse gene, *jumonji,* required for neural tube formation. *Genes Dev* 1995;9:1211–1222.
2. Gregory SL, Kortschak RD, Kalionis B, et al. Characterization of the *dead ringer* gene identifies a novel, highly conserved family of sequence-specific DNA-binding proteins. *Mol Cell Biol* 1996;16:792–799.
3. Herrscher RF, Kaplan MH, Lelsz DL, et al. The immunoglobulin heavy-chain matrix-associating regions are bound by Bright: a B cell-specific *trans-activator* that describes a new DNA-binding protein family. *Genes Dev* 1995;9:3067–3082.
4. Peterson CL, Herskowitz I. Characterization of the yeast *SWI1, SWI2,* and *SWI3* genes, which encode a global activator of transcription. *Cell* 1992;68:573–583.
5. Takeuchi T. A gene trap approach to identify genes that control development. *Dev Growth Differ* 1997;39:127–134.
6. Motoyama J, Kitajima K, Kojima M, et al. Organogenesis of the liver, thymus and spleen is affected in jumonji mutant mice. *Mech Dev* 1997;66:27–37.
7. Kitajima K, Kojima M, Nakajima K, et al. Definitive but not primitive hematopoiesis is impaired in *jumonji* mutant mice. *Blood* 1999;93(1):87–95.
8. O'Brien T, Lee KJ, Chien KR. Positional specification of ventricular myosin light chain 2 expression in the primitive murine heart tube. *Proc Natl Acad Sci USA* 1993; 90:5157–5161.

20

Myocardialization: A Novel Mechanism of Cardiac Septation

A.F.M. Moorman, PhD, M.J.B. van den Hoff, MD,
F. de Jong, MD, D. Franco, MD, W.H. Lamers, MD,
A. Wessels, PhD, and R.R. Markwald, PhD

Cardiac septation remains to be a reluctant topic, particularly in relation to the understanding of the structure of hearts with deficient atrioventricular septation.[1] If we are to understand the process of cardiac septation, it is indispensable to have at our disposal molecular markers that can serve as anatomic hallmarks during development.[2] Key to the understanding of this process is the proper appreciation of the position of the primary foramen in between the embryonic left and right ventricle (Fig. 1). Owing to the expression of the GlN2-epitope in the myocardium encircling this foramen in the human heart[3,4] this area will form both the lower rim of the right atrium just above the right atrioventricular orifice, and the left ventricular, subaortic outflow myocardium. Equally important is the appreciation that atrial and ventricular chambers develop by a process of bulging from the "primary myocardial tube," rather than being segments of this tube[4–6] (Fig. 1). Given these two prerequisites cardiac septation can be simply considered as a logical assembly of two types of components, (1) the original muscular septa of the chambers, the inter-

atrial and interventricular septa, and (2) the initially mesenchymal endocardial swellings of the primary heart tube. Here we report that with development these mesenchymal structures become septa and become largely invaded by cardiomyocytes. We have dubbed this process of myocyte invasion myocardialization.

The original muscular septa of the chambers develop in different ways.[4] The primary atrial septum forms by local myocardial proliferation. In mammals the secondary atrial septum forms by folding of the atrial myocardium.[1] The primary ventricular septum develops by apposition of new cells in between the pouches of the developing left and right ventricles and constitutes the first compact ventricular myocardium to be formed[6,7]. These muscular septa are connected with the endocardial cushions that are modeled so that fusion of these cushions directly results in a physical separation of left and right blood flows. This fusion does not change the flow pattern essentially, as flow in the embryonic circulation is laminar.[8,9]

As a consequence of the fusion of the cushions upstream and downstream of the primary foramen at the ventricular crest, demarcated by expression of the GlN2 epitope, membranous septal components are to be expected in between right ventricle and left ventricular outflow, in between left ventricle and right atrium,

From Clark EB, Nakazawa M, Takao A (eds.): Etiology and Morphogenesis of Congenital Heart Disease: Twenty Years of Progress in Genetics and Developmental Biology. Armonk, NY: Futura Publishing Co., Inc.; © 2000.

and in between both atria at the lower rim of the primary and secondary atrial septum (Fig. 1).

In chicken this is not the case.[10] Figure 1 illustrates the in vivo process of myocardialization in sections of chicken embryonic hearts, both at the ventricular and at the atrial level. Also in mammals these septal components are largely muscular. They comprise the muscular outflow septum, the muscular atrioventricular septum and the lower part of the muscular interatrial septum. Only a small interventricular and atrioventricu-

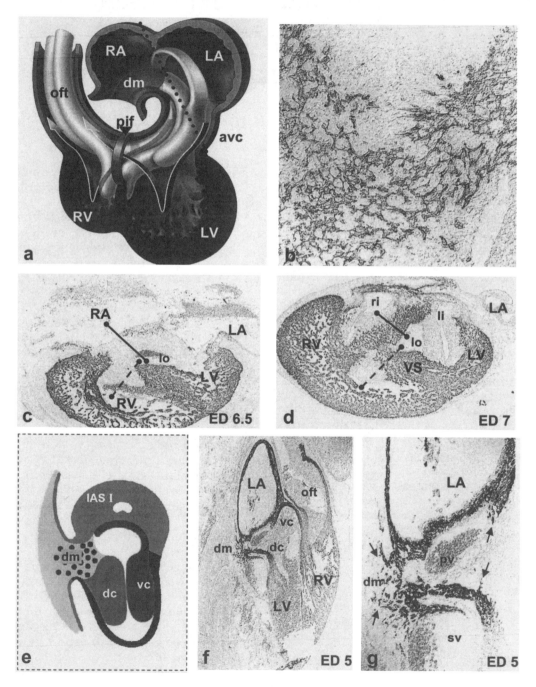

lar septal component, and the central fibrous body remain membranous.[1] The mechanism underlying the myocardialization of the endocardial swellings is fundamental to our understanding of normal and deficient cardiac septation.

As a first approach to unravel this mechanism we have set up an in vitro myocardialization assay. This assay allows the assessment of the distinct myocardialization potencies of the disparate segments of the embryonic heart. Explants from chicken cardiac segments were cultured for 1 week on collagen gels, essentially as described.[11] Myocardial cells were visualized by immunofluorescence staining for myosin heavy chain expression, and analyzed by confocal microscopy. Cardiac explants were prepared at stage H/H 26. When taken from the venous pole of the heart, from the inner curvature or from the outflow tract, these explants displayed extensive myocardialization (Fig. 2a, b, c, d). Explants from the venous pole of the heart displayed highest, and from the arterial pole lower myocardialization. Explants from the ventricular component did not reveal any myocardialization provided apical ventricular tissue was taken only (Fig. 2e). Explants taken from the ballooning embryonic atria, showed a considerably lower extent of myocardialization, than

explants taken from the "primary heart tube" (Fig. 2 f). Limited myocardialization was observed at the periphery of the explant at localized spots, where strands of cardiomyocytes migrated over and into the collagen gel. Myocardialization never appeared all around the explant. Because it is difficult to dissect embryonic atrial myocardium without concomitant contamination of "primary heart tube" at the place of the dorsal mesocardium, we tend to interpret the atrial in vitro myocardialization as the consequence of contamination with dorsal primary myocardium. Explants from stages younger than H/H 20 did not reveal significant myocardialization upon 1 week of culture. However, when cultured in conditioned medium, even H/H 16 explants taken from the arterial pole, could be induced to myocardialize. This conditioned medium consisted of the culture medium from one week cultures of explants taken from "primary heart tube" explants of H/H stage 26 (e.g., arterial or venous poles that demonstrate extensive myocardialization upon culture). Ventricular explants could not be induced by conditioned medium. Interestingly, conditioned medium from nonmyocardial distal outflow tracts permitted the myocardialization of H/H 16 outflow tract explants.

Figure 1. In vivo myocardialization in chicken cardiac development. The cartoons are based on De Jong and coworkers (1997).[4] **a.** Cartoon of the looping embryonic heart, showing the ballooning right and left atria (RA, LA), and left and right ventricles (LV, RV) from the "primary heart tube" (avc: atrioventricular canal; oft: outflow tract; pif: primary interventricular foramen). In the primary heart tube the endocardial swellings (atrioventricular cushions and truncus ridges) are indicated. The dotted line indicates the plane of sectioning of the cartoon shown in panel e. **b.** Detail of the boxed area in panel d showing extensive myocardializtion. **c, d.** Immunohistochemically (ventricular myosin) stained sections at the level of the primary interventricular foramen showing the formation of the muscular interventricular (dashed line) and atrioventricular septa (solid line) by myocardialization from embryonic day 6.5 (**e**) to embryonic day 7 (**f**). li, left inlet; lo, left outlet; ri, right inlet; vs, ventricular septum. **e.** Cartoon of a cross-section through the embryonic heart, showing the relationship between the primary interatrial septum (IAS I), the dorsal mesocardium (dm) and the dorsal and ventral atrioventricular cushions (dc, vc). The black dots indicate the myocardialization of the mesenchyme of the dorsal mesocardium. The sections shown in f and g are left lateral from this cartoon section. **f, g.** (detail **f**) Immunohistochemically (atrial myosin) stained section at the level of the dorsal mesocardium of a chicken heart of 5 days' incubation, showing the extensive myocardialization in this area. pv, pulmonary vein; sv, sinus venosus.

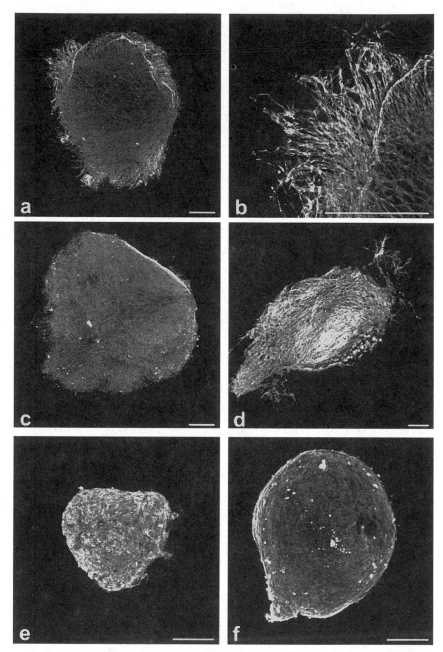

Figure 2. In vitro myocardialization of chicken cardiac explants of H/H stage 26. Explants were cultured for 1 week at 37°C on 3-mm thick rat tail collagen I gels in M199 culture medium (Life Technologies) supplemented with 1% chicken serum and ITS (insulin, transferrin, and selenium; Collaborative Research Inc.). Explants were fixed in ethanol and incubated with MF20 a monoclonal antibody against myosin (Hybridoma-bank) and antibody binding was visualized using a FITC-labeled rabbit anti-mouse serum (Nordic). Myocardialization was assessed in explants from (**a**) venous pole; (**b**) detail a; (**c**) inner curvature myocardium; (**d**) outflow tract; (**e**) atrium (auricles); (**f**) ventricle. Bar represents 0.5 mm.

Taken together, our results may indicate that the "primary heart tube" secretes a myocardialization inducer from H/H stage 20 onward. The inducer may be produced by the non-myocardial component of the primary heart tube. In vivo the first signs of myocardialization are evident at H/H stage 21 at the venous pole and at stage 29 at the arterial pole downstream from the primary interventricular foramen. The primary myocardium is already competent from H/H stage 16 onward, which was the youngest stage analysed. Ventricular working myocardium is not competent and does not produce inducer. The nature of this inducer is currently being analyzed.

Acknowledgments: M.J.B. van de Hoff was supported by the Netherlands Heart Foundation (NHS grant no: 96.002); D. Franco by NHS grant no. 97.206, and by NWO (Medigon), grant no:902-16-219; A. Wessels by grant no NIH-HL 33756 and 52813 and by an NWO NATO-TALENT stipend; and R.R. Markwald by grant no NIH-HL 33756.

References

1. Anderson RH, Ho SY. In: Clark EB, Takao A, eds. *Developmental Cardiology. Morphogenesis and Function*. Mount Kisco, NY: Futura Publishing; 1990:575–592.
2. Lamers WH, Wessels A, Verbeek FJ, et al. New findings concerning ventricular septation in the human heart. Implications for maldevelopment. *Circulation* 1992;86:1194–1205.
3. Wessels A, Vermeulen JLM, Verbeek FJ, et al. *Anat Rec* 1992;232:97–111.
4. de Jong F, Virágh S, Moorman AFM. *Cardiology Young* 1997;7:131–146.
5. de Vries PA, de CM Saunders JB. *Contrib Embryol* 1962;37:87–114.
6. O'Rahilly R, Müller F. Developmental stages in human embryos *Carnegie Inst. Washington;* 1987.
7. Franco D, Jing Y, Wagenaar GTM, et al. In: Ost'ádal B, Nagano M, Takeda N, et al., eds. *The Developing Heart*. New York: Lippincott Raven; 1997:51–60.
8. Meier GEA. *Embryol Hefte* 1987;1:1–19.
9. Yoshida H, Manasek F, Arcilla RA. Intracardiac flow patterns in early embryonic life. A reexamination. *Circ Res* 1983;53:363–371.
10. de Jong F, Lamers WH, Moorman AFM. *Proceedings of the 3rd Bilthoven Symposium* 15; 1992.
11. Runyan RB, Potts JD, Weeks DL. TGF-beta 3-mediated tissue interaction during embryonic heart development. *Mol Reprod Dev.* 1992;32:152–159.

21

Developmentally Regulated Neonatal Skeletal Myosin Heavy Chain Is Expressed in Myocardium and Cardiac Conduction Tissue in the Developing Chick Heart

Shuichi Machida, MD, Setsuko Noda, PhD,
Eriko Hiratsuka, BSc, Shinji Oana, MD, PhD,
Yoshiyuki Furutani, BSc, Atsuyoshi Takao, MD,
Kazuo Momma, MD, and Rumiko Matsuoka, MD

The formation of distinct atrial and ventricular chambers is a critical step during normal heart development. Lineage-specific markers, such as myosin, are essential for examining the mechanisms of cardiac development. The myosin heavy chains (MHCs) are encoded by a multigene family, and express several isoforms in mammalian cardiac and skeletal muscles. The expression of the MHC isoforms is regulated in both a tissue-specific and a developmental stage-specific manner. In chick heart, atrial[1, 2] and ventricular[3,4] MHC genes have been isolated and characterized. The atrial and ventricular MHC genes continue to be predominantly expressed in each tissue from the early embryonic to the adult stage.[3,4,5] However, immunohistochemical studies have demonstrated that several unrecognized MHC isoforms are expressed in developing chick heart.[6,7,8] These studies have suggested that the presence of distinct cardiac MHC genes are developmentally regulated during development of the chick heart. In addition, in chick heart, conduction cells express unique myosin proteins, distinct from the atrial or ventricular types found in ordinary adult cardiac myocytes.[9,10] These studies have indicated that some skeletal-type MHC isoforms exist in the developing chick conduction tissue. The question then arises as to whether or not the developmentally regulated or skeletal-type MHC genes are expressed in chick heart. However, to our knowledge, the developmentally regulated or skeletal-type MHC genes have not yet been isolated from the chick heart cDNA library. We recently isolated a MHC cDNA, CV11E1, from a cDNA library of embryonic chick heart. According to the amino acid sequence[11] and developmental expression pattern of CV11E1 mRNA in skeletal (pectoralis) muscle (Fig. 1), we confirmed that the CV11E1 cDNA encodes the chick neonatal skeletal MHC mRNA. We also determined the full sequence of the chick neonatal skeletal

From Clark EB, Nakazawa M, Takao A (eds.): Etiology and Morphogenesis of Congenital Heart Disease: Twenty Years of Progress in Genetics and Developmental Biology. Armonk, NY: Futura Publishing Co., Inc.; © 2000.

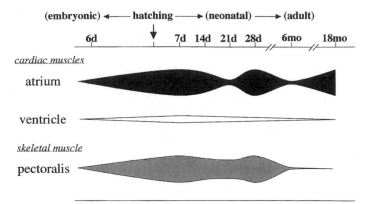

Figure 1. Developmental expression of neonatal skeletal myosin heavy chain gene in cardiac and skeletal muscles. Results of S1-nuclease mapping analyses using CV11E1 probe are displayed in a semiquantitative manner.

MHC gene. To understand the role of the neonatal skeletal MHC gene in chick cardiac muscle development, we investigated the gene expression and protein localization of neonatal skeletal MHC in developing chick heart using the CV11E1 cDNA as a probe or a monoclonal antibody. Whole-mount in situ hybridization demonstrated that diffuse expression of the neonatal skeletal MHC mRNA appeared first in the heart tube at Hamburger and Hamilton[12] stage 10. During the heart tube looping, the mRNA was expressed in the whole heart tube. Then, the expression of the mRNA in the ventricle was downregulated, whereas expression in the atrium was upregulated. After the embryonic heart had achieved a four-chambered configuration, S1-nuclease mapping analysis showed that the expression of neonatal skeletal MHC mRNA in the atria appeared to increase gradually during the embryonic stage until shortly after birth. It then diminished dramatically, and there was only a trace or no expression in the adult. However, transient expression pattern of neonatal skeletal MHC gene occurred during the neonatal and adult stages (Fig. 1). In the ventricle, only a trace of the expression of neonatal skeletal MHC mRNA was detected throughout embryonic life or in the adult. It was observed only after long exposure to X-rays. However, transient expression of the mRNA in the ventricle was observed, post-hatching (Fig. 1). Evans et al.[7] have proposed the presence of developmentally regulated isoform in the developing avian heart. Therefore, we consider that the neonatal skeletal MHC gene is a developmentally regulated gene for both the ventricle and atria. At the present time, the role of the neonatal skeletal MHC gene in developing chick heart is not known. However, based on the expression pattern of this study, the neonatal skeletal MHC gene may play an important role during cardiogenesis and cardiac muscle development.

To determine the localization of neonatal skeletal MHC protein in the developing chick heart, we used a monoclonal antibody, 2E9, specific for neonatal skeletal myosin.[13,14] During the embryonic stage, the atrial myocardium was stained diffusely with 2E9, whereas the ventricles showed weak reactivity with 2E9. At the late embryonic and newly hatched stages, 2E9-positive cells were located clearly in the subendocardial layer, and around the blood vessels of the atrial and ventricular myocardium (Fig. 2). Double-immunofluorescent staining showed that the 2E9-positive cells also reacted strongly with desmin. An immunoelectron microscopic study showed that the myofibrils stained with 2E9 were close to connective tissue or between the connective tissue and ordinary myocardium, and con-

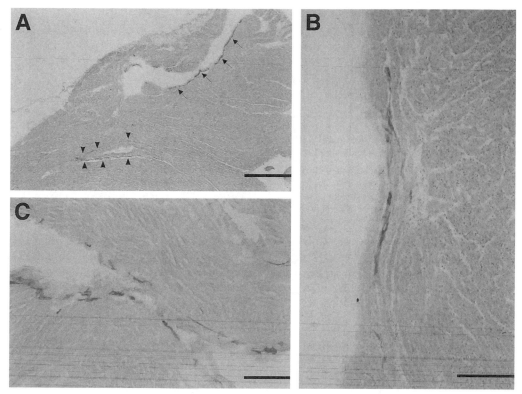

Figure 2. Immunohistochemical analyses of frozen sections of chick heart labeled with 2E9 antibody. Sections from neonatal day (ND) 0 (**A** and **B**), and ND 7 (**C**) were incubated with 2E9 antibody and antibody binding was visualized with a horseradish peroxidase-linked secondary antibody. During the neonatal period, intensely stained 2E9-positive cells were clearly located in the subendocardial layer (**A**, shown by arrows and **C**) and in the blood vessels (**A**, shown by arrowheads) of the atrial myocardium and in the subendocardial layer of the ventricular myocardium (**B**). Bars: 500 μm. See color appendix.

tained numerous mitochondria. This histological feature is known as conduction tissue.[15] These immunohistochemical studies indicated that neonatal skeletal MHC protein is located in developing conduction tissue. On the other hand, the neonatal skeletal MHC could not be detected in the adult conduction cells using the present techniques. From these data, we consider that neonatal skeletal MHC protein is a developmentally regulated MHC for conduction cells of the atria or ventricle and concluded that neonatal skeletal MHC appears during early cardiogenesis and is then localized in the cardiac conduction cells. Gonzalez-Sanchez and Bader[10] have reported that conduc-

tion tissue cells in the both the atria and ventricle expressed a slow skeletal MHC protein at adult. Sweeny et al.[16] and De Groot et al.[17] also showed that the cells within the adult atrial subendocardium reacted with anti-ventricular MHC antibody. According to the previous studies.[10,16-18] and our results, we speculate that developing chick conduction cells express multiple MHC isoforms, including neonatal skeletal and other MHC types, and then a developmental switch occurs, and the neonatal skeletal MHC isoform is downregulated.

In summary, we propose that neonatal skeletal MHC may be a common, developmentally regulated MHC in chick atria, ventricle, and conduction tissue.

Materials and Methods

Animals

White Leghorn chickens and fertilized eggs were used in this study. Embryos were staged according to Hamburger and Hamilton.[12]

Isolation of CV11E1

A CV11E1 was also isolated from a cDNA library, using rat embryonic skeletal MHC cDNA clone [CVM1 (538 bp) kindly provided by Dr. T. Masaki, National Cardiovascular Research Institute]. The λgt10 expression cDNA library from embryonic day (ED)-15 chick ventricular muscle was prepared, as previously described.[1]

S1-Nuclease Mapping Analysis

RNA-DNA hybridization was carried out in the DNA probe (CV11E1), and in an excess of up to 15 µg of the total RNA, as previously described.[1,5]

Whole-Mount in Situ Hybridization

In situ hybridization procedures were carried out, as previously described.[1,5]

Immunocytochemistry

To determine the localization of neonatal skeletal MHC protein, we used mouse anti-MHC monoclonal antibody 2E9 immunoglobulin (Ig) G (kindly provided by Dr. Bandman, University of California, Davis), which reacts specifically with the chick neonatal skeletal MHC isoform but which does not react with the embryonic or adult types MHC isoforms.[13,14] For double immunofluorescence labeling, we used both the 2E9 and desmin antibodies. A rabbit anti-chick desmin polyclonal antibody (Chemicon International Inc., Temecula, Calif) was used to identify myocytes and conduction tissue cells.[19]

Immunoelectron Microscopic Study

For the electron microscopic examination, the above-mentioned immunostained sections were osmicated in 2% OsO4 in phosphate-buffered saline for 1 hour, dehydrated in a series of graded ethanols (70% to 100%), and embedded in Quetol 812. Ultrathin sections were examined with a JEM-120EM II electron microscope without staining with uranyl acetate or lead citrate.

Acknowledgements: We thank Dr. Masaki (National Cardiovascular Center Research Institute, Japan) for providing the CVM1 cDNA clone, and Dr. Bandman (University of California, Davis, Calif) for providing the 2E9 antibody. We thank Ms. B. Levene for reading the manuscript.

References

1. Oana S, Matsuoka R, Nakajima H, et al. Molecular characterization of a novel atrial-specific myosin heavy-chain in the chick embryo. *Eur J Cell Biol* 1995;67:42–49.
2. Yutzey KE, Rhee JT, Bader D. Expression of the atrial-specific myosin heavy chain AMHC1 and the establishment of anteroposterior polarity in the developing chicken heart. *Development* 1994;120:871–883.
3. Bisaha JG, Bader D. Identification and characterization of a ventricular-specific avian myosin heavy chain, VMHC1: Expression in differentiating cardiac and skeletal muscle. *Dev Biol* 1991;148:355–364.
4. Stewart AFR, Camoretti-Mercado B, Perlman D, et al. Structural and phylogenetic analysis of the chicken ventricular myosin heavy chain rod. *J Mol Evol* 1991;33:357–366.
5. Oana S, Machida S, Hiratsuka E, et al. The complete sequence and expression

patterns of the atrial myosin heavy chain in the developing chick. *Biol Cell* 1998; 90(9):605–613.

6. Masaki T, Yoshizaki C. Differentiation of myosin in chick embryos. *J Biochem* 1974; 76:123–131.

7. Evans D, Miller JB, Stockdale FE. Developmental patterns of expression and coexpression of myosin heavy chains in atrial and ventricles of the avian heart. *Dev Biol* 1988;127:376–383.

8. Cantini M, Sartore S, Schiaffino S. Myosin types in cultured muscle cells. *J Cell Biol* 1980;85:903–909.

9. Sartore S, Pierobon-Bormioli S, Schiaffino S. Immunohistochemical evidence for myosin polymorphism in the chicken heart. *Nature* 1978;274:82–83.

10. Gonzalez-Sanchez A, Bader D. Characterization of a myosin heavy chain in the conductive system of the adult heart and developing chicken heart. *J Cell Biol* 1985; 100:270–275.

11. Moore LA, Arrizubieta MJ, Tidyman WE, et al. Analysis of the chicken fast myosin heavy chain family. Localization of isoform-specific antibody epitopes and regions of divergence. *J Mol Biol* 1992;225: 1143–1151.

12. Hamburger V, Hamilton HL. A series of normal stages in the development of the chick embryo. *J Morphol* 1951;88:49–92.

13. Bandman E. Continued expression of neonatal myosin heavy chain in adult dystrophic skeletal muscle. *Science* 1985;227: 780–782.

14. Cerny LC, Bandman E. Expression of myosin heavy chain isoforms in regenerating myotubes of innervated and denervated chicken pectoral muscle. *J Cell Biol* 1986; 103:2153–2161.

15. Manasek FJ. Electron microscopic contributions to conduction development. In *Proceedings of the Conduction Development Conference.* Bethesda, Md: National Heart and Lung Institute, NIH; 1970:3–28.

16. Sweeney LJ, Zak R, Manasek FJ. Transitions in cardiac isomyosin expression during differentiation of the embryonic chick heart. *Circ Res* 1987;61:287–295.

17. De Groot IJM, Hardy GPMA, Los JA, et al. The conducting tissue in the adult chicken atria. *Anat Embryol* 1985;172: 239–245.

18. Moorman AFM, Lamers WH. Molecular anatomy of the developing heart. *Trends Cardiovasc Med* 1994;4:257–264.

19. Thornell E, Eriksson A, Johansson B, et al. Intermediate filament and associated proteins in heart purkinje fibers: A membrane-myofibril anchored cytoskeletal system. *Ann NY Acad Sci* 1985;455: 213–240.

22

Role of Transforming Growth Factor-β3 During the Formation of Endocardial Cushion Tissue in Chick Heart Development

Yuji Nakajima, MD, Toshiyuki Yamagishi, MD,
Hiroaki Nakamura, MD, Vladimir Mironov, MD, PhD,
Edward L. Krug, PhD, and Roger R. Markwald, PhD

Endothelial-to-mesenchymal transformation is a critical event to generate endocardial cushion tissue, the primordia of valves and septa in the adult heart, and is regulated spatiotemporally by unknown myocardially derived inductive signals.[1,2] Abnormal development of endocardial cushion tissue is linked to many congenital heart diseases.[3,4] Transforming growth factor (TGF)-βs are 25-kDa dimeric peptide growth factors thought to regulate cellular proliferation and differentiation at different stages of embryogenesis. The tissue distribution pattern of several TGFβs and their receptors in developing organs suggest that they may have signaling roles in epithelial-mesenchymal interaction.[5] In the present paper, we examined the tissue distribution of TGFβ3 and roles of this growth factor in the formation of endocardial cushion tissue in embryonic chick heart.

In situ hybridization analysis of the stage 14 hearts (before the onset of endocardial cushion tissue formation) showed little or no detectable TGFβ3 transcript in the myocardium and endocardium of the primitive atrium and atrioventricular (AV) region. However, a strong signal was observed in the myocardium at the distal extreme of the outflow tract (OT) region. On the protein level only a very low level of immunoreactivity for TGFβ3 was observed in the stage 14 heart. By stage 18, some of the endothelial cells in both OT and AV regions have changed from an epithelial morphology to become mesenchymal cells that invade the subjacent cardiac jelly, resulting in the formation of endocardial cushion tissue. In addition, ventricular muscle layer has begun to form ventricular trabeculae, which requires loss of its epithelial morphology as well. At this stage, TGFβ3 mRNA was detectable throughout the heart. In the OT and AV region of stage 18 heart, TGFβ3 mRNA was found in myocardium, endocardium, and its associated endocardial cushion mesenchyme. The strongest signal was found in the ventricular myocardium. Immunostaining showed that TGFβ3 protein was distributed in endocardium, myocardium, and mesenchymal cells. There was no detectable staining for TGFβ3 in the extracellular matrix of the cardiac jelly under these fixation conditions.[6]

From Clark EB, Nakazawa M, Takao A (eds.): Etiology and Morphogenesis of Congenital Heart Disease: Twenty Years of Progress in Genetics and Developmental Biology. Armonk, NY: Futura Publishing Co., Inc.; © 2000.

It has been reported that immunoreactivity for TGFβ1/3 in cultured premigratory OT/AV endothelial cells can be upregulated by embryonic cardiocyte conditioned medium (CCM), which contains transformation inductive signals.[7] Whether this represented new synthesis by the target endocardial cells or the acquisition of TGFβ protein from CCM was not determined conclusively, however, no immunoreactive TGFβ1/3 was detectable in the CCM. In order to evaluate the more likely scenario, that TGFβ mRNA is upregulated in the target endocardial cells, AV endothelial monolayers were prepared on collagen gels and pretreated with antisense oligodeoxynucleotides (ODN) specific for TGFβ3. After 12 hours in culture, CCM was added as a source of transformation-promoting activity. As has been reported previously,[8] control and missense ODN-treated AV endothelial monolayers seeded invasive mesenchymal cells into the collagen gel in the presence of CCM. However, pretreatment of AV endothelial monolayers with antisense ODN to TGFβ3 blocked mesenchymal formation in response to CCM. AV endothelial monolayers, pretreated with antisense ODN to TGFβ3 followed by the treatment of CCM, did not show anti-TGFβ3 immunoreactivity.[6] These inhibitory effects of antisense ODN were reversed when CCM was supplemented with recombinant TGFβ3 (Table 1).

In order to further assess the role of endocardially derived TGFβ3 in the epithelial-mesenchymal transformation, stage 14⁻ AV endothelial monolayers cultures were evaluated for their morphological response to exogenous TGFβ3. As shown in Table 2, the addition of recombinant TGFβ3 did not elicit invasive mesenchymal formation after 24 hours in culture. However, TGFβ3 addition did result in significant cell:cell separation and cellular hypertrophy, as well as migratory cells on the surface of the gel at the periphery of monolayer. By 48 hours, 3–5 cells per monolayer had invaded into the collagen gel lattice in the TGFβ3 treated culture. In contrast, premigratory AV endothelial monolayer treated with CCM generated 4 to 7 times the number of invasive mesenchymal cells. Control monolayers treated with CM199 alone did not show any phenotypic change of epithelial-mesenchymal transformation. Because TGFβ2 has been reported in the developing chicken heart,[9] we tested the hypothesis that TGFβ2 and -β3 could act synergistically to affect complimentary events necessary for cushion tissue formation. However, neither TGFβ2 alone nor in combination with TGFβ3 resulted in mesenchyme formation from stage 14⁻ AV endothelial monolayers. In both situations, results were similar to treatment with TGFβ3 alone (Table 2).

TGFβs are known to be potent inducers of mesodermal differentiation and to promote differentiation of endothelial cells into smooth muscle-like cells.[10,11]

Table 1

Perturbation of TGFβ3 in Premigratory AV Endothelial Cells Repressed CCM-Inducible Endothelial-Mesenchymal Transformation in Culture

Culture Conditions		Mesenchyme Formed by 48 Hours	
Pretreatment	Bioassay	Frequency[a]	Mesenchymal cells per monolayer[b]
CM199	CM199	0/8 (0%)	—
CM199	CCM	8/10 (80%)	17 ± 1
CM199 + TGFβ3 ODN	CCM	0/11 (0%)	< 2
CM199 + TGFβ3 ODN	CCM + TGFβ3	4/5 (80%)	21 ± 3
CM199 + missense ODN	CCM	7/9 (78%)	20 ± 2

Stage 14-minus AV endocardial monolayers were prepared on collagen gel lattice and pretreated for 12 hours with CM199 alone, CM199 containing 1 μM antisense oligodeoxynucleotides (ODN) specific to TGFβ3, or missense ODN. The resulting monolayers were then subjected to various culture conditions including CM199, cardiocyte conditioned medium (CCM), or CCM containing 5 ng/mL of chicken recombinant TGFβ3. [a] Number of monolayers forming mesenchyme after 48 hours. [b] Mean number of mesenchymal cells formed per monolayer ± SE.

Table 2
Addition of TGFβs Protein Initiated Initial Characteristics of Endothelial-Mesenchymal Transformation in Culture

Culture Conditions		Endothelial-Mesenchymal Transformation (24–48 hours)	
Bioassay	Conc. Protein	Initial Phenotypic Changes[a]	Mesenchymal Cells[b]
CM199		−	0
TGFβ2	5–50 ng/ml	+	< 5
TGFβ3	0.5–50 ng/ml	+	< 5
TGFβ2 + 3	5–50 ng/ml	+	< 5
CCM		+	15–25

Stage 14-minus AV endothelial monolayers were prepared on collagen gel lattice. Resulting cells were treated with either various concentration of TGFβs in CM199, or cardiocyte conditioned medium (CCM). After 24 and 48 hours in incubation, cultures were assessed for endothelial-mesenchymal transformation under the Hoffman modulation optics. [a] Initial phenotypic changes of endothelial-mesenchymal transformation include cellular hypertrophy, loss of cell:cell contact, migratory appendage formation, and expression of alpha smooth muscle actin. [b] Number of mesenchymal cells invaded into the collagen gel lattice per monolayer.

Based on these activities, we examined the immunolocalization of this isoactin during the cushion tissue formation, using a monoclonal antibody specific to vascular alpha smooth muscle actin (SMA). Both transforming endothelial and migrating mesenchymal cells expressed SMA beneath the cytoplasmic membrane in the presence of CCM. These cells showed a reduction of the endothelial specific marker antigen QH1.[12] Endothelial cells that remained epithelial did not express SMA. Similar SMA staining patterns were observed in TGFβ3 treated AV monolayers, whereas cells cultured in CM199 alone did not (Table 2).[12,13]

Results from this and related studies indicate that: (1) AV endocardium expresses TGFβ3 in response to a myocardially derived signal that is not TGFβ3, (2) AV endocardial TGFβ3 functions in an autocrine fashion to elicit a subset of characteristics of endothelial-mesenchymal transformation, such as loss of cell:cell contact, cellular hypertrophy, migratory appendage formation as well as expression of SMA, but which is insufficient to facilitate formation of invasive mesenchyme in culture. Thus, we propose that there exist at least two signaling pathways to initiate/elicit endothelial-mesenchymal transformation: first, a myocardially derived signal stimulates the progenitor cells of future cushion mesenchyme in OT and AV endocardium to express TGFβ3, which subsequently initiates the initial characteristics necessary for cushion tissue formation. Second, there are additional myocardially derived factors (e.g., ES proteins) that complete the transformation process. Recently, we have found that bone morphogenetic protein (BMP)-2, which is expressed in the stage 18 OT/AV myocardium, enhanced the TGFβ3-inducible initial phenotypic changes of endothelial cell cytodifferentiation in culture, however, BMP2 alone fails to initiate any of these transformation processes.[13] Further experiments are needed to elucidate the inductive mechanisms that complete this embryonic transformation process during the endocardial cushion tissue formation.

References

1. Markwald RR, Mjaatvedt CH, Krug EL. Induction of endocardial cushion tissue formation by adheron-like, molecular complexes derived from the myocardial basement membrane. In: Clark EB, Takao A, eds. *Developmental Cardiology: Morphogenesis and Function.* Mount Kisco NY: Futura Publishing; 1990:191–204.
2. Mjaatvedt CH, Krug EL, Markwald RR. An antiserum (ES1) against a particulate form of extracellular matrix blocks the transformation of cardiac endothelium into mesenchyme in culture. *Dev Biol* 1991;145:219–230.
3. Yasui H, Nakazawa M, Morishima M, et al. Morphological observations on the

pathogenetic process of transposition of the great arteries induced by retinoic acid in mice. *Circulation* 1995;91:2478–2486.

4. Nakajima Y, Morishima M, Nakazawa M, et al. Inhibition of outflow cushion mesenchyme formation in retinoic acid-induced complete transposition of the great arteries. *Cardiovasc Res* 1996;31:E77–E85.

5. Akhurst RJ. The transforming growth factor β family in vertebrate embryogenesis. In: Nilsen-Hamilton M, ed. *Growth Factors and Signal Transduction in Development.* Wiley-Liss, New York; 1994:97–122.

6. Nakajima Y, Yamagishi T, Nakamura H, et al. An autocrine function for transforming growth factor (TGF)-β3 in the transformation of atrioventricular canal endocardium into mesenchyme during chick heart development. *Dev Biol* 1998;194:99–113.

7. Nakajima Y, Krug EL, Markwald RR. Myocardial regulation of transforming growth factor beta expression by outflow tract endothelium in the early embryonic chick heart. *Dev Biol* 1994;165:615–626.

8. Krug EL, Mjaatvedt CH, Markwald RR. Extracellular matrix from embryonic myocardium elicits an early morphogenetic event in cardiac endothelial differentiation. *Dev Biol* 1987;120:348–355.

9. Potts JD, Vincent EB, Runyan RB, et al. Sense and antisense TGFβ3 mRNA levels correlate with cardiac valve induction. *Dev Dyn* 1992;193:340–345.

10. Saint-Jeannet J-P, Levi G, Girault J-M, et al. Ventrolateral regionalization of *Xenopus laevis* mesoderm is characterized by the expression of α-smooth muscle actin. *Development* 1992;115:1165–1173.

11. Arciniegas E, Sutton AB, Allen TD, et al. Transforming growth factor beta 1 promotes the differentiation of endothelial cells into smooth muscle like cells in vitro. *J Cell Sci* 1992;103:521–529.

12. Nakajima Y, Mironov V, Yamagishi T, et al. Expression of smooth muscle alpha-actin in mesenchymal cells during formation of avian endocardial cushion tissue: A role for transforming growth factor β3. *Dev Dyn* 1997;209:296–309.

13. Ramsdell AF, Markwald RR. Induction of endocardial cushion tissue in the avian heart is regulated, in part, by TGFβ-3-mediated autocrine signaling. *Dev Biol* 1997;188:64–74.

14. Yamagishi T, Nakajima Y, Miyazono K, et al. Bone morphogenetic protein (BMP)-2 expression in chick heart development: possible synergistic effect with transforming growth factor β3. Chapter in Clark EB, Nakazawa M, Takao A (eds): Etiology and Morphogenesis of Congenital Heart Disease. Twenty Years of Progress in Genetics and Developmental Biology. Armonk, NY. Futura Publishing Co. 2000. pp. 147–150.

23

BMP-2 Expression in Chick Heart Development: Possible Synergistic Effect With TGFβ3

Toshiyuki Yamagishi, MD, Yuji Nakajima, MD,
Kohei Miyazono, MD, T. Kuber Sampath, PhD,
and Hiroaki Nakamura, MD

Bone morphogenetic proteins (BMPs) are members of the transforming growth factor β (TGFβ) superfamily and play a critical role in early developmental processes, including cellular proliferation, differentiation, and epithelial-mesenchymal interaction.[1-4] BMP-2, -4, and -6 (Vgr-1) are transcribed in the embryonic mouse heart, but we do not know the exact role of BMPs during early heart development. Endocardial cushion tissue, which develops in the outflow tract (OT) and atrioventricular (AV) canal regions of the embryonic heart, is a primordia of valves and septa of the adult heart, and elicited by embryonic processes of endothelial-mesenchymal transformation in a spatio-temporal restricted manner.[5] Maldevelopment of the cushion tissue causes various types of congenital heart disease.[6] In vitro trials have shown that this endothelial-mesenchymal transformation is prompted by unknown signals produced by the subjacent AV myocardium.[7] During chick endocardial cushion tissue formation, TGFβ3 is expressed in transforming endothelial and invading mesen-

chymal cells, and the initial phenotypic changes of this embryonic phenomenon are induced by exogenously administered TGFβ3 in culture.[8,9] In the present paper, we cloned BMPs from embryonic chick hearts and analyzed the role of BMP-2 during the formation of endocardial cushion tissue.

Using reverse transcription-polymerase chain reaction (RT-PCR),[10] we cloned three BMP genes from an early chick embryonic heart (BMP-2, -7, and dorsalin-1). In situ hybridization showed an intense signal of BMP-2 message in the myocardium of the OT and AV at stage 14–18, at which time endothelial-mesenchymal transformation is extensively carried out. After cushion tissue formation BMP-2 transcripts were seen in the AV myocardium until the end of the embryonic stage (stage 33). A weak signal of the dorsalin-1 message was also found in the OT and AV myocaldium. BMP-7 was transcribed in the entire myocardium of the looped heart. There was no detectable signal for these BMPs in the endocardium or endocardial cushion mesenchyme. The results of the tissue distributions of BMPs suggested that BMP-2 may have a critical role in the regulation of endothelial-mesenchymal transformation. Furthermore, heterodimeric peptides of BMP-2/7 may have a significant biological effect

From Clark EB, Nakazawa M, Takao A (eds.): Etiology and Morphogenesis of Congenital Heart Disease: Twenty Years of Progress in Genetics and Developmental Biology. Armonk, NY: Futura Publishing Co., Inc.; © 2000.

regulating embryonic events in vivo.[11,12] To examine whether BMP-2 was required for the generation of the endothelial-mesenchymal transformation, we cultured AV explants from a stage 14⁻ heart on collagen gel lattice and treated them with antisense oligodeoxynucleotides (ODN) specific for BMP-2 (antisense ODN complementary to positions 1–16 of chick BMP-2, 5'-GGGTGGCGGCAACCAT-3'; sense ODN, 5'-ATGGTTGCCGCCACCC-3'; Table 1). After 48 hours in culture with CM199 or sense ODN (1 μM), mesenchymal cell invasion into the gel lattice was observed. When explants were cultured with antisense BMP-2-ODN (1 μM), mesenchymal cell invasion into the gel lattice was inhibited. This inhibitory effect was reversed by the addition of recombinant BMP-2 (1 μg/mL). Whole-mount in situ hybridization showed that BMP-2 mRNA was present in similar amounts in all explants tested. We next examined mRNA expression for Msx1 (Hox-7), a homeobox-containing gene, in the cultured explants with or without the presence of perturbation, because it has been reported that Msx1 is regulated by BMP-2 and is expressed in the transforming AV endothelial/mesenchymal cells.[13,14] Quantitative RT-PCR showed that the amount of Msx1 mRNA in the perturbed explants was significantly suppressed in comparison with that of control explants. When the explants were cultured with antisense BMP-2-ODN and BMP-2 protein, the amount of mRNA for Msx1 was reversed. These results suggested that the antisense ODN to the BMP-2 affects the translation of BMP2 message rather than its transcription. The reduced expression of MSX1 may be due to the reduction in the BMP-2 protein. To test the biological effect of BMP-2 on AV endothelial cells, premigrated stage 14⁻ AV endothelial monolayers were prepared on collagen gel lattice and cultured with CM199, BMP-2, or combined administration of BMP-2 and TGFβ3 (Table 2). AV endothelial monolayers cultured with BMP-2 (1 μg/mL) did not elicit any phenotypic changes of endothelial-mesenchymal transformation. As we had shown previously, endothelial cells treated with TGFβ3 (50 ng/mL) showed initial phenotypic changes of endothelial-mesenchymal transformation such as cell:cell separation, cellular hypertrophy, migratory appendage formation on the gel surface, and a few mesenchymal cells into the gel lattice (less than 2). In contrast, endothelial cells cultured with both TGFβ3 (50 ng/mL) and BMP-2 (1 μg/mL) generated endothelial cell migration on the gel surface and seeded many mesenchymal cells into the gel lattice.

In the present paper, we cloned three BMP genes (BMP-2, -7, and dorsalin-1) from the chick embryonic heart and examined the role of BMP-2 in the formation of endocardial cushion tissue. The results showed that (1) an intense signal for BMP-2 transcripts was found in the myocardium of the AV canal and OT at the onset and during endothelial-mesenchymal transformation; (2) antisense ODN specific for BMP-2 inhibited the AV endothelial-mesenchymal transformation in culture; and (3) although BMP-2 did not induce any phenotypic change of AV endothelial cells, it did enhance TGFβ3-induced phenotypic changes among endothelial cells. These observations suggest that BMP-2 is an essential

---

Table 1

AV Explant Culture in the Presence or Absence of Antisense ODN to BMP-2

Culture Conditions	No. of Invaded Mesenchymal Cells (mean ± SE)
CM199 (N = 22)	124 ± 9
Sense BMP-2 ODN 1 μM (N = 12)	118 ± 11
Antisense BMP-2 ODN 1 μM (N = 27)	53 ± 7
Antisense BMP-2 ODN 1 μM + BMP-2 1 μg/mL (N = 10)	126 ± 20

AV explants were prepared from stage 14⁻ embryonic hearts and cultured under various conditions in a three-dimensional collagen gel culture system. Antisense ODN to BMP-2 inhibited mesenchymal cell transformation (P < 0.05, Mann-Whitney U test). Addition of recombinant BMP-2 reversed the inhibitory effect of antisense BMP-2-ODN. CM199, medium 199 containing 1% chick serum; N, number of explants; No., number.

Table 2
Effects of BMP-2 Protein on Preactivated AV Endothelial Monolayers

Culture Conditions	Endothelial Cell Phenotypic Changes*		No. of Invaded Mesenchymal Cells (mean ± SE)	
	24-hours	48-hours	24-hours	48-hours
CM199 (N = 15)	−	−	0	0
CM199 + BMP-2 1 μg/mL (N = 12)	−	−	0	0
CM199 + TGFβ3 50 ng/mL (N = 14)	+	+	≤2	≤2
CM199 + TGFβ3 50 ng/mL + BMP-2 1 μg/mL (N = 16)	++	+++	6 ± 1	22 ± 3

Four different types of AV endothelial cultures were analyzed to examine the effects of BMP-2. AV endothelial monolayers were obtained from stage 14⁻ hearts and cultured with CM199, BMP-2, TGFβ3, or TGFβ3 + BMP 2. When the endothelial cells were cultured with CM199 alone or BMP-2, neither mesenchymal cell invasion into the gel lattice nor endothelial outgrowth was observed. In contrast, when cells were cultured with TGFβ3 (50 ng/mL), cell:cell separation on the gel lattice and invasion of a few mesenchymal cells into the gel lattice was observed. Endothelial cells cultured with both TGFβ3 (50 ng/mL) and BMP-2 (1 μg/mL) showed invasion by a greater number of mesenchymal cells into the gel lattice and greater endothelial phenotypic changes. * "endothelial phenotypic changes" indicates cellular hypertrophy, cell:cell separation, appendage formation, and migration into the collagen gel lattice.

molecule in the regulation of endothelial-mesenchymal transformation and acts synergistically with TGFβ3 during cushion tissue formation. We also hypothesize that BMP-2 may be one of the myocardially derived inductive molecules considered to regulate endothelial-mesenchymal transformation. However, BMP-2 alone did not induce phenotypic changes characteristic in the endothelial-mesenchymal transformation in cultured preactivated AV endocardium. Thus, another signal(s) secreted by the AV and OT myocardium is likely necessary to complete this embryonic phenomenon.

References

1. Yamagishi T, Nishimatsu S, Nomura S, et al. Expression of BMP-2, 4 genes during early development in *Xenopus. Zool Sci* 1995;12:355–358.
2. Mishina Y, Suzuki A, Ueno N, et al. *Bmpr* encodes a type I bone morphogenetic protein receptor that is essential for gastrulation during mouse embryogenesis. *Genes Dev* 1995;9:3027–3037.
3. Hogan BLM. Bone morphogenetic proteins: Multifunctional regulators of vertebrate development. *Genes Dev* 1996;10:1580–1594.
4. Zhang H, Bradley A. Mice deficient for BMP2 are nonviable and have defects in amnion/chorion and cardiac development. *Development* 1996;122:2977–2986.
5. Markwald RR, Mjaatvedt CH, Krug EL. Induction of endocardial cushion tissue formation by adheron-like, molecular complexes derived from the myocardial basement membrane. In: Clark EB, Takao A, eds. *Developmental Cardiology: Morphogenesis and Function.* New York: Futura; 1990:191–204.
6. Nakajima Y, Hiruma T, Nakazawa M, et al. Hypoplasia of cushion ridges in the proximal outflow tract elicits formation of a right ventricle-to-aortic route in retinoic acid-induced complete transposition of the great arteries in the mouse: Scanning electron microscopic observations of corrosion cast models. *Anat Rec* 1996;245:76–82.
7. Mjaatvedt CH, Krug EL, Markwald RR. An antiserum (ES1) against a particulate form of extracellular matrix blocks the transition of cardiac endothelium into mesenchyme in culture. *Dev Biol* 1991;145:219–230.
8. Nakajima Y, Mironov V, Yamagishi T, et al. Expression of smooth muscle alpha-actin in mesenchymal cells during formation of avian endocardial cushion tissue: A role for transforming growth factor β3. *Dev Dyn* 1997;209:296–309.
9. Nakajima Y, Yamagishi T, Nakamura H, et al. An autocrine function for transforming

growth factor (TGF)-β3 in the transformation of atrioventricular canal endocardium into mesenchyme during chick heart development. *Dev Biol* 1998;194:99–113.

10. Basler K, Edlund T, Jessell TM, et al. Control of cell pattern in the neural tube: Regulation of cell differentiation by dorsalin-1, a novel TGFβ family member. *Cell* 1993;73:687–702.

11. Hazama M, Aono A, Ueno N, et al. Efficient expression of a heterodimer of bone morphogenetic protein subunits using a baculovirus expression system. *Biochem Biophys Res Commun* 1995;209:859–866.

12. Suzuki A, Kaneko E, Maeda J, et al. Mesoderm induction by BMP-4 and -7 heterodimers. *Biochem Biophys Res Commun* 1997;232:153–156.

13. Chan-Thomas PS, Thompson RP, Robert B, et al. Expression of homeobox genes Msx-1 (Hox-7) and Msx-2 (Hex-8) during cardiac development in the chick. *Dev Dyn* 1993;197:203–216.

14. Barlow AJ, Francis-West PH. Ectopic application of recombinant BMP-2 and BMP-4 can change patterning of developing chick facial primordia. *Development* 1997;124:391–398.

Section IV

24

Overview: Extracellular Matrix: Nature Versus Nurture in Cardiac Development

Thomas K. Borg, PhD, Robert Thompson, PhD, Timothy Fitzharris, PhD, Louis Terracio, PhD, and Wayne Carver, PhD

The concept that the extracellular matrix (ECM) plays an important role in cardiac development is borne out by the dynamic nature of the composition and organization of the ECM and its ability to regulate the fundamental biological properties of the cellular components in the heart. The ECM was originally described as having a passive role in both the structure/function relationships of development and the onset of disease in the adult heart.[1] The complex components of the ECM were originally thought to provide a scaffold upon which the cells underwent differentiation to form the heart. Terms like "cardiac jelly" were used to describe the material between the myocardium and endocardium in the developing heart tube. The increased deposition of cardiac jelly in the endocardial cushions represented something that the transforming epithelial cells had to migrate through as they became mesechymal cells. The ECM was thought to be more of a barrier rather than a complex set of macromolecules that played an active role in morphogenesis of the cardiac valves.

Current research now indicates that the ECM is a complex, 3-dimensional organization of several classes of macromolecules that play an integral role in the regulation of heart development.[2,3] A fundamental tenet of any living system is the ability to respond to external stimuli. As the cellular components of the heart are undergoing differentiation, morphogenesis, or maintaining homeostasis as adult cells, they maintain a constant and dynamic interaction with components of the ECM. The concept that cells make and respond to components of the ECM is a critical experimental paradigm of cardiac development.

Components and Organization of the ECM

The ECM contains a diverse set of components that are arranged in a precise 3-dimensional organization. This organization is not always apparent as methods used to visualize the ECM distort or solubilize these components. The ECM is usually divided into 4 classes of molecules: collagens, proteoglycans, glycoproteins and proteases (Table 1).

Collagens represent a unique class of abundant structural components that are critical to heart development. Collagen is composed of unique α chains, arranged in

From Clark EB, Nakazawa M, Takao A (eds.): Etiology and Morphogenesis of Congenital Heart Disease: Twenty Years of Progress in Genetics and Developmental Biology. Armonk, NY: Futura Publishing Co., Inc.; © 2000.

Table 1
Components of the Extracellular Matrix of the Heart

Collagens		
Fibrillar		Location
I		Interstitium, valves
II		Transient expression in development
III		Interstitium, valves
V		Surrounding vasculature
Basement membrane		
IV		Surrounds myocytes, basal layer of endothelium
Facit		
VI		Associated with endocardial cushions
Noncollagenous glycoproteins		
Laminin		Basement membrane
Nidogen/entactin		Basement membrane
Fibulin		Basement membrane
Fibronectin		Interstitium
Tenascin		Interstitium
Fibrillins		Interstitium
Elastin		Interstitium
Flexin		Interstitium
Matrilin		Interstitium
Proteoglycans		
Small leucine-rich proteoglycans (SLRP)		
Decorin		
Biglycan		
Lumican		
Nonhyaluronan-binding proteoglycans		
Perlecan		
Agrin		
Hyaluronan-binding proteoglycans		
Aggrecan		
Versican		
Proteases		
Aspartic proteases		Cysteine proteinases
Cathepsin D		Cathespin B, L, and S
Serine proteases		Metalloproteases
Tissue plasminogen activator		Gelatinases (MMP 2,9)
Urokinase		Stromelysin (MMP 3)
Plasmin		Matrilysin (MMP 7)
Chymase		Interstitial collagenase (MMP 1)
ADAM proteins (5, 12, 13)		TIMPS

helical structures, which provide a variety of functions in the heart. There are at least 34 distinct α chains and the combination of these chains form at least 19 collagen types.[4,5] However, only a few of these have been identified in the heart.

In the heart, analyses of collagen have focused primarily on types I and III as they are the principal structural components of the cardiac skeleton and valves. Ultrastructural immunohistochemical data indicated that both colla-gen I and III can occur in the same collagen bundle making routine histochemical detection of collagen I and III at the light microscope level difficult. Initial studies documented the expression of types I and III in early heart development, primarily associated with valve formation.[6,7] Several studies have indicated that collagen expression and deposition is associated with increased mechanical tension as the cardiac myocyte undergoes increased fibrillogenesis and the blood volume during development increases.[8,9] The expression of collagen I and III is important as the mechanical properties of these collagens are distinct. Collagen type I is a rigid structure while collagen III is more flexible. The ratio of collagen I and III becomes an important index of compliance[10,11]; however, little is known as to the mechanism of how the fibroblasts regulate the expression of these collagens. Undoubtedly this regulation is a complex of chemical (growth factor, cytokine) and mechanical factors (strain/tension).

During late fetal and early neonatal development, the precise 3-dimensional arrangement of the connective tissue becomes apparent (Fig. 1). The classic layers of endomysium and perimysial collagen develop during neonatal and early adult heart stages. Cellular association with the collagen network has important implications for cardiac function. Alteration of the collagen network in animals having a copper deficiency or treated with the lathyritic agent (BAPN) demonstrated an altered compliance.[12,13] These data demonstrate the essential nature of the collagen network associated with cardiac function.

Collagen is associated with the cell surface of the myocyte in two distinct ways: perpendicular and tangential to the myocyte cell surface. Perpendicular attachments form as collagen is secreted by fibroblasts and attached at precise regions just lateral to the Z band.[14] Ultrastructural studies show fibroblasts align parallel to growing myocytes and secrete collagen in close proximity to the site of attachment on the cardiac myocyte[8] (Fig. 1). The collagen attaches directly to the membrane as demonstrated by stereo high-voltage microscopy.[8] This type of collagen attachment is characteristic of the collagen struts which form the myocyte-myocyte and myocyte-capillary connections. The tangential association of collagen with the cell surface occurs on myocytes, fibroblasts and endothelial cells. These tangential associations appear to vary in strength from dense fibers wrapped around capillaries to loose association with fibroblasts. Other collagens have been noted in the heart and may play important roles in the development of the heart.[15,16]

Immunohistochemical studies have shown that collagen II is transiently ex-

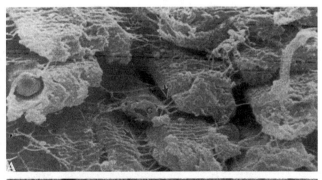
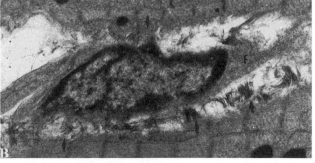

Figure 1. The 3-dimensional organization of the collagenous connective tissue in the heart is seen by scanning electron microscopy (**A**) showing the endomysial weave network (W), myocyte-myocyte and myocyte capillary (C) struts (arrows). Transmission electron microscopy reveals that during the formation of the connective tissue network (**B**), fibroblast (F) lies between myocytes and that the collagen struts (arrows) extend from the fibroblast to them myocyte at sites near the Z bands.

pressed at the time of looping in the regions of the endocardial cushions. However, mice with the collagen II gene knocked out did not show any specific cardiac defect.[17] Collagen type VI is expressed coordinately with the development of the cardiac cushions (11–11.5 ED in mice).[16] At the time of this review, no data were available concerning mice with the collagen VI gene knocked out.

Proteoglycans represent a diverse group of macromolecules that have not been well investigated in cardiac development. Proteoglycans contain conserved core proteins with glycosaminoglycan (GAG) side chains and may be divided into two subfamilies: (1) small leucine rich proteoglycans (SLRP) and (2) large highly glycosylated macromolecules termed modular proteoglycans[4,18] (Table 1). Molecular analysis of the core proteins has demonstrated considerable diversity making it difficult to classify different families of molecules. The SLRP group have small protein cores, amino terminal region for GAG binding, and several regions of leucine clusters. The modular proteoglycans have been divided into two groups based on their ability to bind hylauronan. Members of this group have demonstrated specificity to basement membranes and an interstitial distribution.

While much of the biochemistry and molecular biology of proteoglycans is known, the functional cell biology, especially in the heart, is lacking. Versican has recently been shown to be associated with septation and valvulogenesis as has perlcan[19]; however, these studies are based on expression levels or immunofluorescent localization rather than direct experimentation. It appears that proteoglycans are distinct building blocks of the 3-dimensional nature of the ECM and, by their mere presence, are important components. However, it is still unclear whether they have individual regulatory properties as single entities. Their physical properties are undoubtedly critical in functions of the ECM, in the regulation of movement of molecules and cells through the ECM, and to bind growth factors and cytokines.[20]

Glycoproteins represent a diverse array of components of the ECM. These components have been the subject of numerous studies documenting their importance in regulation of cell migration, adhesion, cell cycle and other critical events in morphogenesis.[3,21] The best described ECM glycoprotein is fibronectin, which has a critical role in the regulation of cell differentiation and morphogenesis. Other non-collagenous glycoproteins that appear to play essential roles include the basement membrane components laminin, nidogen, tenascin, fibrillins, and elastin. Analysis of these molecules yields several common features including: (1) their ability to bind to other molecules in the ECM to become part of the 3-dimensional organization; (2) the different protein chains contain protein motifs that have essential functions as growth factors or adhesion molecules, and (3) they can be alternatively spliced.[21] These features expand the potential of these molecules to regulate biological signaling and cellular function.

Extracellular proteases are now recognized as potentially important components of the ECM and participate in a variety of functions such as turnover of ECM components, modifying extracellular proteins, cell migration, and activation of latent proteins such as growth factors. The extracellular proteases can be divided into 4 basic classes based on the critical functional groups in their catalytic domains[22] (Table 1). While extracellular proteases have been well documented in inflammation and clotting cascades, their role in normal development and homeostasis is only now beginning to be explored. Early studies showed that cathepsins were expressed in the heart as well as proteases necessary for cleaving telopeptides of collagen.[23]

Metalloproteases (MMP) and the serine proteases have been shown to be present and active in the migration of endocardial cushion cells.[24,25] Most proteases are present in the ECM in a latent form that requires activation. How proteases are activated in vivo is not known but in vitro studies have shown that mechanical tension can lead to activation of MMPs.[26] Where examined, it appears that proteases are transcriptionally controlled and associated with their expression are endogenous inhibitors such as Tissue inhibitor of metalloprotease (TIMP). Examination of the expression of MMPs during heart development has shown that MMP-2 and MMP-9 and their associated TIMPs have a distinct temporal and spatial expression.[27] A subclass of the MMPs are the ADAM proteins (a disintegrin and metalloproteases).[28] The ADAM proteins are unique in that they have a metalloprotease domain, an integrin binding site, a transmembrane domain and a cytoplasmic domain. Recent data show that ADAMs are present in the heart during development; however, no functional data is available at this time.[27,28]

The precise interaction between various proteases and the ECM is not clear. There appears to be species variation as well as poorly defined substrate specificity. For example, it is not clear whether substrates for the extracellular proteases are in a soluble or insoluble form. It is likely that the various proteases will be shown to be part of a cascade that requires the activation of several components[29]; however, the exact nature of these cascades remains vague. The biological advantage of such cascades is that there are various check points at which control can be exerted. Limited proteolysis of ECM components may be necessary for a variety of cellular functions but there could be tissue damage if degradation is not tightly controlled.

Receptors for ECM Components

Early studies on the expression and immunohistochemical localization of ECM components revealed precise patterns suggesting that there might be specific receptors for ECM components on the cell surface. Early in vitro investigations of fibronectin resulted in the characterization of focal adhesions where fibronectin showed a precise relationship to distinct regions of cell:ECM interaction.[30–32] These relationships led to the isolation of specific receptors for cell adhesion molecules.[33]

Among the first ECM receptors to be characterized were the integrins named for their ability to "integrate" information from the ECM to the cytoplasm. The integrins are heterodimers composed of an α and β chain which can be subdivided on the basis of the association of the α chains with different β chains (Fig. 2). Early investigations documented that there could be several α chains associated with the same ECM component, such as collagen or laminin. It is now thought that these associations are related to different functions such as adhesion versus migration, where the affinity of the receptor is a critical feature.[34]

The role of integrins in regulating cell behavior is well documented.[34] Integrins participate in a variety of developmental events including cell adhesion, basement membrane formation, angiogenesis, cell migration, and force generation.[35] In addition, it has been proposed that the $\alpha5\beta1$ integrin functions in a process termed anoikis which triggers apoptosis when this integrin is released from ECM binding.[36] Integrins are essential components in heart development as several integrin knockout mice result in early embryonic death due to cardiovascular abnormalities.[37] These data point out not only the essential nature of these receptors but also the importance of cell:ECM interactions in cardiac development.

Receptor tyrosine kinases (RTK) represent a relatively new class of receptors that have been detected in the heart but we know little of their function[38] (Fig. 2). They are similar to integrins in that they have an extracellular domain that binds to ECM components such as collagen, a transmembrane domain, and a cytoplasmic domain that contains tyrosine kinase domains. The RTKs have been shown to be important in cell adhesion.

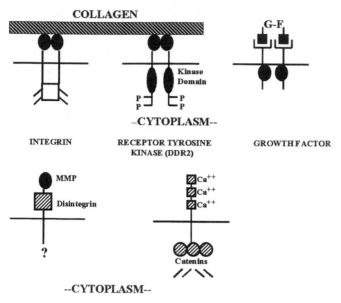

Figure 2. Diagramatic representation of the various types of receptors for extracellular matrix components in the heart.

Cadherins are members of a large group of cell:cell adhesion molecules.[39] These molecules exhibit homotypic binding with their external domains while their cytoplasmic domains associate with a unique class of signalling molecules, the catenins.[39] They are traditionally associated with the formation of the intercalated disk in cardiac myocytes, which is a critical structural event. In addition, they could be important in other aspects of cardiac development such as myofibrillogenesis, cell phenotype and cell polarity. These molecules, along with members of the cell adhesion molecules (CAMS) are critical to cardiac morphogenesis.[40] It is likely that future investigations will reveal other receptors that play important roles in the cell:cell and cell:ECM interaction of cardiac development.

Function of the ECM

Morphological studies have clearly documented the role of the ECM in forming a structural framework of the heart. The formation of collagenous structures like the cardiac skeleton and valves have

been well described as have the defects that can occur in abnormal formation.[41,42] The ECM, as a 3-dimensional structure, is critical to the histoarchitechture of the heart during development and in the adult. The formation of the connective tissue elements into the layers of the perimysium and endomysium are critical to cardiac function[8,12,13] (Fig. 2). The endomysium consists of a woven network surrounding myocytes and collagenous struts that connect adjacent myocytes and capillaries. These latter structures are important in insuring blood flow and myocyte alignment.[14,43] The availability and arrangement of the individual components is dynamic and is constantly undergoing change and turnover. In development of the heart, this process is quite rapid especially at critical times such as cardiac looping and neonatal growth. The structural nature of the ECM is also important in the adaptability of the heart to physiological and pathological stimuli in the adult.[44,45] The processes of growth (hypertrophy) and fibrosis are important at all stages of development.

Besides structural organization, the ECM is known to be important in a wide variety of cellular functions including regulation of phenotype, adhesion, migration, differentiation and response to mechanical stimulation. In vitro studies have documented that the organization of collagen is critical to the establishment of the rod-shaped phenotype of cardiac myocytes.[46] This process is mediated by the $\alpha_1\beta_1$ integrin which regulates myocyte adhesion to the collagen. Other studies have shown that there is a coordinated expression of various ECM components and their receptors which are critical in regulating cellular events in cardiac morphogenesis.[2] In the early stages of cardiac development, cell adhesion to fibronectin is believed to be a critical event in the signaling of cellular commitment.[47] These studies indicate that receptor: ECM interaction is an essential feature of cell signaling. Once internalized, these signals enter a maze of interactive pathways that result in the expression and regulation of a wide variety of proteins.

Another property of the ECM involves the localization and binding of growth factors/cytokines as well as the movement of these molecules within the ECM. The ECM is clearly important in signaling of differentiation. The signaling of an adherent cell population to migrate, such as in the endocardial cushions, is a complex event which must involve signaling from the ECM. In a series of elegant experiments using collagen gels as a migratory substrate, mesenchymal cells from cardiac cushions have been shown to migrate due to some signal from the myocardium (Fig. 3). Variables such as age of the tissue, barriers to signal transmission, and source of the tissue showed that the myocardium was responsible for producing a diffusible substance that caused migration of the cells through the matrix. These studies and others have raised the question as to whether the substance(s) represent a diffusable protein that can selectively bind to components in mi-

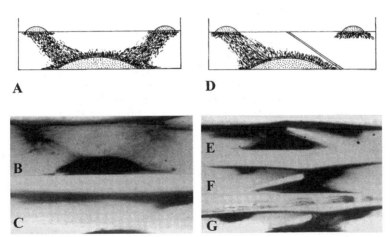

Figure 3. Experiments on the role of the ECM in directing endocardial transformation and growth. The experimental paradigm diagrammed in (**A**) shows the myocardial explant at the base of a 1 mm gel layer 3 days after seeding potent endocardial cushions to the upper surface. In (**B**), cells from the endocardium penetrate and migrate toward a live, beating myocardium, but not toward a killed myocardium (**C**), nor limb bud targets (data not shown). The right panel (**D–G**) shows how directed migration towards live myocardium target is interrupted by barriers embedded in the gel as diagrammed in (**D**). The barriers include impermeable coverslip (**E, F**) or permeable nitrocellulose membrane (**G**). These results suggest that the directed migration is similar to that observed in vivo. The important parameters of the ECM include its deformation (collagen alignment) and the action of diffusible factors in the ECM from the myocardium.

crodomains within the ECM and indicates a potential role for extracellular proteases.

The paradigm that most ECM components are large molecular weight molecules while the signalling molecules such as growth factors/cytokines are small molecular weight components, raises the question as to the potential role of extracellular proteases. Studies using tryptic digestion of ECM components such as fibronectin and laminin have shown that the fragments of proteolysis have distinct biological activities such as EGF signaling, cell adhesion and others.[48] Studies showing localization of MMPs on the leading edge of migrating cells and that MMPs are required for migration leads to the hypothesis that extracellular proteases produce signalling molecules by proteolysis of specific ECM components.[26] The modification of components in the ECM may release or activate signals bound in microdomains or may cause a gradient of signals that causes cells to respond in a chemotactic or haptotactic manner. The data suggest that mesenchymal cells migrating in cardiac jelly express proteases that enhance migration.[24,25] The potential for proteases such as the ADAM proteins is also important as they possess an MMP domain as well as an integrin binding domain. The MMP domain could be responsible for ECM modification while the integrin binding domain might prevent adhesion by binding to integrins on the migrating cell.[49,50]

Summary and New Directions

This brief review has attempted to point out that the 3-dimensional organization of the ECM is a critical and dynamic event in cardiac morphogenesis. We are just beginning to understand the integration of signals from the ECM to the various cellular components of the heart. In future studies it will be essential to understand how these signals are perceived, what proteins are involved, the molecular response to these signals and the result of the molecular response. Clearly signaling will go in both directions as it is the cells that make the ECM. Understanding the ECM as a 3-dimensional entity will be important. The reductionist investigations on single components are important, but it will be equally important to understand how the temporal and spatial organization of the components result in cardiac differentiation and morphogenesis. To this end, it will be essential to examine how microdomains of the ECM are involved in the "storage" of information, its potential release by extracellular proteases, and the perception and response by the individual cellular components of the heart.

References

1. Piez KA. History of extracellular matrix: a personal view. *Matrix Biol* 1997;16:85.
2. Carver W, Terracio L, Borg TK. *Development of Cardiovascular Systems: Molecules to Organisms.* Cambridge University press; 1996.
3. Little CD, Rongish BJ. The extracellular matrix during heart development. *Experimentia* 1995;51:873.
4. Aumailley M, Gayraud BJ. Structure and biological activity of the extracellular matrix. *Mol Med* 1998;76:253.
5. Williams CJ, Vanderberg P, Prockop DJ. *Textbook of Rheumatology.* Philadelphia, Pa: W.B. Saunders; 1997.
6. Borg TK, Terracio L. *Issues in Biomedicine.* Basel, Switzerland, Karger Press; 1990.
7. Thompson RP, Fitzharris TP, Denslow S, et al. Collagen synthesis in the developing chick heart. Texas Repts. *Biol Med* 1979;39:305.
8. Borg TK. Development of the connective tissue network in the neonatal hamster heart. *Am J Anat* 1982;165:435.
9. Carver W, Terracio L, Borg TK. Expression and accumulation of interstitial collagen in the neonatal rat heart. *Anat Rec* 1993;187:445.
10. Borg TK, Gay R, Johnson LD. Changes in the distribution of fibronectin and collagen during development of the neonatal rat heart. *Coll Rel Res* 1982;2:211.

11. Weber KT, Janicki JS, Shroff SG, et al. Collagen remodeling of the pressure-overloaded, hypertrophied nonhuman primate myocardium. *Circ Res* 1988;62:757.

12. Borg TK, Klevay LM, Gay RE, et al. Alteration of the connective tissue network of striated muscle in copper deficient rats. *J Cell Mol Cardiol* 1985;17:1173.

13. Borg TK, Caulfield JB. Collagen in the heart. Texas Repts. *Biol Med* 1979;39:321.

14. Caulfield JB, Borg TK. The collagen network of the heart. *Lab Invest* 1979;40:364.

15. Swiderski RE, Daniels KJ, Jensen KL, et al. Type II collagen is transiently expressed during avian cardiac valve morphogenesis. *Dev Dyn* 1994;200:294.

16. Klewer SE, Krob SL, Kolker SJ, et al. Expression of type VI collagen in the developing mouse heart. *Dev Dyn* 1998;211:248.

17. Vuorio E, Elima K, Peralak M, et al. *Connective Tissue Biology: Integration and Reductionism*. Portland Press, Portland; 1998.

18. Iozzo RV, Murdoch AD. Proteoglycans of the extracellular environment: clues from the gene and protein side offer novel perspectives in molecular diversity and function. *FASEB J* 1996;10:598.

19. Henderson DJ, Copp AJ. Versican expression is associated with chamber specification, septation, and valvulogenesis in the developing mouse heart. *Circ Res* 1998;83:523.

20. Rubin K, et al. *Structure and Function of the Extracellular Matrix of Connective Tissues. Part II. Molecular Components* New York: Harwood Academic Press; 1995.

21. Trelstad RL. *Textbook of Rheumatology*. Philadelphia, Pa: W.B. Saunders; 1997.

22. Nagase H, Okada Y. Textbook of Rheumatology. Philadelphia, Pa: W.B. Saunders; 1997.

23. Samarel A, Parmacek MS, Decker ML, Lesch M, et al. Lysosomal changes during thyroxine-induced left ventricular hypertrophy in rabbits. *Am J Physiol* 1986;250:C589.

24. Nakagawa M, Terracio L, Carver W, et al. Expression of collagenase and IL-1 alpha in developing rat hearts. *Dev Dyn* 1992;195:87.

25. McGuire PG, Orkin RW. Urokinase activity in the developing avian heart: a spatial and temporal analysis. *Dev Dyn* 1992;193:24.

26. Borg KT, et al. *Cardiovasc Pathol* 1997;6:261.

27. Borg TK, et al. *The Fifth International Symposium on Etiology and Morphogenesis of Congenital Heart Disease*. Fifth International Symposium on Etiology and Morphogenesis of Congenital Heart Disease: Twenty Years' Progress, December 7–9, 1998, Tokyo, Japan.

28. Wolfsberg TG, White JM. ADAMs in fertilization and development. *Dev Biol* 1996;180:389.

29. He CS, Wilhelm SM, Pentland AP, et al. Tissue cooperation in a proteolytic cascade activating human interstitial collagenase. *Proc Natl Acad Sci U S A* 1989;86:2632.

30. Couchman JR, Hook M, Rees DA, et al. Adhesion, growth, and matrix production by fibroblasts on laminin substrates. *J Cell Biol* 1983;96:177.

31. Rees DA, et al. *Philos Trans R Soc Lond* 1983;299:169.

32. Rubin K, Hook M, Obrink B, et al. Substrate adhesion of rat hepatocytes: mechanism of attachment to collagen substrates. *Cell* 1981;24:463.

33. Hynes RO. Integrins: versatility, modulation, and signaling in cell adhesion. *Cell* 1992;69:11.

34. Albelda AM, Buck CA. Integrins and other cell adhesion molecules. *FASEB J* 1990;4:2868.

35. Ingber DE. Cellular basis of mechanotransduction. *Biol Bull* 1998;194:323.

36. Frisch SM, Ruoslahti E. Integrins and anoikis. *Curr Opin Cell Biol* 1997;9:701.

37. Hynes RO. Targeted mutations in cell adhesion genes: what have we learned from them? *Dev Biol* 1996;180:402.

38. Schlessinger J. Direct binding and activation of receptor tyrosine kinases by collagen. *Cell* 1997;91:869.

39. Uemura T. The cadherin superfamily at the synapse: more members, more missions. *Cell* 1998;93:1095.

40. Crossin KL, Hoffman S. Expression of adhesion molecules during the formation and differentiation of the avian endocardial cushion tissue. *Dev Biol* 1991;145:277.

41. Gittenberger-de Groot AC, et al. *Circ Res* 1998;82:1043.

42. DeRuiter MC, Poelmann RE, VanMunsteren JC, et al. Embryonic endothelial cells transdifferentiate into mesenchymal cells expressing smooth muscle ac-

tins in vivo and in vitro. *Circ Res* 1997; 80:444.

43. Borg TK, Ranson WF, Moslehy FA, et al. Structural basis of ventricular stiffness. *Lab Invest* 1981;44:49–54.

44. Terracio L, Rubin K, Gullberg D, et al. Expression of collagen binding integrins during cardiac development and hypertrophy. *Circ Res* 1991;68:734.

45. Jalil JE, Doering CW, Janicki JS, et al. Fibrillar collagen and myocardial stiffness in the intact hypertrophied rat left ventricle. *Circ Res* 1989;64:1041.

46. Simpson DG, Terracio L, Terracio M, et al. Modulation of cardiac myocyte phenotype in vitro by the composition and orienta-

tion of the extracellular matrix. *J Cell Physiol* 1994;161:89.

47. Gannon M, Bader D. Avian cardiac progenitors: methods for isolation, culture, and analysis of differentiation. *Methods Cell Biol* 1997;52:117.

48. Ruoslahti E, Hayman EG, Engvall E, et al. Alignment of biologically active domains in the fibronectin molecule. *J Biol Chem* 1981;256:7277.

49. Werb Z, Yan Y. A cellular striptease act. *Science* 1998;283:1279.

50. Peschon JJ, Slack JL, Reddy P, et al. An essential role for ectodomain shedding in mammalian development. *Science* 1998; 283:1281.

25

Adhesion-Mediated Morphoregulatory Mechanisms of Early Cardiogenesis

Kersti K. Linask, PhD

In vivo signals that affect differentiation of an apparently homogeneous, undifferentiated mesoderm into myocardiocytes are beginning to be defined. The problem of cardiac cell differentiation and cell modeling into a functional organ, however, is not one of only regulatory gene activation or growth factor stimulation, it involves also morphoregulatory signals emanating from cell-cell and cell-matrix interactions. My laboratory has focused on the adhesion-mediated events that coordinate differentiation of myocardiocytes with morphogenesis to form a looping, tubular heart. In the chick, these events occur between 17 to 29 hours after fertilization in an anterior-posterior (A/P) progression. The A/P progression means that at different levels along the heart field, cells are at different stages of differentiation: anteriorly, already stably committed and differentiating; posteriorly, still uncommitted. Therefore, an explant of the heart-forming region removed at stage 5 and put into culture is quite different in its percentage of differentiated cells, than an explant removed at stage 6 or at stage 7. Even though the cells may not look that different, they cannot be lumped all together as "precardiac" mesoderm. By stage 8 most of the cells are committed, differentiating myocardiocytes and endocardiocytes.

Regulatory factors, such as Nkx 2.5[1] and the GATAs[2-4], and growth factors, such as FGF-2,[5] TGF-β2, bone morphogenetic protein (BMP)-2 and BMP-4[6], are involved in cardiac cell specification. In situ hybridization patterns of these factors often show gene expression ubiquitously throughout the mesoderm of the cardiogenic crescent. Some factors, as Nkx 2.5, are expressed also in the overlying ectoderm and underlying endoderm.[6] Yet, the heart forms from only a subpopulation of the mesoderm of the lateral plate, i.e., from the ventral mesoderm cells. The specific questions we are addressing include: What specifies the boundary of the cardiac compartment within the homogenous appearing mesoderm? What signaling appears to be involved? To what extent do matrix and adhesion molecules regulate the early cardiac developmental processes?

Adhesion-Mediated Specification of the Dorsal Boundary of the Cardiac Compartment

The expression of the Ca^{2+}-dependent cell adhesion molecule N-cadherin and its intracellular binding molecule β-catenin becomes restricted to membrane surfaces in the central regions of the lateral plate

From Clark EB, Nakazawa M, Takao A (eds.): Etiology and Morphogenesis of Congenital Heart Disease: Twenty Years of Progress in Genetics and Developmental Biology. Armonk, NY: Futura Publishing Co., Inc.; © 2000.

mesoderm in an A/P progression.[7,8] These localized regions designate cells' sorting out to form the dorsal, somatic mesoderm, which forms the pericardial coelom lining, and the ventral, splanchnic mesoderm, which forms the cardiac compartment (Fig. 1). The ventral cells immediately undergo a mesenchymal to epithelial transformation remaining joined to each other via N-cadherin mediated apical adherens junctions. Cells remain associated with fibronectin on their basal surfaces; N-CAM localizes to the lateral cell membranes.[7] During this epithelialization process, the cells become "locked-in" place. The cell shape change is accompanied by phenotypic changes characteristic of myocardiocytes: myofibrillogenesis and electrical activity. Myofibrillogenesis is subsequently detected on the apical side of the cells in association with N-cadherin. This N-cadherin mediated cardiac compartmentalization and myofibrillogenesis can be arrested by exposure to an N-cadherin perturbing antibody both in vivo and in vitro.[8,9] The inhibitory affects on myofibrillogenesis are also seen in the *N-cadherin null* embryo,[10] in which only a weakly contractile heart is formed. The embryos die around day 9 of gestation, a stage when heart function becomes vital. That the cardiac compartment does form at all in the *null* embryo is rather surprising and may indicate that in the mouse weaker interactions provided possibly by other cadherins may compensate in guiding compartmentalization during morphogenesis.

We have proposed a model whereby the bilateral, anterior mesoderm initially is pluripotent (Fig. 2). Subsequently, at stages 4/5, boundary development specified by N-cadherin/β-catenin defines three populations of cells: the dorsal, somatic cells; the cells at the boundary that form phenotypic myocardiocytes as they epithelialize; and the more ventral cells excluded from the myocardiocyte compartment and localizing nearest the fibronectin rich endoderm surface will differentiate into endocardiocytes and down-regulate N-cadherin.[8]

Calcium signaling may be involved in activation pathways leading to cardiac cell differentiation. Between stages 5 and 7, ouabain, an inhibitor of Na/K-ATPase and a marker of the cardiac cell polarized phenotype, reversibly inhibits cardiac cell sorting, arrests coelom formation, heart development, and differentiation.[11] At stage 8, this inhibition is no longer observed. Ouabain is known to exert its effects by increasing intracellular Ca^{2+} levels. To visualize relative calcium levels in the heart field we preloaded stage 5 to 7 chick embryos using Fluo-3-AM (acetoxymethyl) ester fluorescent calcium indicator (Molecular Probes, Inc., Eugene, Ore) and subsequently stimulated the embryos with either acetylcholine or 5 mM Ca^{2+}. During stimulation, cells of the undifferentiated heart forming regions, visualized with a Leica scanning UV confocal microscope over a 60-sec period after stimulation, were observed to have higher intracellular Ca^{2+} levels than cells in neighboring areas (unpublished observations). The latter together with observance of ouabain arrest suggest that Ca^{2+} concentration based signaling is also involved in cardiac differentiation. In corroboration it was reported that *Nkx 2.5* and *Hox d-3* expression is decreased in ouabain treated cardiogenic explants, if removed at early stages, but not after stage 7/8.[12] Additionally, in the embryo N-cadherin mediated adhesion may be associated with the observed increased intracellular calcium concentrations: during neurite growth, N-cadherin signaling involves cell type-specific Ca^{2+} changes in responding cells.[13]

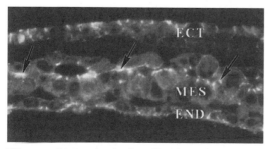

Figure 1. β-catenin localization shown. See arrows.

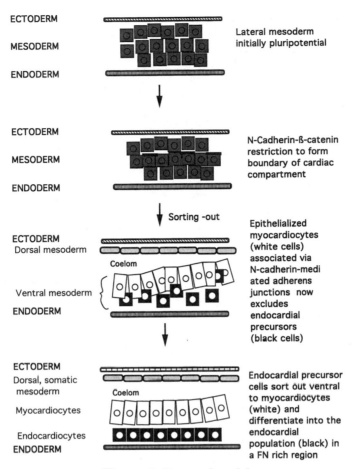

Figure 2. Proposed model.

Cell-Matrix Interactions and Heart Looping

Fibronectin (FN) is one of the first extracellular matrix (ECM) molecules to be detected in the stage 5 chick embryo at the precardiac mesoderm/endoderm interface at the same time period described above.[14] During compartmentalization FN is present in an A/P gradient across the chick heart fields. That a similar gradient is not readily visualized in the mouse does not mean that it never existed. Due to a much steeper gradient of heart development in the mouse, such a gradient may not be as easily detectable, as it is in the chick. No sooner have the cells epithelialized in the chick, then asymmetry of the ECM is detected in the heart fields by the expression of flectin (FL), a newly identified ECM molecule, localizing primarily in the left heart-forming compartment.[15] FL is also secreted at the myocardial/endoderm interface colocalizing with FN. The asymmetry of flectin is maintained throughout the looping stages. Flectin appears to be synthesized chiefly by myocardial cells, as are many other components of the cardiac jelly ECM.[16] In the mouse, flectin is initially symmetrical and only during looping becomes asymmetrical (see chapter 8; see also Reference 17).

Subsequently, the cardiac jelly matrix becomes highly organized. FL-FN interactions often colocalize. If FN-cell interactions are perturbed using RGD-synthetic peptides, then FL expression is repressed in the cardiac jelly and heart looping becomes randomized (see Chapter 8). FN appears to stabilize flectin within specific regions of the ECM due to protein-protein interactions, as transcription of flectin is not changed.

In summary, our studies indicate that cell adhesion and matrix molecules, themselves products of gene signaling, are in turn critical to coordinate signaling during differentiation of cardiomyocytes and morphogenesis of the heart. Among the vertebrates the same molecules tend to be involved in these processes, but their spatiotemporal patterning may show modifications.

References

1. Schultheiss TM, Xydas X, Lassar AB. Induction of avian cardiac myogenesis by anterior endoderm. *Development* 1995;121: 4203–4214.
2. Kelley C, Blumberg H, Zon LI, et al. GATA-4 is a novel transcription factor expressed in endocardium of the developing heart. *Development* 1993;118:817–827.
3. Laverriere AC, MacNeill C, Mueller C, et al. GATA-4/5/6, a subfamily of three transcription factors transcribed in developing heart and gut. *J Biol Chem* 1994;269: 23177–23184.
4. Molkentin JD, Kalvakolanu DV, Markham BE. Transcription factor GATA-4 regulates cardiac muscle-specific expression of the alpha-myosin heavy-chain gene. *Mol Cell Biol* 1994;14:4947–4957.
5. Sugi Y, Lough J. Activin-A and FGF-2 mimic the inductive effects of anterior endoderm on terminal cardiac myogenesis in vitro. *Dev Biol* 1995;168:567–574.
6. Schultheiss TM, Burch JB, Lassar AB. A role for bone morphogenetic proteins in the induction of cardiac myogenesis. *Genes Dev* 1997;11:451–462.
7. Linask KK. N-cadherin localization in early heart development and polar expression of Na+,K(+)-ATPase, and integrin during pericardial coelom formation and epithelialization of the differentiating myocardium. *Dev Biol* 1992;151:213–224.
8. Linask KK, Knudsen KA, Gui YH. N-cadherin-catenin interaction: necessary component of cardiac cell compartmentalization during early vertebrate heart development. *Dev Biol* 1997;185:148–164.
9. Imanaka-Yoshida K, Knudsen K, Linask KK. N-cadherin is required for the differentiation and initial myofibrillogenesis of chick cardiomyocytes. *Cell Motil Cytoskeleton* 1998;39:52–62.
10. Radice GL, Rayburn H, Matsunami H, et al. Developmental defects in mouse embryos lacking N-cadherin. *Dev Biol* 1997; 181:64–78.
11. Linask KK, Gui YH. Inhibitory effects of ouabain on early heart development and cardiomyogenesis in the chick embryo. *Dev Dynamics* 1995;203:93–105.
12. Searcy RD, Yutzey KE. Analysis of Hox gene expression during early avian heart development. *Dev Dynamics* 1998;213:82–91.
13. Bixby JL, Grunwald GB, Bookman RJ. Ca2+ influx and neurite growth in response to purified N-cadherin and laminin. *J Cell Biol* 1994;127:1461–1475.
14. Linask KK, Lash JW. Precardiac cell migration: fibronectin localization at mesoderm-endoderm interface during directional movement. *Dev Biol* 1986;114: 87–101.
15. Tsuda T, Philp N, Zile MH, et al. Left-right asymmetric localization of flectin in the extracellular matrix during heart looping. *Dev Biol* 1996;173:39–50.
16. Manasek FJ. Glycoprotein synthesis and tissue interactions during establishment of the functional embryonic chick heart. *J Mol Cell Cardiol* 1976;8:389–402.
17. Tsuda T, Majumder K, Linask KK. Differential expression of flectin in the extracellular matrix and left-right asymmetry in mouse embryonic heart during looping stages. *Dev Genetics* 1998;23(3):203–214.

26

The Role of the Extracellular Proteases in Cardiac Development

*Thomas K. Borg, PhD, Stephanie Baer, BS,
Taj Burnside, BS, and Wayne Carver, PhD*

The development, organization, and function of organ systems are dependent upon the interaction of both intrinsic and extrinsic factors. Among the extrinsic factors critical to these processes are the components of the extracellular matrix (ECM). Previous studies by our laboratory and others have demonstrated that there is a coordinated regulation of the expression of ECM components, their specific receptors on the cell surface, and the growth and differentiation response by the different cellular systems of the heart.[1,2]

The ECM is composed of a diverse complex of macromolecules including collagens, proteoglycans, noncollagenous glycoproteins, growth factors, and proteases. Initially, studies indicated that the ECM merely provided mechanical scaffolding as a frame work for organogenesis; however, it is now recognized that the ECM exists in a dynamic equilibrium with cellular growth and function.[3]

Many of the ECM components exist as large macromolecules (> 200 kDa) yet signaling molecules tend to be much smaller in size (< 40 kDa). Proteolytic action on the large, latent macromolecules is necessary to release biologically active fragments. This principle was first

shown with fibronectin.[4] When fibronectin was treated with trypsin, smaller molecular weight biologically active fragments were released. These peptides stimulated cell adhesion, DNA binding, and cell binding regions. Active fragments have also been observed in other ECM molecules including laminin and collagen. Growth factors, such as transforming growth factor β, are another class of ECM macromolecules that require activation.

Candidate molecules for the proteolytic action on ECM macromolecules are the extracellular proteases. There are basically 4 classes of proteolytic enzymes that are involved in degradation of ECM substrates including: (a) serine; (b) cysteine; (c) asparate; and (d) metalloproteases. These proteases are secreted as latent forms and require proteolytic action to express the active form. Coordinate secretion of associated inhibitors of these proteases is thought to also be important to their regulation.

Both serine proteases (tissue plasminogen activator, tPA and urokinase plasminogen activator uPA) and the metalloproteases (MMP) have been demonstrated to have potential importance in the morphogenesis of the heart.[5,6] In addition, another class of molecules known as the A disintegrin and metalloprotease (ADAMs) are a family of at least 22 membranes of membrane bound proteases that have been shown to be important in cell-

From Clark EB, Nakazawa M, Takao A (eds.): Etiology and Morphogenesis of Congenital Heart Disease: Twenty Years of Progress in Genetics and Developmental Biology. Armonk, NY: Futura Publishing Co., Inc.; © 2000.

ECM interactions in development. In the present study we have examined the expression of the MMPs, associated tissue inhibitor of metalloprotease (TIMP), and ADAMS by reverse-transcriptase polymerase chain reaction (RT-PCR), in situ hybridization, and immunofluorescence microscopy.

MMP-2 and MMP-9 were expressed in the cardiac cushions and myocardium respectively. TIMP showed a similar pattern with the MMP expression. These data are similar to that reported in neonatal cells in which myocytes expressed primarily MMP-9 and fibroblasts MMP-2.[7] Expression of these MMPs suggests that they could be active in the proteolysis of ECM that could be important in the regulation of morphogenesis. Inhibition of the MMP-2 in vitro has been shown to block cellular functions such as migration and collagen gel contraction.

RT-PCR for the ADAM proteins showed that ADAM-2, -6, -10, and -12 were present in the myocardium by 10.5 days of gestation. Because ADAM-12 has previously been shown to be related to skeletal muscle development, we examined its expression during cardiac development. ADAM-12 was present as early as 10.5 and continued through day 5 of neonatal development. Examination of normal adult rodent heart showed that the expression was markedly lower than at these times of development. In situ hybridization and immunofluorescence microscopy showed that ADAM-12 was primarily associated with the myocardium and that there was very little expression on the atrioventricular or outflow tract cushions.

These studies document the expression of extracellular proteases that appear to be coordinated with cardiac development. Further studies will be necessary to determine substrate specificity and to analyze the biological activity of the proteolytic action of these proteases.

References

1. Borg TK, Terracio L, Rubin K, et al. The cell biology of the cardiac interstitium. *Trends Cardiovasc Med* 1995;6:65–70.
2. Rubin K, Gullberg D, Tomasini-Johansson B, et al. In: Comer WD, ed. *Structure and Function of the Extracellular Matrix of Connective Tissue. Part II. Molecular Components.* Harwood, NY: Academic Press; 1996.
3. Borg TK, Nakagawa M, Carver W, et al. Extracellular matrix, receptors and heart development. In: Clark EB, Markwald RR, Takao A, eds. *Developmental Mechanisms of Heart Disease.* Armonk, NY: Futura Publishing; 1995.
4. Ruoslahti E, Bierschbacher M, Engvall E, et al. Molecular and biological interactions of fibronectin. *J Invest Dermatol* 1982; 79(suppl 1):65s–68s.
5. Nakagawa M, Terracio L, Carver W, et al. Expression of metalloprotease and IL-1α in the developing rat heart. *Dev Dynamics* 1992;195:87–99.
6. McQuire PG, Orkin RW. Urokinase activity in the developing avain heart: A spatial and temporal analysis. *Dev Dynamics* 1992;193:24–33.

27

Role of NFATc in Semilunar Valve Development

Bin Zhou, MD, PhD, Ann Ranger, PhD, Laurie Glimcher, PhD, and H. Scott Baldwin, MD

Although factors regulating atrioventricular valve formation have been extensively studied,[1] relatively little is known about factors regulating development of the semilunar valves. Many of the studies to date have focused on morphological alterations in the outflow tract resulting in leaflet and sinuous formation. These include studies of restricted endothelial cell proliferation overlying the conotruncal ridges, endothelial cell death in the expanding endothelial ridge of the arterial face of the outflow tract and remodeling of the extracellular matrix to form the fibrous skeleton of valve leaflets.[2-4] Another major distinction of outflow tract morphogenesis is the potential contribution of cardiac neural crest.[5] However, little is known about the molecular regulation of aortic and pulmonary valve formation. The following summarizes some of our recent studies implicating nuclear factor of activated T cells (NFATc) as a critical factor in this important developmental event.

From Clark EB, Nakazawa M, Takao A (eds.): Etiology and Morphogenesis of Congenital Heart Disease: Twenty Years of Progress in Genetics and Developmental Biology. Armonk, NY: Futura Publishing Co., Inc.; © 2000.

NFATc Is a Transcription Factor With Multiple Functions and Diffuse Expression

NFATc is a member of NFAT family, which are well-known transcription factors involved in the upregulated expression of multiple cytokines in activated T cells.[6] Four isoforms of NFAT with a high degree of homology to each other are known: NFATc, NFATp, NFAT4/x/c3, and NFAT3. In quiescent T cells, NFATs exist as a phosphorylated form in the cytoplasm, upon activation through the T cell receptor, it is dephosphorylated in response to increased intracellular calcium levels and activation of the phosphatase, calcineurin, and then translocated to the nucleus. In the nucleus, NFAT forms complexes with AP-1 family members on purine-rich enhancer elements of specific genes, leading to transcription activation of various cytokine and growth factors. The phosphatase activity of calcineurin is blocked by the immunosuppressive drugs, cyclosporine A (CSA) and FK506,[7,8] thereby preventing the nuclear translocation of NFAT and subsequent activation of cytokine gene transcription. It is the inhibition of NFAT nuclear translocation that is thought to provide the major immunosuppressive effect of these drugs. The first evidence for the existence of NFATs was derived from analysis of antigen-responsive enhancer elements in the cytokine IL-2 gene promoter in lymphocytes[9] and expression of the NFATs was initially thought to be restricted to the immune system. However, NFAT expression and function has been described in several types of non-lymphoid cells[10,11] including vascular endothelial cells,[12,13] vascular smooth muscle cells,[14] and skeletal muscle cells.[15,16] Thus, NFATc may play important roles in signal transduction and gene expression in nonimmune tissues in vivo. Indeed, constitutive expression of calcineurin causes heart failure, where another membrane of NFAT family, NFAT3, has been documented to activate a subset of hypertrophic response genes.[17] Conversely, FK506, a calcineurin inhibitor, may prevent cardiac hypertrophy.[18]

NFATc-1 Is Required for Semilunar Valve Formation

To determine whether the NFATc1 protein had unique functions in vivo, the NFATc gene was disrupted in embryonic stem cells by homologous recombination replacing the Rel homology domain with a neomycin resistance gene resulting in a frame shift mutation.[19] Two different embryonic stem (ES) cell clones (141 and 112) resulted in successful targeting. Following blastocyst injection, mice heterozygous for the disrupted allele were intercrossed to generate NFATc(−/−) mice. Of 181 pups born, no homozygous and a slightly lower number of heterozygous than expected were obtained, suggesting that NFATc is required for survival. Serial timed matings revealed the expected mendelian ratios (+/+), (+/−), and (−/−) animals between E 8.5 and

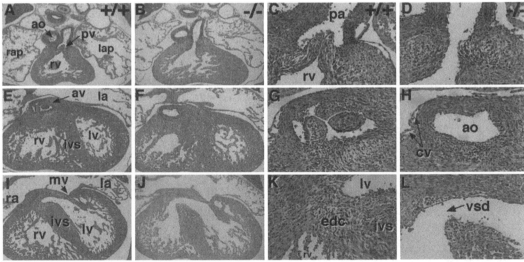

Figure 1. Histological analysis of E14.5 wild-type and NFATc mutant embryos. **A, B.** Show low-power magnification of comparable cross-sections through the right ventricular outflow tracts (rv) of wild-type (**A**) and mutant (**B**) embryos. **C, D.** Show high-power magnification of comparable cross-sections through the left ventricular outflow tract (lv) of wild-type (**E**) and null-mutant (**F**) embryos. High-power magnifications document severe defects in formation of the aortic valve leaflets (av) in the null-mutant embryos (**H**) when compared to control (**G**). Defects were also seen in the interventricular septum of mutant (**J, L**) but not wild-type (**I, K**) embryos. Ao, aorta; pv, pulmonary vein; aps, aorticopulmonary septum; pa, pulmonary artery; cv, coronary vessels; ra, right atrium; rap, right atrial appendage; la, left atrium; lap, left atrial appendage; mv, mitral valve; edc, endocardial cushion. See color appendix.

12.5. However, from E13.5-E17.5 increasingly fewer live (–/–) embryos and no (–/–) live births were detected. By E14.5 (–/–) embryos appeared pale and edematous with frequent pericardial effusions and abdominal hemorrhages. The timing of demise and appearance suggested a primary cardiac abnormality.[20] A thorough examination of mutant embryos at E13.5 and E14.5 revealed a consistent pattern of defects which included conspicuous absence of both the pulmonary and aortic valve leaflets (Fig. 1) with normal formation of aorticopulmonary septum resulting in a clearly defined right ventricular/pulmonary outflow separated from the left ventricular or aortic outflow. In addition, there was a defect in the superior margin of the intraventricular septum. Of note, there were no defects in formation of the compact ventricular myocardium, ventricular trabeculation, epicardial morphogenesis, or coronary vascularization. A complementary set of experiments by de la Pampa and colleagues revealed similar observations documenting the pivotal role of NFATc in outflow tract morphogenesis.[21]

NFATc Is Expressed in AVC Endothelial Cells but not Required for Mitral or Tricuspid Valve Formation

In order to define the temporal and tissue specific distribution of NFATc during cardiovascular development, we utilized a monoclonal antibody (mAb) specific for the endothelial cell adhesion molecule PECAM-1[22] and a mAb specific for NFATc1 (generous gift of Dr. Gerald

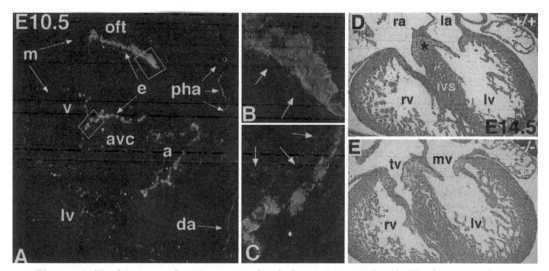

Figure 2. Dual-immunofluorescent confocal photomicrographs (**A–C**) of a sagittal section through the heart of an E10.5 embryo utilizing a monoclonal antibody to PECAM-1 (green, FITC-labeled secondary antibody) in combination with a monoclonal antibody to NFATc1 (red, Cy5-labeled secondary antibody). NFATc expression is restricted to the endocardium of the heart (a, ventricle; avc, atrioventricular canal; v, ventricle; oft, outflow tract) and was not detected in endothelial cells outside the heart (lvr, liver; da, dorsal aorta; pha, pharyngeal arch). A higher-power magnification of the oft (**B**) and avc (**C**) documents the nuclear localization of NFATc in the endocardium and the down regulation of NFATc in endothelial cells that have undergone mesenchymal transformation (arrows). Photomicrographs through the mitral (mv) and tricuspid (tv) valve region of an E14.5 wild type (**D**) and null mutant (**E**) embryo demonstrating no qualitative defects in valve formation. (ra, right atrium; la, left atrium; rv, right ventricle; lv, left ventricle). See color appendix.

Crabtree) for double immunofluorescent labeling of wild-type and mutant embryos during critical periods of valve formation in the E10.5 embryo. As summarized in Figure 2A–C, coimmunolocalization of PECAM-1 (green) and NFATc (red) demonstrated conclusively that NFATc expression was restricted to the endocardium of the heart. Although there was an accentuation of NFATc expression in the endocardium of the outflow tract and atrioventricular canal (AVC) region, attenuated expression was also seen in the endocardium lining the ventricular trabeculae. In addition, no NFATc was detected in endothelium outside the heart as demonstrated by the absence of detectable fluorescence in the pharyngeal arch arteries, dorsal aorta, and liver.

Of particular importance, *no* expression was detected in the endothelial cells that had transformed into mesenchyme and begun invasion of the extracellular matrix (Fig. 2B, C) suggesting that NFATc is not primarily involved in maintenance of the mesenchymal phenotype. Further, it can be seen that although PECAM expression is limited to the cell membrane, NFATc expression is clearly nuclear, suggesting that it is in an active, dephosphorylated form. Histological evaluation of the outflow tract endocardial cushions (or conotruncal ridges) of wild type and mutant embryos at E11.5 (data not shown) confirmed that there were no qualitative defects in endothelial transformation, migration, or proliferation of mesenchyme within the extracellular matrix of the conotruncal ridges. Furthermore, examination of the AVC at E14.5 (Fig. 2D, E) revealed no gross abnormalities of the mitral or tricuspid valve in mutant embryos when compared to the wild type litter mates. Unlike our studies, del la Pompa and colleagues detected subtle abnormalities in AVC endocardial cushion formation.[21] Although this discrepancy could reflect strain variability, the exact reason for the difference in phenotypic alterations has not yet been determined.

NFATc Expression Is Restricted to the Endocardium and Present at the Onset of Endocardial Differentiation

To determine the timing of NFATc expression during cardiac development we performed dual fluorescence confocal microscopic analysis on E8.5 (straight heart tube stage) embryos as described above. As in the E10.5 embryo above, NFATc expression was restricted to the endocardium of the heart and no expression was detected in other endothelial cell populations. Of note, NFATc expression was localized to the nucleus consistent with dephosphorylated active form at least 24 hours prior to the first detectable evidence of valve formation as noted by endothelial transformation. Further RT-PCR analysis with NFATc specific primers demonstrated expression in the embryo at E7.5, the period of initial endocardial and myocardial differentiation from the mesoderm.[23] This burst of NFATc expression was temporally restricted to active cardiac development and could not be detected in the E13.5 heart by RT-PCR or immunohistochemistry (not shown). To our knowledge, the observations document NFATc to be the only endocardial specific transcription factor identified to date.

Known Targets of NFATc Activation Are Not Expressed in the Developing Heart During Semilunar Valve Formation

To determine if there were alterations in the expression of known targets of NFATc activation in null mutant embryos that might explain the defects observed, we utilized a multiprobe RNAse protection assay. This assay contained templates to most of the known downstream targets of NFATc activation that have be described in the adult immune system.[6] For these studies, RNA was extracted from the outflow tracts of E12.5 wild type, heterozygote, and NFATc null mutant embryos as well as outflow tracts from a mouse strain not used in development of the targeting construct or generation of null mutant mice. Much to our surprise, there was *no* detectable expression in many of these NFATc targets in the developing out flow tract at this critical time point in semilunar valve formation. In addition, whereas expression of all TGFβ isoforms was easily identified, there were no substantive alterations in expression in either heterozygous or null mutant NFATc mutant embryos when compared with wild type controls. Because TGFβ expression in the developing conotruncus has been implicated as a potential regulator of outflow tract morphogenesis,[24] detectable expression served as an intrinsic positive control for these reactions. These data would suggest that target(s) of NFATc1 activation responsible for the defects in semilunar valve morphogenesis observed in the null mutant embryos are either novel proteins or are known proteins not previously documented to be effected by NFATc.

Summary

These observations document that NFATc is required for normal semilunar valve development and suggest that molecular regulation of valve formation in the outflow tract is distinct from that in the AVC as mitral and tricuspid valve formation were not severely affected in the null mutation. However, the mechanism of NFATc dependent valve formation remains obscure. Preliminary evidence suggests that both the activation of NFATc as well as its down stream targets are different than those delineated in the immune system and may indeed be unique to the developing heart. In addition, these experiments establish NFATc as a unique marker of endocardial differentiation and suggest that the endocardium develops as a distinct subpopulation of vascular endothelium from the onset of mesodermal differentiation. Experiments to define the critical components of NFATc mediated endocardial differentiation and semilunar valve formation are currently underway.

References

1. Eisenberg LM, Markwald RR. Molecular regulation of atrioventricular valvuloseptal morphogenesis. *Circ Res* 1995;77:1–6.
2. Maron BJ, Hutchins GM. The development of the semilunar valves in the human heart. *Am J Pathol* 1974;74:331–334.
3. Hurle JM, Colvee E, Blanco AM. Development of mouse semilunar valves. *Anat Embryol Berl* 1980;160:83–91.
4. Ya J, van den Hoff MJB, de Boer PAJ, et al. The normal development of the outflow tract in the rat. In: Normal and Abnormal Development of the Outflow Tract of the Embryonic Heart. Dept. of Anatomy and Embryology, Amsterdam. (thesis) 1997: 64–94.
5. Noden DM, Poelmann RE, Gittenberger-de Groot AC. Cell origins and tissue boundaries during outflow tract development. *Trends Cardiovasc Med* 1995;5:69–75.
6. Rao A, Luo C, Hogan PG. Transcription factors of the NFAT family: Regulation and function. *Annu Rev Immunol* 1997;15:707–747.
7. Flanagan WM, Corthesy B, Bram RJ, et al. Nuclear association of a T-cell transcription factor blocked by FK-506 and cyclosporin A. *Nature* 1991;352:803–807.
8. Beals CR, Clipstone NA, Ho SN, et al. Nuclear localization of NFATc by a calcineurin-dependent, cyclosporin-sensitive intramolecular interaction. *Genes Dev* 1997;11:824–834.
9. Durand D, Shaw J, Bush M, et al. Characterization of antigen receptor response elements within the interleukin-2 enhancer. *Mol Cell Biol* 1988;8:1715–1724.
10. Weiss DL, Hural J, Tara D, et al. Nuclear factor of activated T cells is associated with a mast cell interleukin 4 transcription complex. *Mol Cell Biol* 1996;16:228–235.
11. Ho AM, Jain J, Rao A, et al. Expression of the transcription factor NFATp in a neuronal cell line and in the murine nervous system. *J Biol Chem* 1994;269:28181–28186.
12. Cockerill GW, Bert AG, Ryan GR, et al. Regulation of granulocyte-macrophage colony-stimulating factor and E-selectin expression in endothelial cells by cyclo-

sporin A and the T-cell transcription factor NFAT. *Blood* 1995;7:2689–2698.

13. Boss V, Wang X, Koppelman LF, et al. Histamine induces nuclear factor of activated T cell-mediated transcription and cyclosporin A-sensitive interleukin-8 mRNA expression in human umbilical vein endothelial cells. *Mol Pharmacol* 1998;54:264–272.

14. Boss V, Abbott KA, Wang X-F, et al. Expression of the cyclosporin A-sensitive factor NFAT in cultured vascular smooth muscle cells: Differential induction of NFAT-mediated transcription by phospholipase C-coupled cell surface receptors. *J Biol Chem* 1998;273:19664–19671.

15. Abbot KL, Friday B, Thaloor D, et al. Activation, and cellular localization of the cyclosporine A-sensitive transcription factor NFAT in skeletal muscle cells. *Mol Biol Cell* 1998;9:2905–2916.

16. Chin ER, Olson EN, Richardson JA, et al. A calcineurin-dependent transcriptional pathway controls skeletal muscle fiber type. *Genes Dev* 1998;12:2499–2509.

17. Molkentin JD, Lu JR, Antos CL, et al. A calcineurin-dependent transcriptional pathway for cardiac hypertrophy. *Cell* 1998;93:215–228.

18. Sussman MA, Lim HW, Gude N, et al. Prevention of cardiac hypertrophy in mice by calcineurin inhibition. *Science* 1998; 281:1690–1693.

19. Ranger AM, Grusby MJ, Hodge MR, et al. The transcription factor NFATc is essential for cardiac valve formation. *Nature* 1998 12;392(6672):186–90.

20. Copp AJ. Death before birth: Clues from gene knockouts and mutations. *Trends Genetics* 1995;11:87–93.

21. de la Pompa JL, Timmerman LA, Takimoto H, et al. Role of the NFATc transcription factor in morphogenesis of cardiac valves and septum. *Nature* 1998;392:182–186.

22. Baldwin HS, Shen HM, Chung A, et al. Platelet endothelial cell adhesion molecule-1 (PECAM-1/CD31): Alternatively spliced, functionally distinct isoforms expressed during mammalian cardiovascular development. *Development* 1994;120:2539–2553.

23. Baldwin HS, Jensen KL, Solursh M. Myogenic cytodifferentiation of the precardiac mesoderm in the rat. *Differentiation* 1991; 47:163–172.

24. Dickson MC, Slager HG, Duffie E, et al. RNA and protein localisations of TGF beta 2 in the early mouse embryo suggest an involvement in cardiac development. *Development* 1993;117:625–639.

28

Cell-Cell and Cell-Matrix Adhesions During Formation and Arrangement of Developing Cardiac Myofibrils

Isao Shiraishi, MD, Tetsuro Takamatsu, MD, Zenshiro Onouchi, MD, and Thomas K. Borg, PhD

We have previously studied three-dimensional observation of myofibrillogenesis and expression of N-cadherin, fibronectin before and during looping of the whole-mounted chicken embryonic heart tubes by using a confocal scanning laser microscope.[1-4] From the early stage of myofibrillogenesis, myofibrils connected at cell membranes. They constituted random networks in the outer layer of myocardial cells and circumferential alignments at the bottom of the inner myocardial layer cells facing the cardiac jelly. N-cadherin constituted cell-cell junctions of developing myofibrils. Fibrils of fibronectin, together with thick actin bundles at the bottom of the inner layer, temporally aligned in the circumferential direction of the heart tube. These findings indicate that the arrangement of myofibrils develops in association with changing cell-cell and cell-matrix adhesions.

The phosphorylation of tyrosine residues on proteins (P-Tyr) is thought to participate in regulating cell-cell and cell-matrix adhesion and to organize the cytoskeletal actin bundles.[5] A high concentration of P-Tyr is detected during embryogenesis and may play an integral role in cell growth, division, and differentiation.[6] However, the precise localization and role of P-Tyr during initial cardiac myofibrillogenesis of normal embryonic tissue is uncertain. We discussed here the temporal and spatial immunolocalization of P-Tyr during myofibrillogenesis of the chicken embryonic heart tube by means of confocal laser scanning microscopy.[7]

Six- to Seven-Somite Stages

Along the apical region of outer myocardial cells, continuous "belt-like" sites of P-Tyr were present. "Punctate" immunolocalization of P-Tyr was also observed along the "belt-like" sites and other cell-cell boundaries of the outer and inner layer cells. Along the basal surface of the inner myocardial cells facing the cardiac jelly, faint staining of "punctate" P-Tyr was diffusely present. This was coincident with cortical fine actin filaments.

Eight- to Ten-Somite Stages

Along the "belt-like" sites of P-Tyr localization and other cell-cell boundaries of both layers, the "punctate" immunostaining of P-Tyr become more intense and constitutes a "clumped" expression

From Clark EB, Nakazawa M, Takao A (eds.): Etiology and Morphogenesis of Congenital Heart Disease: Twenty Years of Progress in Genetics and Developmental Biology. Armonk, NY: Futura Publishing Co., Inc.; © 2000.

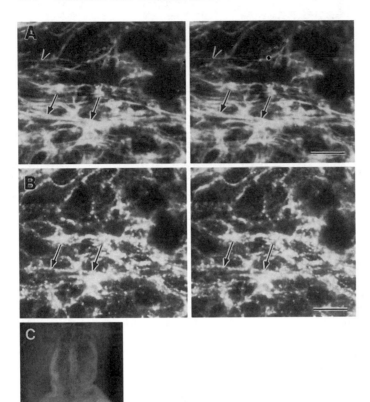

Figure 1. A and **B.** Stereoscopic images at the bottom of the inner myocardial cell layer of a 9-somite stage embryo stained with phalloidin (**A**) and anti-P-Tyr antibody (**B**). Particulate P-Tyr immunolabeling (**B**, arrows) are aligned with thick actin bundles (**A**, arrows). Note that serial particulate P-Tyr immunolabeling cannot be detected at the site of immature myofibrils with small periodic dots (**A**, arrowheads), which represents a more advanced phase of myofibril formation than thick actin bundles. **C.** Non-confocal image of the heart tube. Bars 8 μ. (Reproduced with permission from Reference 7.)

pattern. Along the basal surface of the inner myocardial cell layer, the "punctate" P-Tyr immunostaining also become more intense. Some sites of P-Tyr immunolabeling, together with thick actin bundles, were serially oriented circumferentially around the heart tube. However, immature myofibrils with incomplete striation were not accompanied by intense P-Tyr staining (Fig. 1).

Eleven- to Thirteen-Somite Stages

The "belt-like" pattern and the "clump-type" arrangement of P-Tyr at the cell-cell boundaries become more intense. These P-Tyr "clumps" constituted intercalated disks terminating striated myofibrils. Along the basal surface of the inner layer cells facing the cardiac jelly, serially aligned "particulate" P-Tyr immunostain-

ing decreased, although mature striated myofibrils increased.

Tyrosine Phosphorylation at Sites of Cell-Cell Adhesion

Co-localization of P-Tyr with F-actin in continuous "belt-like" patterns at the apical region of the outer layer cells corresponds to the adhesion belt. Dominant phosphorylated substrates at the adhesion belt, nonjunctional cell contact, and early intercalated disks are thought to be catenins, which modulate the binding of cadherin-containing complexes to actin filaments.[8] The tight junction protein ZO-1[9] at adhesion belt, gap junction protein connexins[10] are also phosphorylated on tyrosine residues during differentiation. P-Tyr at the junctional complex appears to be involved in maintaining the sheet-like appearance of the outer layer cells during the period of rapid differentiation.

"Punctate" P-Tyr immunolocalization at cell-cell boundaries, other than the apical region of the outer layer, corresponds to isolated adherens junctions, gap junctions, or nonjunctional cell contacts. "Clumped-type" P-Tyr expression localized at the cell-cell junction of developing myofibrils corresponds to early intercalated disks. P-Tyr at the developing intercalated disks may play a role in modulation of cell-cell junctions and the differentiation and rapid increase in site of nascent myofibrils.

Tyrosine Phosphorylation at Areas of Cell-Matrix Adhesion

The temporal and serially aligned "particulate" P-Tyr at the basal surface of the inner layer cells may play a role in assembling circumferentially-aligned developing myofibrils. The major tyrosine kinase substrates concentrated at cell-matrix adhesions of non-muscle cells are paxillin[11] and focal adhesion kinase.[12] The regulated phosphorylation of tyrosine residues on these proteins may perform a critical role in controlling the rearrangement of cells and tissue cytoarchitecture

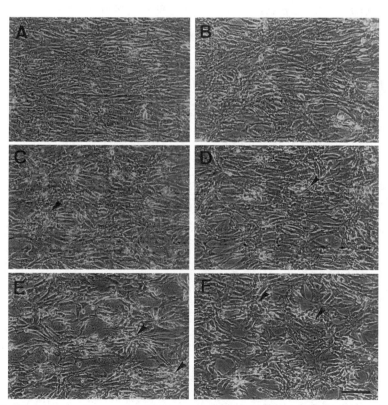

Figure 2. Phenotype of myocytes 72 hours after plating treated without (**A**) or with various sequences of ODNs. Myocytes treated with random sequence ODNs had little significant effect on alignment (**B**). Some myocytes treated with sense-1 (5'-CGA-TGCCAGTGTTTCATACG-3') and antisense-1 (5'-CGTATGAAACACTGGCATCG-3') formed clusters (**C** and **D,** arrowheads). However, parallel alignment of myocytes was basically maintained. Myocytes treated with antisense-2 (5'-GGTGGCATATCTCTCT-TCAG-3') and -3 ODN (5'-CCTTCGCAAGTCTCCTAGTT-3') revealed a disrupted alignment of myocytes (**E, F**). The cluster formation was obvious in these cells (**E** and **F,** arrowheads). Bars, 100μ. (Reproduced with permission from Reference 13.)

during development. Increases in P-Tyr levels at focal adhesions may also induce changes in cytoskeletal rearrangement. In myocytes, proteins at Z-band such as α-actinin, vinculin, talin, the β1 subunit of integrin or other costametric proteins could be temporarily phosphorylated in order to assemble and align developing myofibrils.

Antisense Oligonucleotides Complementary to Vinculin Disrupt Normal Formation and Arrangement of Myofibrils in Fetal Mouse Cardiac Myocytes

To ascertain the function of cell-matrix adhesion during the determination of cell shape and the formation of myofibrils in vitro, various sequences of antisense oligonucleotides (ODNs) complementary to vinculin were used to perturb the expression of the protein during myofibril assembly and arrangement in mouse cardiac myocytes.[13] Two different antisense oligonucleotides altered the formation of the tissue-like phenotype of myocytes cultured on aligned collagen gels[14] (Fig. 2). These antisense ODNs also suppressed vinculin protein expression at 43.5% ± 26.8% and 48.7% ± 20.9%, assembly of thick and thin actin filaments, and formation of Z-bands when compared to myocytes that were not treated. Random sequence 20-mer oligonucleotides used as controls had little detectable effect on vinculin protein expression (94.2% ± 14.8%), cell shape, normal alignment or assembly of myofibrils. This experiment indicates that vinculin-mediated cell-matrix adhesion is a critical component that functions in the determination of cell shape and the arrangement and organization of developing myofibrils.

Conclusions

Dynamic changes of cell-cell and cell-matrix adhesions play important roles during formation and arrangement of developing cardiac myofibrils.

References

1. Shiraishi I, Takamatsu T, Minamikawa T, et al. 3-D observation of actin filaments during cardiac myofibrinogenesis in chick embryo using a confocal laser scanning microscope. *Anat Embryol* 1992;185:401–408.
2. Shiraishi I, Takamatsu T, Fujita S. 3-D observation of N-cadherin expression during cardiac myofibrillogenesis of the chick embryo using a confocal laser scanning microscope. *Anat Embryol* 1993;187:115–120.
3. Shiraishi I, Takamatsu T, Fujita S. Three-dimensional observation with a confocal scanning laser microscope of fibronectin immunolabeling during cardiac looping in the chick embryo. *Anat Embryol* 1995;191:183–189.
4. Shiraishi I, Takamatsu T, Fujita S. In: Clark EB, Markwald RR, Takao A, eds. *Developmental Mechanisms of Heart Disease.* New York: Futura Publishing; 1995:471.
5. Burridge K, Turner CE, Romer LH. Tyrosine phosphorylation of paxillin and pp125FAK accompanies cell adhesion to extracellular matrix: a role in cytoskeletal assembly. *J Cell Biol* 1992;119:893–903.
6. Takata K, Singer SJ. Phosphotyrosine-modified proteins are concentrated at the membranes of epithelial and endothelial cells during tissue development in chick embryos. *J Cell Biol* 1988;106:1757–1764.
7. Shiraishi I, Takamatsu T, Fujita S. Temporal and spatial patterns of phosphotyrosine immunolocalization during cardiac myofibrillogenesis of the chicken embryo. *Anat Embryol* 1997;196:81.
8. Takeichi M. Cadherin cell adhesion receptors as a morphogenetic regulator. *Science* 1991;251:1451.
9. Kurihara H, Anderson JM, Farquhar MG. Increased Tyr phosphorylation of ZO-1 during modification of tight junctions between glomerular foot processes. *Am J Physiol* 1995;268:F514–24.
10. Musui LS, Cunningham BA, Edelman

GM, et al. Differential phosphorylation of the gap junction protein connexin43 in junctional communication-competent and -deficient cell lines. *J Cell Biol* 1990;111: 2077–2088.

11. Turner CE. Paxillin is a major phosphotyrosine-containing protein during embryonic development. *J Cell Biol* 1991;115: 201–207.

12. Schaller MD, Borgman CA, Cobb BS, et al. pp125FAK a structurally distinctive protein-tyrosine kinase associated with fo-

cal adhesions. *Proc Natl Acad Sci U S A* 1992;89:192–196.

13. Shiraishi I, Simpson DG, Carver W, et al. Vinculin is an essential component for normal myofibrillar arrangement in fetal mouse cardiac myocytes. *J Moll Cell Cardiol* 1997;29:2041.

14. Simpson DG, Terracio L, Price RL, et al. Modulation of cardiac myocyte phenotype in vitro by the composition and orientation of the extracellular matrix. *J Cell Physiol* 1994;161:89.

29

Effects of Bis-diamine on Cardiovascular Development in an Early Rat Embryo: In Vivo and in Vitro Morphologic Analyses

Masao Nakagawa, MD, Hidetoshi Fujino, MD,
Setsuko Nishijima, MD, Takashi Hanato, MD,
Masanori Kondo, MD, Nobuhiko Okamoto, MD,
Thomas K. Borg, PhD, and Louis Terracio, PhD

Bis-diamine administration to pregnant rats induces conotruncal anomalies including truncus arteriosus communis and tetralogy of Fallot.[1-4] These anomalies are often clinically associated with anomalous coronary arteries. However, the developmental anatomy of the coronary circulation system or the pathologic mechanisms of anomalous coronary arteries associated with these conotruncal defects have not been fully demonstrated. To determine whether bis-diamine induces abnormal coronary arterial development, we performed morphological analysis of coronary arteries in bis-diamine treated rat embryos. Furthermore, to examine the patho-pharmacologic effects of bis-diamine on an early developing heart, we analyzed rat embryos cultured in a medium containing bis-diamine.

The embryos treated with bis-diamine demonstrated truncus arteriosus communis in 69% and tetralogy of Fallot in 23%. Anomalous coronary arteries in-

From Clark EB, Nakazawa M, Takao A (eds.): Etiology and Morphogenesis of Congenital Heart Disease: Twenty Years of Progress in Genetics and Developmental Biology. Armonk, NY: Futura Publishing Co., Inc.; © 2000.

cluding single or extremely hypoplastic coronary arteries were seen in all embryos with these conotruncal anomalies (Fig 1). No abnormal coronary arteries were detected in the bis-diamine treated embryos with no cardiac anomaly. All embryos treated with bis-diamine also exhibited a defect of the left diaphragm.

bFGF and V-CAM were first detected in the embryonic day 13 control heart on the myocardium and epicardium. In the embryonic day 15 control heart, they were widely observed in the myocardial layers. These immunoreactivities were localized on the trabeculae and endocardial endothelial cells in the embryonic day 17 heart. On the other hand, the immunoexpressions of bFGF and V-CAM in the hearts of bis-diamine-treated embryos were reduced in each developmental stage.

Because we previously showed the usefulness of the rat whole embryo culture system to study several critical periods in mammalian heart development,[5] atrial septation and truncal looping that occurred during the culture periods were examined. No significant difference in the yolk sac diameter, crown-rump length, number of somites, or morphologic scores were detected between control and bis-

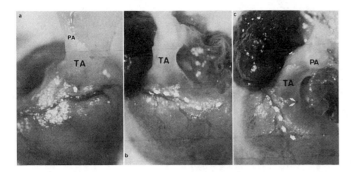

Figure 1. Truncus arteriosus communis induced by bis-diamine. Pulmonary artery (PA) is observed to originate from aorta (TA). Right coronary artery (large arrows in **a–c**) is traced by India ink injection, however, left coronary artery can not be traced. Only the ostium of the left coronary artery (small arrows) is stained with India ink.

diamine-treated embryos. However, an enlarged and dilated ventricle or winding and elongated outflow tract were observed in 19 of 23 (82.6%) bis-diamine exposed embryos (Fig. 2), but in none of the controls. Five embryos (21.7%) exhibited anomalous otic pit. Some bis-diamine-treated embryos had a hyperplastic maxilla and mandible when compared with controls.

These results indicate that bis-diamine disturbs normal development of several organs including the heart, ears, and diaphragm in the early embryonic stage. Okagawa et al.[6] showed a continuous chain of N-CAM expression between the neural crest and the fourth aortic arch via the neural plexus near the foregut in a normal embryonic day 13.5 rat embryo. Fujino et al.[7] demonstrated delayed closure of the neural tube and discontinuity of N-CAM immunoreactive chain from the neural crest to the fourth aortic arch in an embryonic day 13.5 embryo treated with bis-diamine on gestational day 10.5. Furthermore, they detected reduced N-CAM immunoreactivities in the splanchnic mesenchymal tissue around the sixth aor-

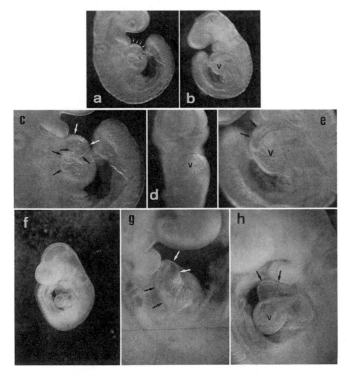

Figure 2. a–e. An embryo cultured with a medium containing bis-diamine. Elongated outflow tract (arrows) was noticed when compared with control (**f–h**). V, ventricle.

tic arch. These results suggest that bis-diamine reduced the amount of neural crest cells that appeared to participate in the aortic arch formation or truncal septation and subsequently induced cardiac defects such as persistent truncus arteriosus communis and tetralogy of Fallot. An enlarged and dilated ventricle or winding and elongated outflow tract observed in the bis-diamine exposed embryos in vitro showed early morphological changes induced by this chemical. As the coronary arteries had not appeared at this developmental stage, coronary arterial malformations may have been partly induced by abnormal truncal division. Hood and Rosenquist[8] and Poelman et al.[9] suggested the possible contribution of the neural crest cells to the coronary vascular development. Although we could not obtain evidence of neural crest cell contribution to coronary arterial formation, bis-diamine may have disrupted the role directly or indirectly by abnormal truncal division. Another important finding in the present study was the high incidence of the absent diaphragm in the bis-diamine-treated embryos. As the distributional patterns of bFGF and V-CAM were found to be different between control and bis-diamine-treated embryos, the transverse septum and epicardium were suggested to play an important role in cardiac vascular formation as suggested by Spirito et al. and Tomanek et al.[10,11] These results indicated that poor development of the transverse septum and subsequent epicardium also induced abnormal distribution of coronary arteries.

Methods

Morphological and Histological Analysis of Bis-diamine-treated Rat Embryos

A single dose of 200 mg bis-diamine was administered to pregnant Wistar rats at 10.5 days of gestation. The embryos were removed on gestational day 20 and used for anatomic analysis of hearts and coronary arteries. Special attention was paid to the number and site of coronary arterial ostium in the aorta and running patterns of coronary arteries. Immuno-distributional patterns of anti-bFGF and anti-V-CAM antibodies were histologically examined in the hearts of 13, 15, 17, and 20 embryonic day rat embryos from mothers treated with bis-diamine on gestational day 10.5. The immunolocalizations of bFGF and V-CAM were compared with control embryos at the same developmental stages.

Morphological Analysis of Rat Embryos Cultured With Bis-diamine

Wistar rat embryos carefully removed from mother rats on embryonic day 10.5 were transferred into a 50-mL culture bottle containing 4 mL of rat serum, 1 mL of Tyrode's solution containing NaCl (0.137 M), KCl (2.7 mM), $NaH_2PO_4 \cdot H_2O$ (3.6 mM), d-glucose (27 mM), $NaHCO_3$ (3.6 mM), $CaCl_2$ (1.36 mM), $MgCl_2$ (0.5 mM), streptomycin (0.13 mM), and 1 mg of bis-diamine. One embryo was cultured per bottle. After the embryos were exposed to bis-diamine for several hours, they were transferred into another bottle containing 4 mL of rat serum and 1 mL of Tyrode's solution. The embryos were gassed for 2 minutes in the culture bottles using a mixture of 20% O_2, 5% CO_2, and 75% N_2, and were then incubated at 37°C in a Natural Incubator (Model NIB-90, IWAKI, Funahashi, Japan). They were cultured for 24 hours following the procedures described by Cockroft and New.[12] Control embryos were cultured for 24 hours without exposure to bis-diamine. During incubation, the culture bottles were continuously rotated at 30 rpm (Rotator Model RT-50, TAITEC, Koshigaya, Japan) and were re-gassed for 2 minutes every 12 hours with a mixture of 20% O_2, 5% CO_2, and 75% N_2.

References

1. Taleporos P, Salgo MP, Oster G. Teratogenic action of a bis (dichloroacetyl) dia-

mine on rats: Patterns of malformations produced in high incidence at time-limited periods of development. *Teratology* 1978; 18:5–16.

2. Okamoto N, Satow Y, Lee JY, et al. Morphology and pathogenesis of the cardiovascular anomalies induced by bis-(dichloroacetyl) diamine in rats. In: Takao A, Nora JJ, eds. *Congenital Heart Disease: Causes and Processes.* Armonk NY: Futura Publishing Co; 1984:199–221.

3. Momma K, Ando M, Takao A. Fetal cardiac morphology of tetralogy of Fallot with absent pulmonary valve in the rat. *Circulation* 1990;82:1343–1351.

4. Kuribayashi T, Roberts WC. Teratology of Fallot, truncus arteriosus, abnormal myocardial architecture and anomalies of the aortic arch system induced by bis-diamine in rat fetuses. *J Am Coll Cardiol* 1993;21: 768–776.

5. Nakagawa M, Price RL, Chintanawonges C, et al. Analysis of heart development in cultured rat embryos. *J Mol Cell Cardiol* 1997;29:369–379.

6. Okagawa H, Nakagawa M, Shimada M. Immunolocalization of N-CAM in the heart of the early developing rat embryo. *Anat Rec* 1995;243:261–271.

7. Fujino H, Nakagawa M, Okagawa H, et al. Immunochemical distribution of N-CAM in normal and bis-diamine treated rats. *Circulation* 1996;94(suppl 1):482.

8. Hood LC, Rosenquist TH. Coronary artery development in the chick: Origin and deployment of smooth muscle cells, and the effects of neural crest ablation. *Anat Rec* 1992;234:291–300.

9. Poelman RE, Gittenberger de Groot AC, Mentink MMT, et al. Development of the cardiac coronary vascular endothelium, studied with antiendothelial antibodies, in chicken-quail chimeras. *Circ Res* 1993;73: 559–568.

10. Spirito P, Fu YM, Yu ZX, et al. Immunohistochemical localization of basic and acidic fibroblast growth factors in the developing rat heart. *Circulation* 1991;84: 322–332.

11. Tomanek RJ, Haung L, Suvarna PR, et al. Coronary vascularization during development in the rat and its relationship to basic fibroblast growth factor. *Cardiovasc Res* 1996;31:E116–E126.

12. Cockroft DL, New DAT. Abnormalities induced in cultured rat embryos by hyperthermia. *Teratology* 1978;17:277–284.

30

Possible Roles of the Tenascin Family in Early Heart Development

Kyoko Imanaka-Yoshida, MD and Teruyo Sakakura, MD

The tenascins are a family of extracellular matrix proteins. Tenascin-C, the first member of this family, is expressed in a spatiotemporally restricted pattern during morphogenesis and embryogenesis.[1] To clarify the possible roles of tenascin-C during heart development, we examined the expression of the gene using mouse lines containing the *lacZ* gene targeted to the tenascin-C locus by homologous recombination in ES cells.[2] Heterozygous mutant mice were developmentally normal, exhibited no distinct phenotypes, and expressed both *lacZ* and tenascin-C. The staining pattern of *lacZ* clearly reflected the endogenous pattern of the tenascin-C gene.

Tenascin-C initially appeared in a presomite mouse embryo at the heart forming region (Fig. 1a). At this stage, precardiac mesoderm is delineated from somatic mesoderm by the formation of the pericardial cavity. This process is dependent on the patterning of N-cadherin and catenins.[3] During cavity formation, precardiomyocytes undergo a mesenchymal epithelial transformation and differentiate into cardiomyocytes. Concomitantly, endocardial cells are delaminating from precardiac cells. The histological section of the *lacZ*-stained heart forming region demonstrated that the mesoderm cells forming the pericardial cavity were posi-

tive for *lacZ* staining. No expression was detected in the endoderm (Fig. 1b). When precardiomyocytes differentiated to express sarcomeric proteins, the expression of *lacZ* was downregulated, whereas endocardial cells continued to be positive.

The differentiating precardiac mesoderm cells form a primitive single heart tube composed of the myocardium and endocardium separated by a thick cell-free expanse of extracellular matrix (ECM) termed cardiac jelly. A subset of the endocardium of the atrioventricular canal and proximal outflow tract undergo epithelial mesenchymal transformation and invade the cardiac jelly.[4,5] Endocardial cells lined the endocardial tube and migrating cushion mesenchymal cells expressed *lacZ*. During this stage, cardiomyocytes of the outflow tract also express *lacZ*.

When the heart tube forms an S-shaped loop, cells in the septum transversum form villous projections.

Cell aggregates at apices of mesothelial projections detach and adhere to the surface of the heart tube and spread over the heart to become epicardium.[6] These epicardial cells are considered to be progenitors of coronary vessels or interstitial fibroblasts.[7,8] *LacZ* expression was observed in the mesenchymal cells of the projections of the septum transversum (Fig. 1c), however, the expression was diminished in the epicardial cells on the heart surface.

From Clark EB, Nakazawa M, Takao A (eds.): Etiology and Morphogenesis of Congenital Heart Disease: Twenty Years of Progress in Genetics and Developmental Biology. Armonk, NY: Futura Publishing Co., Inc.; © 2000.

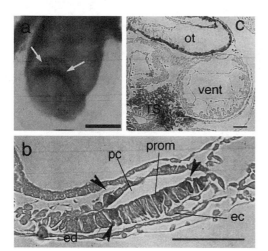

Figure 1. Whole-mount *lacZ* staining of the heterozygous mouse embryo at the presomite stage (**a**). *LacZ* staining is seen in the heart forming region (arrows). Histological section of the heart forming region (**b**) shows that mesodermal cells forming pericardial coelom are positive for *lacZ* staining (arrow heads). At E9, endocardial cells, migrating cushion mesenchymal cells, cardiomyocytes of outflow and mesenchymal cells of the projections of septum transversum express *lacZ* (**c**). Bars: 0.5 mm (**a**); 50 μm (**b** and **c**). pc, pericardial coelom; prom, procardiomyocyte; ec, endocardial cells; ed, endoderm; ot, outflow tract; vent, ventricle; TS, septum transversum

Thus, tenascin-C is transiently expressed at important steps at cardiogenesis: (1) differentiation of cardiomyocytes from the mesoderm, (2) formation of cushion tissue, (3) development of the outflow tract, and (4) migration of precursor cells of coronary arteries. These findings strongly suggest key roles of tenascin-C during early heart development. However, tenascin-C knockout mice do not show a distinct phenotype.[2] A possible explanation for this is that another member of the family compensates for the lack of tenascin-C.

A new member, tenascin-X, is ubiquitously expressed in various tissues but is most abundant in the heart and skeletal muscles. The expression of tenascin-X and tenascin-C are often reciprocal.[9] We analyzed the expression pattern of tenascin-X during heart development in normal mouse embryos by immunohistochemical examination and compared it with that of tenascin-C. Whole-mount immunohistochemistry showed that tenascin-X appears as scattered small spots on the surface of the embryonic heart on day 11. These spots increased in number and fused each other to form a network pattern which covered the surface of the heart on day 12 (Fig. 2b). Immunostaining of the histological sections of the heart demonstrated positive staining of anti-tenascin-X around epicardial cells that form vascular channels and migrate into the myocardium (Fig. 2c).

In the tenascin-C null embryo, the expression pattern of *lacZ* was identical to that of tenascin-C in wild and heterozygous embryos observed by in situ hybridization and immunostaining. Indeed, no staining for tenascin-C was seen in the tenascin-C null embryo. The expression pattern of tenascin-X was the same as that of the wild type. We did not detect the expression at *lacZ* positive sites where tenascin-C must be essentially expressed.

The reciprocal expression pattern of tenascin-C and tenascin-X suggests that different functions and collaboration of tenascins are necessary for coronary vasculogenesis; tenascin-C may play an important role in the initiation of migration of

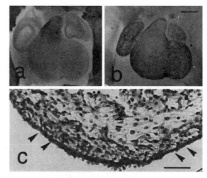

Figure 2. Whole-mount immunostaining of the hearts of a 12-day-old mouse embryo for tenascin-C (**a**) and tenascin-X (**b**). Immunostaining for tenascin-X of the histological section (**c**). Positive staining is seen at the epicardial layer (arrow heads). Bars: in (**b**) 0.5 mm for (**a**); in (**c**) 50 μm.

proepicardial cells (= precursors of coronary vessels) from the mesenchyme of the septum transversum to the surface of the primitive heart, while tenascin-X may be involved in the formation of the vascular channel by epicardial cells.

Our findings did not suggest that tenascin-X compensates for the loss of tenascin-C. Another unidentified gene may substitute for tenascin-C. Mammals likely have several compensatory pathways that effectively counterbalance deficits of matrix proteins during important processes such as embryogenesis.

Methods

Antibody

Antibodies used in this study were: polyclonal rabbit anti-tenascin-C[10]; and anti-tenascin-X.[10]

Immunohistochemistry

Whole-mount antibody staining was performed as described.[11] The rabbit anti-tenascin-C antibody was used at 1:1000 dilution, and the anti-tenascin-X antibody was used at 1:1000. Secondary antibody was peroxidase conjugated anti-rabbit IgG (MBL, Nagoya, Japan) and was used at 1:500. Immunostaining of tissue sections was performed as described.[10,12]

References

1. Chiquet-Ehrismann R, Mackie EJ, Pearson CA, et al. Tenascin: an extracellular matrix protein involved in tissue interactions during fetal development and onco-genesis. *Cell* 1986;53:383–390.

2. Saga Y, Yagi T, Ikawa Y, et al. Mice develop normally without tenascin. *Genes Dev* 1992;6:1821–1831.

3. Linask KK, Knudsen KA, Gui Y-H. N-cadherin-catenin interaction: necessary component of cardiac cell compartmentalization during early vertebrate heart development. *Dev Biol* 1997;185:148–164.

4. Markwald RR, Fitzharris TP, Smith A. Structural analysis of endocardial cytodifferentiation. *Dev Biol* 1975;42:160–180.

5. Markwald RR, Fitzharris TP, Manasek FJ. Structural development of endocardial cushions. *Am J Anat* 1977;148(1):85–119.

6. Komiyama M, Ito K, Shimada Y. Origin and development of the epicardium in the mouse embryo. *Anat Embryol* 1987;176:183–189.

7. Poelmann RE, Gittenberger-de Groot AC, Mentink MMT, et al. Development of the cardiac coronary vascular endothelium, studied with antiendothelial antibodies, in chicken-quail chimeras. *Circ Res* 1993;73:559–568.

8. Mikawa T, Fischman DA. Retroviral analysis of cardiac morphogenesis: discontinuous formation of coronary vessels. *Proc Natl Acad Sci U S A* 1992;89:9504–9508.

9. Matsumoto K, Saga Y, Ikemura T, et al. The distribution of tenascin-X is distinct and often reciprocal to that of tenascin-C. *Cell Biol* 1994;125:483–493.

10. Hasegawa K, Yoshida T, Matsumoto K, et al. Differential expression of tenascin-C and tenascin-X in human astrocytomas. *Acta Neuropathol* 1997; 93:431–437.

11. Kataoka H, Takakura N, Nishikawa S, et al. Expressions of PDGF receptor alpha, c-Kit and Flk1 genes clustering in mouse chromosome 5 define distinct subsets of nascent mesodermal cells. *Dev Growth Differ* 1997;39:729–740.

12. Kalembey I, Yoshida T, Iriyama K, et al. Analysis of tenascin mRNA expression in the murine mammary gland from embryogenesis to carcinogenesis: an in situ hybridization study. *Int J Dev Biol* 1997;41:569–573.

Section V

31

Overview: Cardiac Morphogenesis: Outflow Tract, Aortic Arch, and Conduction System

Adriana C. Gittenberger-de Groot, PhD
and Robert E. Poelmann, PhD

Introduction

Cardiac morphogenesis is a broad developmental field in which we are only grazing the surface in trying to understand the underlying mechanisms and gene regulatory cascades. Unraveling the puzzle is, however, highly intriguing and for this chapter we will try to add new data that show not only the importance of the basic building blocks of the heart being the myocardium and the endocardium but also the relevance of initially extracardiac cell contributions. These seem of particular importance for the late events in cardiac morphogenesis.

Both intra- and extracardiac components interact in aortic arch patterning, cardiac septation, and valve formation, which are essential in the formation of the four-chambered heart. This complex pumping organ is supported by the development of devices that coordinate cardiac function, consisting of the conduction system and the parasympathetic and sympathetic nervous system. Last of all, the growing complexity and increasing wall thickness necessitates the development of a coronary vasculature.

From Clark EB, Nakazawa M, Takao A (eds.): Etiology and Morphogenesis of Congenital Heart Disease: Twenty Years of Progress in Genetics and Developmental Biology. Armonk, NY: Futura Publishing Co., Inc.; © 2000.

As we will show in this chapter none of the aforementioned processes can be brought to a successful functioning substrate without the contribution, at varying points in time, of extracardiac cellular components, such as the neural crest, a newly recognized cell population derived from the ventral half of the neural tube and the cells originating from the epicardial organ. We will concentrate on the cellular contributions and origin and will rely on experimental data from either mechanically removed cells, such as seen in ablation studies, or from perturbation of their function by epigenetic factors and/or gene manipulation to deduct their relevance in normal cardiac morphogenesis.

With regard to the development of cardiac malformations it is becoming more and more clear that different pathways lead to similar malformations. It remains to be investigated whether these pathways take parallel courses, or are intertwined.

Looping and Wedging

The basis for the development of the four-chambered heart in the avian and mammalian, including the human, heart is the process of looping that leads from a not quite straight heart tube to a complex three-dimensional S-shaped heart in which the formation of a tight inner curvature[1] is instrumental.

It is not only the looping that is essential but also the shortening process of the outflow tract that brings the aortic orifice in its typical wedged-in position between the tricuspid and mitral orifice.

The three-dimensional form of the borderline between the myocardially lined outflow tract (or conotruncal region in birds) and the mesenchyme of the vessel wall already brings the future aortic side in a position that extends deeper into the inner curvature as compared to the pulmonary side of the saddle-shaped orifice level. Whether the shortening process is just a matter of growth retardation[2] or also actively under control of apoptosis as was recently shown[3] are points that deserve further study. In our studies we could not find apoptosis in the myocardial

sheath of the outflow tract, only in the endocardial outflow tract ridges without a preference for the inner or outer ridge.[4]

The mechanisms that underlie the looping process of the heart tube have been described in Chapter 16. It is evident that the maturation of the contractile myocardium and the formation of endocardial cushions from the cardiac jelly both at the atrioventricular and outflow tract level are essential in this process.

Disturbance of early myocardial contractile function, which can depend on many factors, leads to incomplete looping. The current literature on both mouse[5,6] and avian models[7–9] shows a great variety of genes that play a crucial role in myocardium-dependent loop formation. The most well-known malformation in animal models caused by such disturbance leads to a double outlet right ventricle

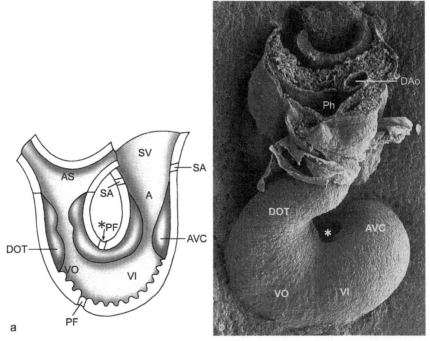

Figure 1. a. Schematic view of the internal surface of a looped heart tube showing the various segments (A, atrium; vi, ventricular inlet; VO, ventricular outlet; AS, aortic sac) and transitional zones (SV, sinus venosus; SA, sinoatrial transition; AVC, atrioventricular canal; PF, primary fold; DOT, distal outflow tract). In the inner curvature (asterisk) the future superior atrioventricular cushion and the dorsolateral outflow tract ridge are continuous. **b.** Scanning electron micrograph of an HH14 chicken embryo heart comparable to the schematic drawing. At this time point the primary fold is not visible externally. Ph, pharynx; DAo, dorsal aorta.

(DORV). This malformation is either lethal in early human development or can develop into other malformations such as isolated ventricular septal defect or transposition of the great arteries with septal defects. The observation of the development of DORV into transposition of the great arteries (TGA) has been made by the late Pexieder,[10,11] who concluded this on the basis of harvesting large series of embryos of successive ages.

The next step in development of a functioning myocardial tube is the maturation of the lining cardiac jelly. For this process a proper interaction between endocardium and myocardium is essential. Therefore, it is often unclear whether faulty endocardial cushion development based upon endocardial-mesenchymal transformation is purely endocardium derived or determined by a myocardial to endocardial interaction disturbance. At least in a number of models it has become clear that early lethality is based on inadequate formation of the endocardial cushions. It is also remarkable that lethality in this respect is more related to abnormal atrioventricular cushions compared to anomalous outflow tract cushions.

In the avian embryo looping of the heart tube (Fig. 1a, b) is a continuing process between day 2 (HH10) to day 4 (HH24) and in those stages it is only partially dependent on extracardiac cell contributions for further cardiac morphogenesis. In the mouse embryo this process is evident between day 8.5 and 12.

Genetic Markers for Cardiac Segments and Transitional Zones

Various genetic markers accompany the formation of the cardiac segmentation compartments and show expression patterns specific for the developmentally designated left and right side.[12] In general, however, these genes are only transiently compartment specific. A similar transient expression can be observed for the transitional or intersegmental zones. The sino-

atrial junction and the primary fold (Figs. 1a and 2a) express several markers, sometimes slightly different in various animal species. In general, these have in common a glycoprotein epitope stained by antibodies such as HNK1, RMO, and NCAM. As it turns out these two zones have a relation to the developing central conduction system.[12]

Three zones stand out with an inner lining of endocardial cushion tissue. For two, the atrioventricular canal and the outflow tract, this has long since been recognized. The loose mesenchymal tissue that lines the underrim of the developing atrial septum, also referred to as spina vestibuli, might also qualify as endocardial cushion(like) tissue (Fig. 2a, b).

It is in the inner curvature of the looped heart tube these endocardial cushion tissue masses (i.e., the spina vestibuli, the superior atrioventricular cushion and the dorsal outflow tract endocardial ridge) coalesce. Fusion of this endocardial tissue mass and subsequent fibrosis leads in the mammalian heart to the formation of the fibrous septum membranaceum.

The particular attention that is currently given to myocardialization of the endocardial cushions during both the atrioventricular and outflow tract cushion fusion is of value in formation of the avian heart.[13,14] In the mouse, rat and human heart this process is mainly relevant in formation of the muscular outflow tract septum.[15]

For clarity the main issues of septation of the atrium and sinus venosus, the inflow tract septation of the main body of the right and left ventricle and the outflow tract septation will be described separately.

Cardiac Septation

In cardiac septation we are dealing with three relatively independent septation processes that must coincide properly for adequate separation of the systemic and pulmonary blood flow. In normal septation both myocardial and endocardial

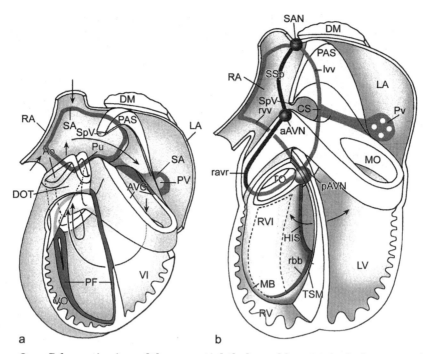

a   b

Figure 2. a. Schematic view of the more tightly looped heart tube before septation. At the atrial level the borderline with the sinus venosus is indicated by the sinoatrial transition (SA) in gray. This transition not only encircles the future superior and inferior caval vein that enter the right atrium (RA) but also surrounds the pulmonary venous pit (PV) that at this stage is positioned at the left atrial (LA) of the developing primary atrial septum (PAS) at the left atrial. It can be appreciated that endocardial cushion like tissue of the spina vestibuli (SpV) by way of the inferior and superior atrioventricular cushion (AVC) is continuous with the dorsolateral endocardial ridge of the outflow tract (DOT). In this inner curvature, where in fact all transitional zones meet, the primary fold (PF) is present between the AVC and the DOT. Before septation the AVC is completely positioned above the trabeculated ventricular inlet segment (VI) and by crossing over the PF the trabeculated ventricular outlet segment (VO) is reached. This segment connects by way of the DOT to the arterial orifice level that already shows an aortic (Ao) and pulmonary (Pu) side. **b.** Schematic view of the heart halfway through atrial and ventricular septation. The primary atrial septum (a separate septum secundum is not shown) almost closes of the ostium primum by fusion with the already fused atrioventricular cushions, that result in a separate tricuspid (TO) and mitral (MO) orifice. Normal ventricular inflow septation is the result of expansion of the dorsal part of the primary fold (PF) by which a newly recognizable right ventricular inlet (RVI) is formed below the tricuspid orifice. Remnants of the primary fold are present as trabecula septomarginalis (TSM), moderator band (MB), and surround the tricuspid orifice, both anteriorly and posteriorly. This septation process is reflected in the position of the primitive conduction system. At atrial level the sinus venosus and sinoatrial transition form the sinoatrial node (SAN). In the embryonic period immuno-histochemically detectable tracts run through the right venous valve (rvv), the left venous valve (lvv), and anteriorly through the septum spurium (ssp). Where these tracts meet the right atrioventricular ring bundle (ravr) derived from the PF, a nodal like structure in seen. This results in a posterior (pAVN) and an anterior (aAVN) Anlage. This latter structure is found in a retroaortic position. In the mature heart primitive conduction tissue is not recognizable anymore in the area of the coronary sinus, the pulmonary veins and in the right atrioventricular ring. It is expected, however, that these sites, that stand out during development, may play a role in pathological circumstances. HIS, common bundle; LV, left ventricle; rbb, right bundle branch; RV, right ventricle.

cushion components are essential. The involved myocardial components derive from the transitional (or intersegmental) zones being the atrial fold between the right and left atrium and the primary fold between the trabeculated ventricular inlet and the ventricular outlet (Figs. 1a and 2a, b).

Neural Crest Contribution

Before the role of neural crest will be described in more detail it is relevant to introduce the concept of the dual gateway to the heart[16] in which extracardiac cells are able to enter the cardiac tube. The most important cellular contribution is derived from the neural tube and consists of a classically described neural crest cell contribution and a more recently discovered population residing in the ventral half of the neural tube.[16]

The part of the neural tube that contributes neural crest cells to the heart and pharyngeal arch arteries has been elegantly described by Kirby and her group.[17] These cells migrate through the arches to reach the circumpharyngeal region and subsequently the vessel wall and heart. In this process the neural crest cells differentiate into a number of cell types such as smooth muscle cells, parasympathetic ganglionic cells, satellite cells and a mesenchymal cell population that predominantly ends up in the heart.[14,16,18,19]

Retrovirally transmitted reporter gene (*lacZ*) tracing revealed an additional contribution to the venous pole of the

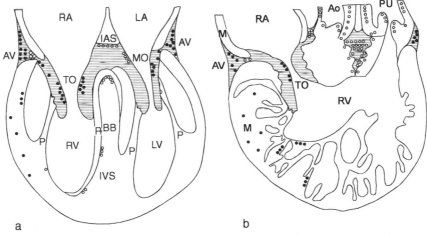

a   b

Figure 3. a. Schematic section through the atrioventricular connection of the heart at inflow level. The cushion mass has been designed to be continuous with the epicardial sulcus tissue (hatched) although they have a different developmental origin. **b.** Schematic section in a different direction showing the inner curvature of the heart with the retroaortic region between the tricuspid orifice (TO) and the aortic orifice (Ao) and thus the outflow level. Both drawings show that neural crest cells (open circles) and epicardial derived cells—so called EPDC (black dots) reach the various parts of the heart (myocardium, atrioventricular cushions and valves, outflow tract cushions, outflow tract septum, semilar valves conduction system) where they can exert a modulating role. The neural crest cells mostly end up in an apoptotic pathway whereas the EPDCs have been traced in a fibroblast and smooth muscle cell differentiation line. The latter may also be instrumental in Purkinje fibre differentiation, whereas the apoptotic neural crest cells encase the developing central conduction system. AV, atrioventricular sulcus; IAS, interatrial septum; IVS, interventricular septum; LV, left ventricle; M, mycardium; MO, mitral orifice; PU, pulmonary orifice; P, papillary muscle; RBB, right bundle branch; RV, right ventricle; TO, tricuspid orifice.

heart whereas the hitherto described results after studies with neural crest quail-chicken chimeras showed the arterial pole as the site of entrance. These *lacZ* studies revealed a neural crest input not only in the endocardial outflow tract cushions up to the level of the superior atrioventricular cushion but also an extension of neural crest (NC)-derived cells in the myocardial cuff surrounding the arterial orifices. This contribution extended into the retroaortic sulcus area. From this site isolated neural crest cells could be followed along the anterior atrial wall and around the right atrioventricular orifice (Fig. 3a, b). Along the posterior rim of this orifice cells have been observed in the posterior atrioventricular cushion and, even more important, in the dorsal mesocardium. A large number of *lacZ*-positive cells are found surrounding the His bundle and scattered cells are seen adjacent to the left and right bundle branches (Fig. 3a). At these sites, the *lacZ*-positive cells surround the myocardium where the future conduction system is seen to develop (Fig. 2b).

Intracardial Neural Crest Cell Targeting and Glycoprotein Epitopes

A still unsolved question pertains to the mechanisms that guide neural crest cells to their final destination. It is remarkable that our more complete homing pattern of neural crest cells confirms our earlier observations that areas that express RMO and HNK1 epitopes are populated by NC cells. Shortly after the NC arrival in these areas, the RMO and HNK1 expression disappears. In this respect it is also of interest to speculate on the role of apoptosis.

Apoptosis: The Intracardiac Fate of Neural Crest Cells

The labeling of the NC by retroviral *lacZ* staining allows the follow-up of this cell population during the complete developmental period of a chicken embryo. In the vessel wall and ganglion destination[18,19] the NC can be followed into their definitive differentiation stage by double staining with a differentiation marker.

The intracardiac mesenchymal NC population does not develop into a cell line that is recognized by any of our known differentiation markers. There is a short time expression of a smooth muscle actin of NC cells in the outflow tract cushions,[14] but this staining is weak and it is not a reliable marker in the chick. However, it was evident that the NC, taking up positions on the borderline of myocardium and endocardium and in the fusion lines of the endocardial cushions, became apoptotic. This phenomenon was found for all areas where the intracardiac NC were encountered, including the surroundings of the developing conduction system.[16] That apoptosis is a prominent finding in the developing heart has been described by several authors[20,21] but without a concomitant marker the real proof that those were NC was lacking. Our experiments with retroviral tracing do not exclude that other cell types such as endocardial cushion mesenchyme or myocardium show apoptosis.

Experiments in chicken embryos in which neural crest cells were ablated and in which outflow tract malformations were induced by rerouting venous return by a clip on a vitelline vein[9] were checked for the fate of NC cells by concomitant flushing with a retrovirally transmitted reporter gene. In the ablation studies it was remarkable that NC did reach the heart but in lower numbers and that these cells were still present at stages when they should already have gone into apoptosis. This was particularly apparent in cases with persistent truncus arteriosus. In the venous clip embryos the full-blown persistent truncus was not found but we encountered ventricular septal defects at and just below orifice level referred to as DORV. It was remarkable that in these malformations the presence of neural crest cells at the interface of endocardial cushions and myocardium did not correlate with reorganization of the myocardial cells to form a normal muscular outflow tract septum. The above findings led us to speculate about the role of apoptosis. One hypothesis is that these NC were misdirected and that they simply disappeared by anoikis. A more likely explanation points towards an active role in which, by the increased permeability of the cell membrane, low molecular substances are released that initiate, e.g., myocardial remodeling, differentiation of the conduction system and valve formation. The TGFβ2 knock out model[6] that shows a number of malformations fitting within the spectrum of neural crest cell disturbance makes TGFβ2 a likely candidate to be activated by the process of NC cell apoptosis.[14]

Epicardial Covering and Epithelial-Mesenchymal Transition

After the first looping stage is completed the myocardial heart tube is covered by a layer of coelomic epithelium forming the epicardium.[22,23] This process takes place both in the avian and mammalian heart and is known to be a prerequisite for subsequent coronary vascular formation.[24,25] Recent quail-chicken chimera studies (Fig. 3a, b) revealed a more extensive role for the epicardium in that the epicardial derived cells (EPDC) have been demonstrated and reach the subepicardium first to infest the myocardium and subendocardium.[26] At a later stage EPDCs migrate through the atrioventricular sulcus into the endocardial cushion where they become dispersed in the cushion. The role of these EPDCs is still to be resolved, but staining with a procollagen antibody points toward a role in cardiac fibroblast differentiation. EPDCs are also found in areas adjacent to the endocardium or to endothelium (as in coronary vessels) in which Purkinje fibers are differentiating. This suggests a role in Purkinje fibre induction, although the

Purkinje fibers themselves differentiate from the myocardium.

The last role for EPDCs turns out to be differentiation into the smooth muscle cells and fibroblasts that surround the developing coronary vasculature. In this process the surface epicardial cells become cuboid, detach from the lining and can be followed in to the wall of the neighboring coronary vessel.[27] The process resembles endocardial mesenchymal transformation as it takes place on the inside of the heart. This finding is supported by the expression of so-called transformation markers (JB3 and ES130) as described by the group of Markwald.[28]

Atrial Septation and Sinus Venosus Incorporation

The septation of the atrial segment has received emphasis in many cardiac embryology books. The basic developmental research is mainly covered by Odgers[29] and Los.[30] Our own investigations on the development of the embryonic vascular network and its connections in the heart in the quail lead to a renewed study of this area.[31] An important finding relates to the location of the so-called pulmonary Anlagen or pulmonary pit that in the quail and in the human (unpublished data) is part of the sinus venosus and as such connected to the dorsal body wall by the dorsal mesocardium (Fig. 2b). This is also the already mentioned site of entrance of the ventral neural tube-derived cells. The endothelial cells that form the precursors of the pulmonary veins in the quail are shown to connect already to the sinus venosus so that an actual outgrowth of pulmonary venous sprouts is not seen.

This finding has implications for the formation of the atrial septum. Initially, the septum primum and septum secundum cannot be distinguished so that we call the ridge that will form the atrial septa the atrial ridge. To the right side, the sinoatrial transition forms the left and right venous valves that encircle the right and left superior and inferior cardinal veins. These are later on referred to as the right and left superior caval vein and coronary sinus. With completion of atrial septation the primary atrial septum with the cushion-like spina vestibuli in its free underrim closes the ostium primum. In this process part of the sinus venosus encircling the pulmonary vein primordium ends up in the posterior wall of the left atrium. The basal part of the atrial septum is most probably formed in part by the sinus venosus tissue that is continuous between the left venous valve and the pulmonary veins. The septum secundum in this view is a secondary structure, consisting of an infolding of the myocardium of the atrial roof, which forms a recognizable ridge on the right side of the atrial septum, being the limbus fossa ovalis. The septum secundum formation is lacking in the avian embryo, however, atrial septation in the avian embryo is not essentially different.

It is remarkable that the septum primum becomes fenestrated and thin like a valve. The ostium secundum is a funnel-like channel between the limbus and the free rim of the septum primum.

Atrial Septation Abnormalities and Abnormal Pulmonary Venous Drainage

Atrial septation abnormalities and abnormal pulmonary venous drainage can be attributed to septum primum, septum secundum, and sinus venosus deficiencies because all three structures have a different origin and differences in their differentiation. The current terminology of atrial septation defects does not adequately cover the differences in morphogenesis. Especially the centrally located, and most common, septum secundum defect can be the result of a nonclosure of the foramen ovale as well as a deficiency in formation of the other atrial septation components. It is evident that when the dorsal and basal part of the atrial septum are of sinus venosus origin that the so-

called sinus venosus defects are often accompanied by pulmonary vein connection anomalies.

The spectrum of abnormal pulmonary vein drainage can be easily understood from both right and left dorsal atrial (actually sinus venosus derived) wall as well as from the persistent left superior caval vein connected to the sinus venosus.

Ventricular Inflow Tract Septation

Inflow tract septation is highly dependent on the so-called primary fold that is positioned between the left and right ventricular segments (Fig. 2a, b). Our interpretation of inflow tract septation differs somewhat from the current descriptions in which the left-sided segment is referred to as the future left ventricle and the right segment as the future right ventricle. This is not solely a matter of semantics. It is based on the assumption that in the ventricular part of the heart tube, initially containing just two segments, the trabeculated apex still has to develop to end up with a ventricle that has three components. These two parts are the right ventricular inflow below the tricuspid orifice and ditto valve and the left ventricular outflow below the aortic orifice. Only when these parts are connected to their respective ventricular segments morphologically completed ventricles are achieved. For the outflow tract we will discuss this under that heading.

Formation of the right ventricular inlet part is essential for normal ventricular septation. In our view this is achieved by splitting (or expansion) of the primary fold in the dorsal wall. In this process a new part of the right ventricular dorsal wall is formed, whereas the lateral boundary of the primary fold can still be seen as the moderator band that continues up to the ventriculoinfundibular fold (Fig. 2a, b). The newly formed ventricular inlet septum is bordered anteriorly by the trabecula septomarginalis. The trabecula septomarginalis connects in a normal heart to the ventriculoinfundibular fold by way of the crista supra ventricularis that forms the underrim of the muscular outflow tract infundibulum.

It is essential that primary fold-derived tissue borders the lateral wall of the right ventricle and encircles the tricuspid orifice, connecting the retroaortic area to the crux of the heart where the dorsal part of the atrial septum is reached (Fig. 2b). Our description is not corroborated by recent molecular differentiation markers and is supported by expression patterns of various markers of the primary fold as described earlier.

Inflow Tract Septum Abnormalities Such as Double Inlet Left Ventricle, Straddling, and Absent Tricuspid Valve and Atrioventricular Septal Defects

In experimental animal models the most common cause of inflow septation abnormalities is linked to incomplete looping. An example is double inlet left ventricle (DILV), the counterpart of DORV. DILV can occur with a common valve and with a bivalvular situation. In case of a common valve we assume that similar to persistent truncus arteriosus, the newly described ventral neural tube-derived cells, that enter the heart by way of the dorsal mesocardium, have not taken part in proper septation. This can lead to situations with complete double inlet anomalies with a right or left dominance of the common atrioventricular valve. Essential in this anomaly is that the atrial septum in looping abnormalities does connect to the crux of the heart, but is not in line with the underlying ventricular septum. This anomaly is actually the basic problem in the trisomy 16 mouse, which has erroneously been associated with an atrioventricular septal defect.[32] In the latter case there is a proper alignment of the atrial and ventricular

septum and the anomaly is mainly focussed on a too small inlet septum that is primarily fold-derived. This implies that in atrioventricular septal defects looping abnormalities do not seem to be the primary problem. This leaves us without an adequate animal model for atrioventricular septal defects.

In DILV hearts with two atrioventricular valves, a variance can be seen from complete double inlet left ventricle to more or less straddling of the tricuspid valve in posterior position.[33] In these cases expansion of the primary fold has taken place but the main body of the inlet septum has moved to the right. Thus the newly formed posterior wall of the ventricle is completely or in part positioned in the left ventricle. The absence of right atrioventricular connection or tricuspid atresia belong within this category.[32,34] This anomaly is again present in the trisomy 16 mouse and was also seen in the TGFβ2 knock-out mouse.[6]

Outflow Tract Septation

To complete ventricular septation it is necessary to have an alignment of the inlet septal component, derived from the primary fold, and the muscular infundibulum, which is formed below the pulmonary orifice and which in part is a septum between the right and left ventricular outlet. The complex three-dimensional architecture in this area leads to a long right ventricular outflow tract (RVOT) and a short left ventricular outflow tract (LVOT). Outflow tract septation and alignment are acquired by essentially two independent processes: looping and wedging. This process has been described earlier and if it does not take place in a sufficient way the outflow segment of the heart tube will remain too much to the right.

Subsequently, the RVOT and LVOT have to become separated as well as the aortic sac and the arterial orifice level above it. For this separation process neural crest cells are essential. They form a mass of condensed mesenchyme at orifice level with two prongs extending into the endocardial outflow tract ridges. The neural crest cells take up a subendocardial position and are also located in the myocardial/endocardial.[4] Both populations eventually go into apoptosis. At the myocardial/endocardial interface myocardial cells are seen to protrude into the cushions and finally muscularize the fused cushions. The resulting shortening of the outflow tract is described through several mechanisms. Thompson[35] explained that the aorticopulmonary septal complex shortened physically, thereby resulting in septation. We think that this concept is still the most promising. It fits with earlier data from our group showing that muscularization of the infundibulum was affected by a sort of bulging-in of myocardium[15] without an active myocardialization process. There is, however, the need for architectural change and we postulate that neural crest cell apoptosis plays an inductive role through most probably TGFβ2 activation.[14] In outflow tract separation several levels can be influenced and although in human and mouse embryos the endocardial outflow tract cushions form a continuous sleeve,[36] in the chicken the cushion mass can be distinguished in a proximal or conal cushion mass and a distal or truncal cushion mass.

Sorting out the nomenclature confusion in this area has been performed very efficiently by our late colleague Tomas Pexieder.[10] Whatever nomenclature is used, it is essential to appreciate that the cushion mass always stays within the myocardial cuff and never extends into the mesenchymal aortic sac area.

Outflow Tract Septation Anomalies Such as DORV, VSD, and Persistent Truncus Arteriosus

The DORV has already been mentioned several times because it forms the most common anomaly in animal experiments. This anomaly is far less common in the human population and surpassed by the incidence of ventricular septal defects.

To describe the morphogenesis of this anomaly it is important to realize that a terminology problem complicates understanding the mechanism. A true DORV has a muscular conus (sleeve of tissue) below both arterial orifices. This anomaly is rare in man. If one takes the definition of the Brompton classification the degree of overriding of an arterial orifice is the basis. This extends the number of DORV extensively and as a consequence we can separate two anomalies, one that has an overriding of the aortic orifice and consequently a subaortic ventricular septal defect (VSD) (an essential part of DORV). This anomaly comes in two forms, one with subpulmonary stenosis and an anterior displacement of the outlet septum leading to a tetralogy of Fallot. The other without a subpulmonary outflow tract stenosis, also called an Eisenmenger VSD, has a subpulmonary defect with an overriding of the pulmonary orifice and belongs to the category of transposition of the great arteries.

To complicate matters further it turns out that species differences exist. In chicken only very rarely, or perhaps never, a subpulmonary position with as a consequence an anterior and rightward positioned aorta is encountered, whereas in the mouse this is far more common. In fact, we encountered both forms in the mouse.

The above explanation is important as we see the descriptions in the literature of the occurrence of DORV very often but it is important to put more emphasis on the details of the defects to sort out the specific disturbances. Most experiments that are described have a combination of looping and outflow tract septation abnormalities. This is the case for neural crest ablation,[37] retinoic acid receptor knock outs,[38] retinoic acid overdosis,[39] hemodynamic interferences such as in the venous clip model[9] and the Pax 3 mutant splotch mouse.[40] There is increasing evidence that the heart should be studied at more timepoints as early lethality may select out those cases that have a combination of both atrioventricular and outflow tract underdevelopment with accompanying decompensation.

Semilunar and Atrioventricular Valve Formation

An intriguing subject concerns the formation of the semilunar and atrioventricular valves. There have been elegant studies by Hurle[41] that describe the formation of the semilunar valves from the distal endocardial outflow tract cushions that become scooped out to transform into the actual valve leaflets. The mechanisms that direct commissure formation or abnormalities such as raphae in bicuspid valves remain obscure. There are few animal models that have been described with recurrent semilunar valve abnormalities such as the Syrian hamster.[42] This animal bears a genetically inherited semilunar valve abnormality coinciding with coronary vessel abnormalities. This coincidence does not have its counterpart in the human population. In hearts after neural crest ablation there are semilunar valves present even if the result is a persistent truncus arteriosus. The interesting finding is that the coronary arteries originate close to the outflow tract ridges, which, as we have recently shown, still contain neural crest cells. In the venous clip model, in which a shear stress dependent gene cascade is postulated, the semilunar valve leaflets are present but clearly abnormal in number and in their morphology of commissures and raphae.[9] The recent report of genes like Sox4,[43] NF-Atc[44] are the first genes that directly link to semilunar valve development because knock out mutants show in a dramatic and lethal way absence of valve formation. This anomaly when encountered in humans leads to intra-uterine death.[45]

The above-mentioned genes seem to extend their influence by way of the endocardial cells lining the endocardial cushions and probably do not act via the neural crest cells that are known to be present in the semilunar valves[14,46] although the role of the latter is still obscure.

Differentiation of the atrioventricular valves remains a still underdeveloped area of research. The formation of the tricuspid and mitral valve and the role of the myocardium was highlighted in the eighties by Wenink and co-workers.[47,48] The underestimated role, at that time, of the contribution of the atrioventricular cushions to the definitive valves has been re-evaluated in that now most authors agree that atrioventricular valves mainly derive from the atrioventricular endocardial cushions.[49-51] A meticulous study of human and mouse material unraveled the formation of the papillary muscle complex especially for the mitral valve[52] showing how these muscles develop from the early myocardial trabeculations. In mitral abnormalities, such as the parachute mitral valve, it was shown that non-fusion of papillary muscles has occurred during development, but rather that the embryonic muscle mass did not separate. Furthermore, it was shown that the mitral valve could attach over a great length to the myocardial wall, a phenomenon that is normal in mouse and rat embryos.[52] The chicken is a less adequate model for atrioventricular valve formation as the tricuspid valve essentially becomes muscular. The genes that are active in semilunar valve development also have their influence on atrioventricular valve development.

Development of the Conduction System

In general it can be postulated that the sinoatrial and the atrioventricular conduction system differentiate from the embryonic transitional zones being the sinus venosus and sinoatrial transition and the primary fold. Interestingly both areas stain in the early embryonic stages with the glycoprotein rich markers like HNK1 (Fig. 2a). Recent studies of our group have concentrated on the description of these markers in the early development of the human heart.

In Figure 2b the tracts are indicated in gray and in general do follow earlier descriptions on this subject. New data concern the tracts in the atrium running between the sinoatrial node and the anterior and posterior part of the right atrioventricular ring bundle. It seems that already during normal development an anterior and a posterior atrioventricular node Anlage are present. Whether these Anlagen fuse to form a regular atrioventricular node or whether the posterior node is the only one to persist, needs to be studied in more detail. At least the anterior node Anlage can explain an anterior node in certain congenital heart malformations. Interestingly the tracts in the atrium that relate to the embryonic sinus venosus also surround the pulmonary veins and the coronary sinus. These areas might reflect the basis for sites of abnormal atrial automaticity as seen in human rhythm disturbances.

In conclusion, the study of genes in animal models is relevant for understanding of mechanistic processes that are taking place in cell-cell and cell-matrix interactions of the various cell types that make up the heart architecture. It is clear that the interplay of myocardium and endocardium is modulated by extracardiac cell sources such as neural crest and epicardium.

A direct link between genes active in human cardiac malformations and those found in animal models is our goal for the next millennium. Current data, however, point towards very complex gene cascades that intrigue us by redundancy, regulating cascades, incomplete penetrance, and eventual heterogeneity. The current nomenclature of classifying human cardiac anomalies is based on clinical use for diagnosis and treatment. A regrouping to a more mechanistically based system as devised by Clark[53] is essential. The latter grouping, however, will also need to be updated while new data pour in and this will at least keep embryologists, developmental biologist and clinicians busy and interactive for the coming years.

References

1. Gittenberger-de Groot AC, Bartelings MM, Poelmann RE. Cardiac morphology and the developmental basis of cardiac defects. Normal and abnormal cardiac outflow tract septation. In: Imai Y, Momma K, eds. *Proceedings of the Second World Congress of Pediatric Cardiology and Cardiac Surgery.* Armonk, NY: Futura Publishing Co; 1998:1025.
2. Pexieder T. Development of the outflow tract of the embryonic heart. *Birth Defects* 1978;14:29–68.
3. Watanabe M, Choudhry A, Berlan M, et al. Developmental remodelling and shortening of the cardiac outflow tract involves myocyte programmed cell death. *Development* 1999;125:3809–3820.
4. Poelmann RE, Mikawa T, Gittenberger-de Groot AC. Neural crest cells in outflow tract septation of the embryonic chicken heart: Differentiation and apoptosis. *Dev Dyn* 1998;212:373–384.
5. Mendelsohn C, Larkin S, Mark M, et al. RARβ isoforms: distinct transcriptional control by retinoic acid and specific spatial patterns of promoter activity during mouse embryonic development. *Mech Develop* 1994;45:227–241.
6. Sanford LP, Ormsby I, Gittenberger-de Groot AC, et al. TGFβ 2 knockout mice have multiple developmental defects that are non-overlapping with other TGFβ knockout phenotypes. *Development* 1997;124:2659–2670.
7. Leatherbury L, Connuck DM, Kirby ML. Neural crest ablation versus sham surgical effects in a chick embryo model of defective cardiovascular development. *Pediatr Res* 1993;33:628–631.
8. Bouman HGA, Broekhuizen MLA, Baasten AMJ, et al. Spectrum of looping disturbances in stage 34 chicken heart after retinoic acid treatment. *Anat Rec* 1995;243:101–108.
9. Hogers B, DeRuiter MC, Gittenberger-de Groot AC, et al. Unilateral vitelline vein ligation alters intracardiac blood flow patterns and morphogenesis in the chick embryo. *Circ Res* 1997;80:473–481.
10. Pexieder T. Conotruncus and its septation at the advent of the molecular biology era. In: Clark EB, Markwald RR, Takao A, eds. *Development Mechanisms of Heart Disease.* Armonk, NY: Futura Publishing Co.; 1995:227–247.

11. Pexieder T, Pfizenmaier-Rousseil M, Prados-Frutos JC. Prenatal pathogenesis of the transposition of great arteries. In: Vogel M, Bühlmeyer K, eds. *Transposition of the Great Arteries. 25 Years after Rashkind Balloon Septostomy*. Darmstadt, Germany: Steinkopf Verlag; 1992: 11–27.

12. Franco D, Kelly R, Lamers WH, et al. Regionalized transcriptional domains of myosin light chain 3f transgenes in the embryonic mouse heart: Morphogenetic implications. *Dev Biol* 1997;188:17–33.

13. de Jong F, Geerts WJC, Lamers WH, et al. Isomyosin expression pattern during formation of the tubular chicken heart: A three-dimensional immunohistochemical analysis. *Anat Rec* 1990;226:213–227.

14. Poelmann RE, Mikawa T, Gittenberger-de Groot AC. Neural crest cells in outflow tract septation of the embryonic chicken heart: Differentiation and apoptosis. *Dev Dyn* 1998;212:373–384.

15. Bartelings MM, Wenink ACG, Gittenberger-de Groot AC, et al. Contribution to the aortopulmonary septum to the muscular outlet septum in the human heart. *Acta Morphol Neerl Scand* 1986;24: 181–192.

16. Poelmann RE, Gittenberger-de Groot AC. A subpopulation of apoptosis-prone cardiac neural crest cells targets to the venous pole: Multiple functions in heart development? *Dev Biol* 1999;207:271–286.

17. Kirby ML. Cellular and molecular contributions of the cardiac neural crest to cardiovascular development. *Trends Cardiovasc Med* 1993;3:18–23.

18. Bergwerff M, Verberne ME, DeRuiter MC, et al. Neural crest cell contribution to the developing circulatory system. Implications for vascular morphology? *Circ Res* 1998;82:221–231.

19. Verberne ME, Gittenberger-de Groot AC, Poelmann RE. Lineage and development of the parasympathetic nervous system of the embryonic chicken heart. *Anat Embryol* 1998;198:171–184.

20. Pexieder T. Cell death in the morphogenesis and teratogenesis of the heart. *Adv Anat Embryol Cell Biol* 1975;51:1–99.

21. Hurle JM, Ojeda JL. Cell death during the development of the truncus and conus of the chick embryo heart. *J Anat* 1979;129: 427–439.

22. Virágh SZ, Gittenberger-de Groot AC, Poelmann RE, et al. Early development of quail heart epicardium and associated vascular and glandular structures. *Anat Embryol* 1993;188:381–393.

23. Vrancken Peeters M-PFM, Mentink MM, Poelmann RE, et al. Cytokeratins as a marker for epicardial formation in the quail embryo. *Anat Embryol Berl* 1995; 191:503–508.

24. Vrancken Peeters M-PFM, Gittenberger-de Groot AC, Mentink MMT, et al. Differences in development of coronary arteries and veins. *Cardiovasc Res* 1997;36:101–110.

25. Vrancken Peeters M-PFM, Gittenberger-de Groot AC, Mentink MMT, et al. The development of the coronary vessels and their differentiation into arteries and veins in the embryonic quail heart. *Dev Dyn* 1997;208:338–348.

26. Gittenberger-de Groot AC, Vrancken Peeters M-PFM, Mentink MMT, et al. Epicardial derived cells, EPDCs, contribute a novel population to the myocardial wall and the atrioventricular cushions. *Circ Res* 1998;82:1043–1052.

27. Vrancken Peeters M-PFM, Gittenberger-de Groot AC, Mentink MMT, et al. Smooth muscle cells and fibroblasts of the coronary arteries derive from epithelial-mesenchymal transformation of the epicardium. *Anat Embryol* 1999;199:367–378.

28. Krug EL, Rezaee M, Isokawa K, et al. Transformation of cardiac endothelium into cushion mesenchyme is dependent on es/130: Temporal, spatial, and functional studies in the early chick embryo. *Cell Mol Biol Res* 1995;41:263–277.

29. Odgers PNB. The formation of the venous valves, the foramen secundum and the septum secundum in the human heart. *J Anat* 1934;69:412–422.

30. Los JA. Embryology. In: Watson H, ed. *Paediatric Cardiology*. London: Lloyd-Luke; 1968:1–28.

31. DeRuiter MC, Gittenberger-de Groot AC, Wenink ACG, et al. In normal development pulmonary veins are connected to the sinus venosus segment in the left atrium. *Anat Rec* 1995;243:84–92.

32. Webb S, Brown NA, Anderson RH. Cardiac morphology at late fetal stages in the mouse with trisomy 16: Consequences for different formation of the atrioventricular junction when compared to humans with trisomy 21. *Cardiovasc Res* 1997;34:515–524.

33. Wenink ACG, Gittenberger-de Groot AC. Straddling mitral and tricuspid valves: Morphologic differences and developmen-

tal backgrounds. *Am J Cardiol* 1982;49: 1960–1971.

34. Wenink ACG, Ottenkamp J. Tricuspid atresia. Microscopic findings in relation to "absence" of the atrioventricular connexion. *Int J Cardiol* 1987;16:57–65.

35. Thompson RP, Sumida H, Abercrombie M, et al. Morphogenesis of human cardiac outflow. *Anat Rec* 1985;213:578–586.

36. Bartelings MM, Gittenberger-de Groot AC. The outflow tract of the heart-embryologic and morphologic correlations. *Int J Cardiol* 1989;22:289–300.

37. Kirby ML, Turnage KL, Hays BM. Characterization of conotruncal malformations following ablation of "cardiac" neural crest. *Anat Rec* 1985;213:87–93.

38. Sucov HM, Dyson E, Gumeringer CL, et al. RXRα mutant mice establish a genetic basis for vitamin A signaling in heart morphogenesis. *Gene Dev* 1994;8:1007–1018.

39. Broekhuizen MLA, Bouman HGA, Mast F, et al. Hemodynamic changes in HH stage 34 chick embryos after treatment with all-trans-retinoic acid. *Pediatr Res* 1995;38: 342–348.

40. Conway SJ, Henderson DJ, Kirby ML, et al. Development of a lethal congenital heart defect in the splotch (Pax3) mutant mouse. *Cardiovasc Res* 1997;36:163–173.

41. Hurle JM, Colvee E, Blanco AM. Development of mouse semilunar valves. *Anat Embryol* 1980;160:83–91.

42. Sans-Coma V, Cardo M, Thiene G, et al. Bicuspid aortic and pulmonary valves in the Syrian hamster. *Int J Cardiol* 1992;34: 249–254.

43. Schilham MW, Oosterwegel MA, Moerer P, et al. Defects in cardiac outflow tract formation and pro-b- lymphocyte expansion in mice lacking sox-4. *Nature* 1996; 380:711–714.

44. De la Pompa JL, Timmerman LA, Takimoto H, et al. Role of the NF-Atc transcription factor in morphogenesis of cardiac valves and septum. *Nature* 1998;392: 182–186.

45. Hartwig NG, Vermeij-Keers C, De Vries HE, et al. Aplasia of semilunar valve leaflets: Two case reports and developmental aspects. *Pediatr Cardiol* 1991;12:114–117.

46. Sumida H, Akimoto N, Nakamura H. Distribution of the neural crest cells in the heart of birds: A three dimensional analysis. *Anat Embryol* 1989;180:29–35.

47. Wenink ACG, Gittenberger-de Groot AC. Embryology of the mitral valve. *Int J Cardiol* 1986;11:75–84.

48. Wenink ACG, Gittenberger-de Groot AC. The role of atrioventricular endocardial cushions in the septation of the heart. *Int J Cardiol* 1985;8:25–44.

49. Wenink ACG, Wisse BJ, Groenendijk PM. Development of the inlet portion of the right ventricle in the embryonic rat heart: The basis for tricuspid valve development. *Anat Rec* 1994;239:216–223.

50. Lamers WH, Virágh SZ, Wessels A, et al. Formation of the tricuspid valve in the human heart. *Circulation* 1995;91:111–121.

51. Oosthoek PW, Wenink ACG, Vrolijk BCM, et al. Development of the atrioventricular valve tension apparatus in the human heart. *Anat Embryol* 1998;198:317–329.

52. Oosthoek PW, Wenink ACG, Macedo AJ, et al. The parachute-like asymmetric mitral valve and its two papillary muscles. *J Thorac Cardiovasc Surg* 1997;114:9–15.

53. Clark EB. Pathogenetic mechanisms of congenital cardiovascular malformations revisited. *Semin Perinatol* 1996;20:465–472.

32

Overview: Understanding CHD Through Dissection of Segmental Cardiac Molecular Pathways

Deepak Srivastava, MD

Congenital defects of the heart most commonly affect a particular chamber or segment of the developing heart rather than affecting the heart globally. This clinical observation suggests that unique and separable molecular pathways must exist that govern development of distinct regions of the heart. The discovery of two members of the basic helix-loop-helix (bHLH) family of transcription factors, dHAND and eHAND, has provided an entry into the molecular pathways regulating segmental development of the heart.[1-3] Analysis of dHAND and eHAND expression and function in distinct mesodermal and neural crest-derived cardiovascular structures has revealed pathways involved in cardiogenesis and congenital heart disease (CHD).

Although co-expressed throughout the developing chick heart, dHAND and eHAND display interesting polarities of expression along all three embryonic axes in mouse embryos (Fig. 1).[4,5] Whereas dHAND and eHAND are expressed symmetrically along the left-right axis of the straight heart tube, they exhibit a striking dorsoventral (D-V) asymmetry with ventral, but not dorsal, expression along the linear heart tube. eHAND is ex-

pressed differentially along the antero-posterior axis of the heart tube with transcripts detectable in the conotruncus, left ventricle, and atrial segments, but not the future right ventricle region. After cardiac looping converts the A-P orientation of the ventricular segments to a L-R orientation, dHAND and eHAND display complementary expression in the right and left ventricles of mouse embryos, respectively. The D-V asymmetry of HAND expression in the straight heart tube is manifested as expression along the more rapidly expanding outer curvature of the looped heart tube, whereas the inner curvature is devoid of HAND transcripts. The asymmetries of dHAND and eHAND expression suggest a role in patterning the embryonic heart along multiple axes.

Targeted deletion of *dHAND* in mice resulted in lethality by embryonic day 11.0 (E11.0).[4] *dHAND*-null embryos began the process of cardiac looping in the rightward direction, but failed to develop the segment of the heart tube that forms the right ventricle, consistent with the predominant expression of dHAND in the right ventricle-forming region. The atrial chamber moves dorsally and to the left as it should during cardiac looping in the mutant, suggesting that the process and direction of cardiac looping were initiated correctly.

Expression of lacZ under control of the right ventricle-specific MLC2V pro-

From Clark EB, Nakazawa M, Takao A (eds.): Etiology and Morphogenesis of Congenital Heart Disease: Twenty Years of Progress in Genetics and Developmental Biology. Armonk, NY: Futura Publishing Co., Inc.; © 2000.

dHAND

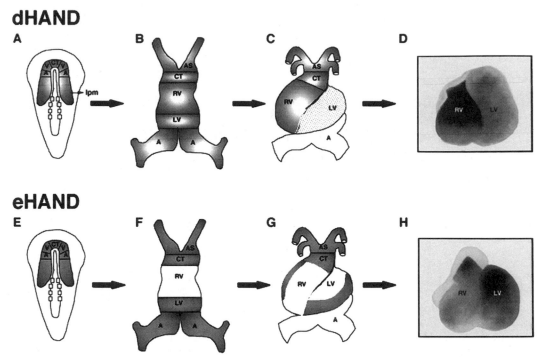

eHAND

Figure 1. *HAND* gene expression during cardiac morphogenesis. The dynamic expression of dHAND and eHAND are shown in cartoon form. Expression is superimposed upon a schematic for the developing heart tube. a, aortic sac; ct, conotruncus; rv, right ventricle; lv, left ventricle; a, atrium; 1pm, lateral plate mesoderm. D and H show expression of dHAND and eHAND by in situ hybridization on embryonic hearts.

moter[6] in the *dHAND*-null background revealed that dHAND was not required in the initial specification of right ventricle cells at the straight heart tube stage. However, in the absence of dHAND, the right ventricle failed to expand between E8.0 and E8.5. Proliferation of cells was unaffected, but cells of the right ventricle segment underwent extensive apoptosis in *dHAND* mutants. In cultured cardiomyocytes, overexpression of dHAND protects cells from serum deprivation-induced activation of the programmed cell death pathway. Thus, dHAND appears to be playing a role in suppressing apoptosis during the period of rapid organ growth.

To investigate the molecular mechanisms through which dHAND functions, we sought to find genes downstream of dHAND by comparing RNA species in wild-type and *dHAND*-null E9.5 embryonic hearts by suppressive subtraction hybridization and differential display.

Through these approaches, a proapoptic *Bcl2* family member, Nip3,[7] was found to be upregulated in *dHAND* mutants. Heterodimerization of Nip3 with Bcl2 is thought to maintain a balance of pro- and antiapoptotic cellular forces. It is possible that dHAND normally represses Nip3 and promotes cell survival during cardiogenesis. Whether eHAND functions in a similar fashion regulating left ventricle survival and growth is unclear secondary to early embryonic lethality of *eHAND* mutants from placental insufficiency.[8,9] Tissue-specific deletion of *eHAND* in the future will provide a more detailed analysis of its role in cardiogenesis.

In addition to the role of dHAND in the cardiac mesoderm, it is expressed and functions in neural crest-derived cells affected in 22q11 deletion syndrome (also known as DiGeorge syndrome or CATCH-22).[10] Children with this syndrome have typical craniofacial defects, thymic and parathyroid hypoplasia, and conotruncal and aortic arch defects.[11] Targeted deletion of the signaling peptide, endothelin-1 (ET-1), and its receptor, ET_A, in mice resulted in a mouse model of 22q11 deletion syndrome.[12,13] ET-1 and ET_A-null mice display defects of craniofacial structures derived from the branchial arches and have conotruncal and aortic arch defects. dHAND and eHAND are downregulated in ET-1 mutants,[10] suggesting that the HAND proteins and endothelins function in a common molecular cascade. However, neither $HAND$ genes or members of the endothelin signaling pathway map to 22q11 in humans.

A 2 Mb region of 22q11 is most commonly detected in 22q11 deletion syndrome and is known as the DiGeorge critical region (DGCR). Nearly 30 genes have been identified in the DGCR by direct sequencing. Although identification of the one or more genes responsible for 22q11 deletion syndrome has been elusive by traditional genetic approaches,[11] dissection of the molecular pathway regulated by dHAND has provided some insight into the potential basis for this syndrome. Through subtraction cloning,[14] a dHAND-dependent gene encoding the mouse homologue of a protein involved in degradation of ubiquitinated proteins in yeast (Ufd1)[15] was identified. Human $UFD1L$ is located in the DGCR (Fig. 2)[16] and was deleted in 182/182 patients with 22q11 deletion, as detected by fluorescent in situ hybridization (FISH).[14]

Ufd1 is expressed specifically in the branchial arches, conotruncus, palatal precursors, frontonasal region, ear, and limb bud of the developing mouse embryo.[14] Within the aortic arch arteries, Ufd1 is expressed at highest levels in the fourth aortic arch artery. The fourth arch artery is responsible for formation of the transverse portion of the mature aortic arch and is undeveloped in one of the defects most commonly associated with 22q11 deletion (interrupted aortic arch, type B). In sum, Ufd1 is expressed in most tissues affected in 22q11 deletion syndrome, suggesting that deletion of a single gene may contribute to many of the phenotypic features observed.

Evidence of a $UFD1L$ mutation or deletion in an individual with cardiac and craniofacial defects who did not have detectable 22q11 deletions would confirm a role for $UFD1L$ in 22q11 deletion syndrome. One individual has been identified with a de novo monoallelic deletion of exons 1 to 3 of $UFD1L$ (Fig. 2), leaving exons 4 to 12 intact. The phenotype of this patient encompassed nearly all features commonly associated with a 2 Mb 22q11 deletion. Four days after birth, she was diagnosed with interrupted aortic arch, persistent truncus arteriosus (PTA), cleft palate, small mouth, low-set ears, broad nasal bridge, neonatal hypocalcemia, T-lymphocyte deficiency, and syndactyly of her toes. Although other chromosome deletions can also result in a similar phenotype,[17] placement of UFD1L in a molecular pathway regulating neural crest development, the patient with $UFD1L$ deletion and the $UFD1L$ expression pattern suggest that $UFD1L$ haploinsufficiency can contribute to many features observed in 22q11 deletion syndrome.

There is substantial variability in the phenotype associated with 22q11 deletions. Thus, it is possible that other genes in this region, including the histone regulatory gene, $HIRA$,[18,19] distant modifier genes or environmental factors could contribute to distinct features of 22q11 deletion syndrome. $CDC45$, the human homologue of a yeast cell cycle protein, is immediately telomeric to $UFD1L$[20] and was used to define the 5′ breakpoint of the deletion in patient JF to the region between exons 5 and 6 of $CDC45$ (Fig. 2). Although the ubiquitous nature of $CDC45$ expression[21] and its normal expression in $dHAND$ mutants[14] make it an unlikely candidate gene for the 22q11 deletion syndrome, it is conceivable that the deletion of $CDC45$ may act as a modifier of patient JF's phenotype.

Yeast lacking $Ufd1$ exhibit a cell survival defect that is incompletely rescued by one allele of $Ufd1$,[15] consistent with the notion that haploinsufficiency of

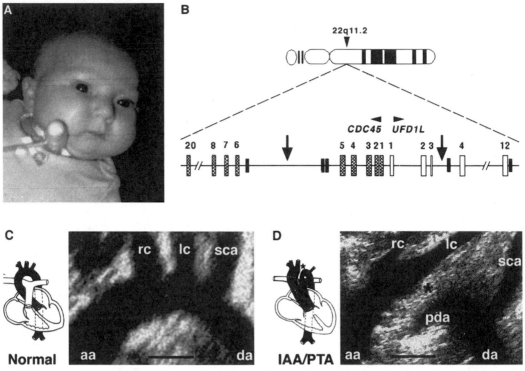

Figure 2. *UFD1L* deletion in human cardiac and craniofacial defects. The dHAND-dependent gene, *UFD1L*, is deleted in a patient with cleft palate and craniofacial features typical of those with 22q11 deletion (**A**) but who did not have the usual 2–3 Mb 22q11 deletion. A small, 20-kb deletion (**B**) encompassing the first 3 exons of *UFD1L* and the first 5 exons of the ubiquitously expressed, gene, *CDC45*, was found in the patient in (**A**). This patient also had an interrupted aortic arch (IAA) between the left carotid (lc) and left subclavian artery (sca), as indicated by the asterisk on the ultrasound image (**D**). Image of a normal aortic arch is shown (**C**). Cartoon depiction of the cardiac defect is seen in inserts with vessels shaded in black. aa, ascending aorta; rc, right carotid; pda, patent ductus arteriosus; da, descending aorta; PTA, persistent truncus arteriosus.

UFD1L may contribute to the phenotype seen in 22q11 deletion syndrome. It is possible that *UFD1L* haploinsufficiency leads to defective survival of cardiac and cranial neural crest cells, resulting in premature thymic apoptosis and loss of cells that contribute to the transverse aortic arch, palate and craniofacial structures. Further mutation analysis of *UFD1L* in humans and elucidation of the cellular pathways regulated by UFD1L may provide new directions in understanding basic mechanisms of neural crest development and congenital cardiac and craniofacial defects.

The use of transcription factors as entry points in dissection of segmental molecular pathways regulating cardiogenesis should be a valuable method in understanding the basis of many congenital heart defects. Here we have shown that elucidation of a dHAND-dependent pathway led to identification of *UFD1L* as the gene likely responsible for many features of 22q11 deletion syndrome. Whether the HANDs or members of their pathways are involved in the pathogenesis of hypoplastic right or left ventricles is under investigation. By utilizing a combination of molecular biology, embryology and human genetic approaches, it should be possible to define the critical factors which govern individual morphogenetic events during cardiac development and ultimately identify those that are mutated in CHD. This effort will represent the first step in providing better genetic counseling for parents and, eventually, in designing novel therapeutic approaches to CHD.

References

1. Srivastava D, Cserjesi P, Olson EN. A subclass of bHLH proteins for cardiac morphogenesis. *Science* 1995;270:1995–1999.
2. Cserjesi P, Brown D, Lyons GE, et al. Expression of the novel basic helix-loop-helix gene eHAND in neural crest derivatives and extraembryonic membranes during mouse development. *Dev Biol* 1995;170: 664–678.
3. Srivastava D. Segmental regulation of cardiac development by the basic helix-loop-helix transcription factors dHAND and eHAND. In: Rosenthal N, Harvey R, eds. *Heart Development*. New York: Academic Press; 1998:143–155.
4. Srivastava D, Thomas T, Lin Q, et al. Regulation of cardiac mesodermal and neural crest development by the bHLH transcription factor, dHAND. *Nat Genet* 1997;16: 154–160.
5. Thomas T, Yamagishi H, Overbeek PA, et al. The bHLH factors, dHAND and eHAND, specify pulmonary and systemic cardiac ventricles independent of left-right sidedness. *Dev Biol* 1998;196:228–236.
6. Ross RS, Navankasattusas S, Harvey RP, et al. An HF-1a/HF-1b/MEF-2 combinatorial element confers cardiac ventricular specificity and established an anterior-posterior gradient of expression. *Development* 1996;122:1799–1809.
7. Chen G, Ray R, Dubik D, et al. The E1B 19K/Bcl-2-binding protein Nip3 is a dimeric mitochondrial protein that activates apoptosis. *J Exp Med* 1997;186: 1975–1983.
8. Firulli AB, McFadden DG, Lin Q, et al. Heart and extra-embryonic mesodermal defects in mouse embryos lacking the bHLH transcription factor Hand1. *Nat Genet* 1998;18:266–270.
9. Riley P, Anson-Cartwright L, Cross JC. The Hand1 bHLH transcription factor is essential for placentation and cardiac morphogenesis. *Nat Genet* 1998;18:271–275.
10. Thomas T, Kurihara H, Yamagishi H, et al. A signaling cascade involving endothelin-1, dHAND and msx1 regulates development of neural-crest-derived branchial arch mesenchyme. *Development* 1998;125: 3005–3014.
11. Emannuel BS, Budarf ML, Scambler PJ. In: Harvey RP, Rosenthal N, eds. *Heart Development*. New York: Academic Press; 1998:463–478.
12. Kurihara Y, Kurihara H, Oda H, et al. Aortic arch malformations and ventricular septal defect in mice deficient in endothelin-1. *J Clin Invest* 1995;96:293–300.
13. Clouthier DE, Hosoda K, Richardson JA, et al. Cranial and cardiac neural crest defects in endothelin-A receptor-deficient mice. *Development* 1998;125:813–824.
14. Yamagishi H, Garg V, Matsuoka R, et al. A molecular pathway revealing a genetic basis for human cardiac and craniofacial defects. *Science* 1999;283(5405):1158–61.
15. Johnson ES, Ma PC, Ota IM, et al. A proteolytic pathway that recognizes ubiquitin as a degradation signal. *J Biol Chem* 1995; 270:17442–17456.
16. Pizzuti A, Novelli G, Ratti A, et al. UFD1L, a developmentally expressed ubiquitination gene, is deleted in CATCH 22 syndrome. *Hum Mol Genet* 1997;6:259–265.
17. Daw SC, Taylor C, Kraman M, et al. A common region of 10p deleted in DiGeorge and velocardiofacial syndromes. *Nat Genet* 1996;13:458–460.
18. Wiilming LG, Snoeren CA, Van Rijswijk A, et al. The murine homologue of HIRA, a DiGeorge syndrome candidate gene, is expressed in embryonic structures affected in human CATCH22 patients. *Hum Mol Genet* 1997;6:247–258.
19. Magnaghi P, Roberts C, Lorain S, et al. HIRA, a mammalian homologue of Saccharomyces cerevisiae transcriptional corepressors, interacts with Pax3. *Nat Genet* 1998;20:74–77.
20. McKie JM, Wadey RB, Sutherland HF, et al. Direct selection of conserved cDNAs from the DiGeorge critical region: Isolation of a novel CDC45-like gene. *Genome Res* 1998;8:834–841.
21. Shaikh TH, Gottlieb S, Sellinger B, et al. Identification and characterization of hCDC45L, a human gene related to yeast CDC45 that is within the 22q11.2 deletion assiciated with DiGeorge and velocardiofacial syndromes. *Am J Hum Genet* 1998; 63:A193.

33

Adenoviral Gene Delivery System Reveals Mechanisms of Cardiac Outflow Tract Morphogenesis

Michiko Watanabe, PhD and Steven A. Fisher, MD

Introduction

The transformation of the primitive heart tube into the complex multichambered heart is likely to involve stage- and region-specific cell proliferation, differentiation, death, and migration. A number of methods have been developed over the years to study the cell and molecular mechanisms that drive these morphogenetic processes. One method that has been particularly useful is to tag the cells so as to identify their positions and their fates as organogenesis proceeds. Early studies relied on various particles or dyes to mark tissues and cells. More recently recombinant retroviral vectors have been employed to express exogenous proteins within cells which are easily detected histochemically, such as β-galactosidase (β-gal), in order to mark the cells and study their fates in a number of developing organs,[1,2] including the heart.[3,4] We have utilized recombinant-replication defective adenovirus to (1) tag cardiomyocytes so as to follow their fates as complex structures of the heart are formed[5,6] and (2) force the expression of proteins which may regulate aspects of cell behavior required for normal morphogenesis.[7]

From Clark EB, Nakazawa M, Takao A (eds.): Etiology and Morphogenesis of Congenital Heart Disease: Twenty Years of Progress in Genetics and Developmental Biology. Armonk, NY: Futura Publishing Co., Inc.; © 2000.

Results and Discussion

We selected the developing chick heart as our experimental model since the embryo develops external to the body and thus is readily accessible for adenoviral injection, yet is similar in its development to the mammalian heart. Under stereoscopic visualization approximately 10^7 plaque forming units (pfu) of recombinant replication-defective adenovirus was injected into the pericardial space of HH stage 13–16 embryos. When the adenovirus contained the Rous sarcoma virus (RSV) LTR promoter driving expression of the marker protein β-gal (AdRSVGal), highly efficient transduction and expression of β-gal was evident in ventricular, atrial, and OFT myocytes (Fig. 1A). β-gal expression was detected by in situ staining as early as 12 hours post application, peaked at 48 hours post injection, and declined to lower levels at 72 and 96 hours.[5] Expression appeared restricted to the myocyte population, as endocardial cells and the atrioventricular (AV) cushion and outflow tract mesenchymal cells that arise from them were β-gal negative, likely due to their internal position. The remainder of the embryo was also β-gal negative, presumably due to epithelial barriers preventing spread and uptake of virus. In embryos injected after stage 17 (18–23) and subsequently stained for β-gal, large patches of the heart were β-gal negative (Fig. 1B), corresponding to

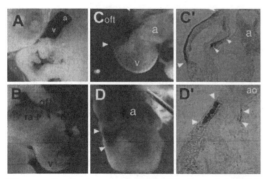

Figure 1. Analyses of AdRSVGal- and AdCM-VGal-infected hearts. Under stereoscopic visualization, 500 nL of recombinant replication-defective adenovirus solution was injected via a 30-micron bore micropipette onto the surface of the heart.[5] Embryos were injected with (**A**) AdRSVGal, stages 13–16; (**B**) AdRSVGal, stage 21; (**C, D**) AdCMVGal stage 13–16 and harvested at (**A–B**) stage 29; (**C**) stage 27; or (**D**) stage 32 and stained for β-gal by standard methods.[5]

regions of the heart, which have been observed by electron microscopy to be covered by epicardium at the stage of virus injection.[8,9] Thus, by staggering the timing of viral injection, the process of epicardialization of the bare myocardium can be re-constructed by the β-gal negative images.

In order to study chamber-specific morphogenic processes, we sought to identify an adenoviral vector that would allow us to tag and follow the fate of select populations of cardiomyocytes. To our surprise, an E1a-deleted recombinant adenovirus expressing β-gal under the control of the human cytomegalovirus (CMV) major immediate early promoter (MIEP, –552 to +51 bp) filled such a role. In contrast to the results with AdRSVGal injections, injection of stage 13–16 embryos with AdCMVGal followed by β-gal staining marked myocytes of the OFT, i.e., there were few or no β-gal-positive cells in the atrial or ventricular compartments (Fig. 1C and Reference 6). Similar results of tissue restricted expression when transgene transcription is driven by a CMV promoter have recently been obtained with a number of delivery systems, including embryonic chick[10] and mouse

adenoviral injections[11] as well as in transgenic mice studies.[12,13] Each of these studies reported comparable as well as distinct sites of transgene (β-gal) expression, likely reflecting the different modes of transgene delivery, e.g., different methods of adenovirus injection. Our study was the first to show that the CMV promoter will specifically drive transcription in the OFT myocardium,[6] though the transgenic studies have demonstrated that the CMV promoter appears to be transcriptionally active in outflow tract structures and silent in the embryonic atria and ventricles. The specific regulatory elements that may mediate the tissue-specific transcriptional activity of the CMV promoter in vivo have not been identified, but candidate regulatory elements include retinoids, cAMP and NFκB response elements (reviewed in Reference 14).

The selective tagging of the myocytes of the tubular OFT with the AdCMVGal vector allowed us to follow their fates during the complex remodeling process of this structure. Analyses of hearts injected with AdCMVGal at stages 13–16 and examined for β-gal-positive cells at 24- to 48-hour intervals indicated that between stages 27–32 there was a dramatic reorganization of the OFT tissue (compare Fig. 1C, C' with 1D, D'). Beginning at stage 27, the distal boundary of the tubular OFT appeared to recede towards the ventricle, so that by stage 32 only a wedge-shaped ring of β-gal-positive OFT tissue adjacent to the ventricles remained. This stained band of tissue was wider in the ventral surface adjacent to the base of the pulmonary artery, comprising a structure referred to as the pulmonic infundibulum, than in the dorsal region below the aorta. Also, the thickness of the stained OFT myocardium appeared to increase between stages 27 and 32. In sections the marked cells were observed to be confined to the myocardial portion of the OFT (Fig. 1). These results demonstrate that the pulmonic infundibulum originates from and is the remnant of the embryonic outflow tract myocardium.

A number of hypotheses have been proposed to account for the developmental remodeling and shortening of the OFT, including migration, compaction, and resorption of myocytes as well as their transdifferentiation into nonmuscle cells (reviewed in Reference 15). To test for resorption of myocytes by apoptosis, two different histological assays were employed. Annexin V binds to phosphatidylserine (PS) residues, which flip to the outer membrane leaflet in apoptosis, and TUNEL staining detects chromosomal fragmentation (reviewed in Reference 16). Results of the two assays were concordant and will be described in a combined fashion. Apoptotic cells were not detected within the heart myocardium until stage 25, but were present in the OFT mesenchyme at stages 23 and 24.[6] By stage 25 and 26, apoptotic cells were detected in the proximal OFT myocardium immediately adjacent to the ventricle, and by stage 27 and 28 appeared aligned in the proximal OFT myocardium adjacent to the epicardium (Fig. 2A, B). They were distributed throughout the OFT myocardial wall between stages 29–32, with particularly dense foci in the distal OFT (Fig. 2C, D). The percentage of apoptotic nuclei per total nuclei at these foci was >50%. At least some of these cells were identified as cardiomyocytes by the observation by confocal microscopy of the presence of the muscle-specific cytoskeletal components

titin and myosin.[6] After stage 35, the incidence of apoptosis in the OFT declined to nearly undetectable levels. In summary, the incidence of apoptotic myocytes within the OFT corresponded to the period when the β-gal-labeled tissue shortened from a tubular to a ring-like configuration, supporting the hypothesis that a mechanism for OFT shortening is the elimination of myocytes by apoptosis.

These cell fate studies have thus suggested a mechanism by which the tubular OFT remodels to form the infundibulum of the mature heart. These observations in this particular experimental system now allow us to explore two important questions: (1) Do perturbations of OFT myocardium apoptosis play a role in the relatively common and life-threatening congenital defects that occur in this region, including tetralogy of Fallot, transposition of the great vessels and double outlet right ventricle? Each of these anatomic defects involves malposition of the conal myocardium.[17] This may be tested by applying specific peptide inhibitors of the enzymatic executioners of the apoptotic cascade, the caspases, which we have shown to be active in the OFT myocardium,[6] and examining the resultant morphology. (2) What are the molecular pathways that result in the selective apoptosis of the OFT myocytes? Although a great deal has been learned about why cells undergo apoptosis in vitro, little is known

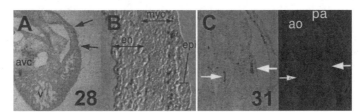

Figure 2. Apoptosis during remodeling of the tubular OFT. Chick embryos were harvested at stages 23–35 fixed in 10% neutral buffered formalin, embedded in paraffin, and sectioned. Serial sagittal sections 7 μm in thickness were collected on coated slides (Plus slides, Fisherbrand, Fisher Scientific, Pittsburgh, Pa). For detection of apoptosis, deparaffinized sections were treated with 2% hydrogen peroxide to quench endogenous peroxide then stained with the in situ apoptosis detection kit (Oncor ApopTag, Gaithersburg, Md) using the TUNEL method and peroxidase as tags. (**A**) Low power and (**B**) high power magnification of apoptotic cells in the OFT myocardium of stage 28 heart. (**C**) Transmitted light shows apoptotic foci in distal OFT of stage 32 heart and (**D**) same section with RITC filter defining the myocardium.

about the regulation of this process in vivo. Investigators have used recombinant viruses to deliver dominant negative forms of various receptors, including members of the TGFβ and BMP receptor families,[18,19] to demonstrate their roles in regulating cell growth and death in, for example, the developing limb bud. It will be of interest to determine the extent to which these signaling pathways play a role in the developmental remodeling of the OFT myocardium.

References

1. Cepko C. Retrovirus vectors and their applications in neurobiology. *Neuron* 1988;1:345–353.
2. Sanes JR, Rubenstein JLR, Nicolas J. Use of a recombinant retrovirus to study post-implantation cell lineage in mouse embryos. *EMBO J* 1986;5:3133–3142.
3. Mikawa T, Borisov A, Brown AMC, et al. Clonal analysis of cardiac morphogenesis in the chicken embryo using a replication-defective retrovirus: I. Formation of the ventricular myocardium.*Dev Dyn* 1992;193:11–23.
4. Mikawa T, Fischman DA. Retroviral analysis of cardiac morphogenesis: discontinuous formation of coronary vessels. *Proc Natl Acad Sci U S A* 1992;89:9504–9508.
5. Fisher SA, Watanabe M. Expression of exogenous protein and analysis of morphogenesis in the developing chicken heart using an adenoviral vector. *Cardiovasc Res* 1996;31:E86–E95.
6. Watanabe M, Choudhry A, Berlan M, et al. Developmental remodeling and shortening of the cardiac outflow tract involves myocyte programmed cell death. *Development* 1998;125:3809–3820.
7. Fisher SA, Siwik E, Branellec D, et al. Forced expression of the homeodomain protein Gax inhibits cardiomyocyte proliferation and perturbs heart morphogenesis. *Development* 1997;124:4405–4413.
8. Ho E, Shimada Y. Formation of the epicardium studied with the scanning electron microscope. *Dev Biol* 1978;66:579–585.
9. Hiruma T, Hirakow R. Epicardial formation in embryonic chick heart: computer-aided reconstruction, scanning, and transmission electron microscopic studies. *Am J Anat* 1989;184:129–138.
10. Yamagata M, Jaye DL, Sanes JR. Gene transfer to avian embryos with a recombinant adenovirus. *Dev Biol* 1994;166:355–359.
11. Baldwin HS, Mickanin C, Buck CA. Adenovirus-mediated gene transfer during initial organogenesis in the mammalian embryo is promoter-dependent and tissue-specific. *Gene Ther* 1997;4:1142–1149.
12. Koedood M, Fichtel A, Meier P, et al. Human cytomegalovirus (HCMV) immediate-early enhancer/promoter specificity during embryogenesis defines target tissues of congenital HCMV infection. *J Virol* 1995;69:2194–2207.
13. Baskar JF, Smith PP, Ciment GS, et al. Developmental analysis of the cytomegalovirus enhancer in transgenic animals. *J Virol* 1996;70:3215–3226.
14. Stinski MF, Macias MP, Malone CL, et al. In: Michelson S, Plotkin SA, eds. *Multidisciplinary Approach to Understanding Cytomegalovirus Disease.* London: Elsevier Science Publishers; 1993:3–12.
15. Ya J, Schilham MW, Clevers H, et al. Animal models of congenital defects in the ventriculoarterial connection of the heart. *J Mol Med* 1997;75:551–566.
16. McCarthy NJ, Evan GI. Methods for detecting and quantifying apoptosis. *Curr Top Dev Biol* 1998;36:259–278.
17. Van Pragh R, Weinberg PM, Matsuoka R, et al. In: Adams FH, Emmanouilides GC, eds. *Heart Disease in Infants, Children, and Adolescents.* Vol. 3. Baltimore: Williams and Wilkins; 1983:422–450.
18. Yamamoto H, Ueno H, Ooshima A, et al. Adenovirus-mediated transfer of a truncated transforming growth factor-beta (TGF-beta) type II receptor completely and specifically abolishes diverse signaling by TGF-beta in vascular wall cells in primary culture. *J Biol Chem* 1996;271:16253–16259.
19. Zou H, Niswander L. Requirement for BMP signaling in interdigital apoptosis and scale formation. *Science* 1996;272:738–741.

34

Novel Mechanisms Used by Cardiac Neural Crest Cells in Supporting Structural and Functional Heart Development

Margaret L. Kirby, PhD, Michael Farrell, PhD, Karen Waldo, MS, Tony L. Creazzo, PhD, Robert E. Godt, PhD, and Linda Leatherbury, MD

Ablation of premigratory cardiac neural crest results in cardiac outflow septation defects.[1] A consistent finding after neural crest ablation has been that altered myocardial development is found at a time prior to the normal entry of neural crest cells into the heart proper (Fig. 1).[2] Prior to its arrival in the outflow tract, cardiac neural crest cells populate the caudal pharyngeal arches.[3]

Myofibrillogenesis and electrical activity begin in the myocardium approximately stage 7.5–8 in the chick,[4–6] with striated myofibrils appearing in scattered cardiomyocytes at approximately stage 10 when the first weak contractions can be seen.[7–10] Anterograde circulation of blood begins at stage 14,[11] coincident with the time when the first myocardial abnormalities can be seen in the absence of cardiac neural crest.

In cardiac neural crest-ablated embryos, characteristic external features of the looping heart included straight outflow limbs, tighter heart loops, and variable dilations.[12] These hearts are readily

From Clark EB, Nakazawa M, Takao A (eds.): Etiology and Morphogenesis of Congenital Heart Disease: Twenty Years of Progress in Genetics and Developmental Biology. Armonk, NY: Futura Publishing Co., Inc.; © 2000.

distinguishable because of their variability although morphometric measurements have yielded no consistent differences. Recent experiments showed that within 24 hours after neural crest ablation, several parameters of myocardial development were abnormal beginning at stage 14.[13] Myocardial intracellular calcium transients were depressed by 30% to 60% indicating impaired excitation-contraction coupling. This was accompanied by increased myocardial proliferation and disorganized myofibrils. The thickness of the cardiac jelly, another indicator of myocardial development, appeared uneven. It is likely that the extreme variability in external morphology after neural crest ablation could be attributed to this uneven distribution of cardiac jelly. In contrast, endocardial development appeared normal as evidenced by normal expression of fibrillin-like protein (JB3 antigen), normal seeding of the cardiac jelly by mesenchyme to form cushions and formation of trabeculae. Formation of trabeculae depends on a heregulin signal from the endocardium. Therefore, the presence of normal trabeculation suggests that endocardial development is unaffected by cardiac neural crest ablation.

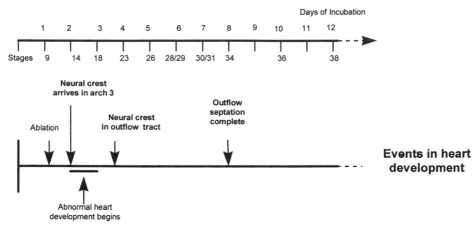

Figure 1. Timeline showing the relationship of neural crest ablation to events in chick heart development with respect to the period when signs of abnormal heart development are first noted.

These signs of abnormal myocardial development suggest that the presence of cardiac neural crest cells in the caudal pharyngeal arches during early heart development is necessary for normal differentiation and function of the myocardium. Many of these early alterations can be attenuated by replacing the cardiac neural crest, suggesting that the early changes are not due to a surgical effect or some other artifact of embryo manipulation.[13]

Cell tracing studies have shown that the neural crest does not interact directly with the myocardium at the stage when these changes are first observed. Furthermore, various individuals in our group have been unable to document any hemodynamic alterations of the aortic arch arteries that could cause such myocardial changes (Leatherbury, Jackson, Stewart, Connuck, unpublished observations). We have, however, observed in cardiac neural crest-ablated embryos, that the pharyngeal endoderm lies in apposition to the myocardium at stages 13 to 15 until mesenchyme derived from the epipharyngeal placodes and lateral plate mesoderm intervenes.[14] Normally the myocardium is well insulated from components of the pharynx by cardiac neural crest.[15] This observation led to the hypothesis that cardiac neural crest cells, which normally interpose between the pharyngeal endoderm and the myocardium, intercept a signal produced by the pharyngeal endoderm that would deleteriously affect further myocardial development. It has been shown previously that endoderm continues to release factors that can induce myocardial development from lateral plate mesoderm long after these signals are needed for heart formation.[16] We have confirmed this finding using stage 14 chick pharyngeal endoderm to induce stage 3 lateral plate mesoderm to differentiate into myocardium.[17]

To determine whether pharyngeal endoderm could be responsible for some of the myocardial changes seen in neural crest-ablated embryos, we cultured stage 12 to 13 myocardium with stage 14 pharyngeal endoderm for 24 hours. Using Fura-2, we were able to show a 26% decrease in the magnitude of the field-stimulated myocardial calcium transient in stages equivalent to 14 (Fig. 2), which is similar to the decrease seen in myocardium from stage 14 neural crest-ablated embryos. FGF-2 caused a 33% decrease in the myocardial calcium transient at stage 14, and anti-FGF neutralizing polyclonal antibody reversed the effect of both FGF-2 and endoderm on the myocardial transient. In contrast, TGF-β caused an

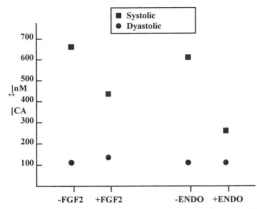

Figure 2. Average diastolic and peak systolic intracellular Ca^{2+} levels in cultured myocardium obtained from stage 14 chick embryos with or without FGF or pharyngeal endoderm for 24 hours.

18% increase in calcium transients and endothelin-1 had no effect.[18]

These results support the view that the cardiac neural crest cells interposed between the pharyngeal endoderm and the myocardium intercept an FGF-like signal that is deleterious to myocardial development. Additional studies indicate that abnormal myocardial development at these early stages is associated with malalignment defects such as dextroposed aorta,[19] and this may provide a common mechanism to explain the presence of these defects in a number of experimental paradigms.

Acknowledgments: This work was supported by PHS grants HL36059, HL51533, and HD17063.

References

1. Kirby ML, Waldo KL. Neural crest and cardiovascular patterning. *Circ Res* 1995; 77:211–215.
2. Creazzo TL, Godt RE, Leatherbury L, et al. Role of cardiac neural crest cells in cardiovascular development. *Ann Rev Physiol* 1998;60:267–286.
3. Waldo KL, Kumiski D, Kirby ML. Cardiac neural crest is essential for the persistence rather than the formation of an arch artery. *Dev Dyn* 1996;205:281–292.
4. Tokuyasu KT, Maher PA. Immunocytochemical studies of cardiac myofibrillogenesis in early chick embryos. II. Generation of alpha-actinin dots within titin spots at the time of the first myofibril formation. *J Cell Biol* 1987;105:2781–2793.
5. Lyons GE. *TCM* 1994;4:70–77.
6. Kamino K, Hirota A, Fujii S. Localization of pacemaking activity in early embryonic heart monitored using voltage-sensitive dye. *Nature* 1981;290:595–597.
7. Hibbs RG. *Am J Anat* 1956;99:17–52.
8. Manasek FJ. Histogenesis of the embryonic myocardium. *Am J Cardiol* 1970;25: 149–168.
9. Han Y, Dennis JE, Cohen-Gould L, et al. Expression of sarcomeric myosin in the presumptive myocardium of chicken embryos occurs within six hours of myocyte commitment. *Dev Dyn* 1992;193:257–265.
10. Hiruma T, Hirakow R. An ultrastructural topographical study on myofibrillogenesis in the heart of the chick embryo during pulsation onset period. *Anat Embryol* 1985;172:325–329.
11. Romanoff AL. In *The Avian Embryo. Structural and Functional Development.* New York: The Macmillan Company; 1960.
12. Leatherbury L, Yun JS, Wolfe R. *Ped Res* 1996;39:62A.
13. Waldo KL, Zdanowicz M, Burch J, et al. Abnormal myocardial development after cardiac neural crest ablation in chick embryos. *J Clin Invest* 1999;103(11):1499–507.
14. Kirby ML. Nodose placode provides ectomesenchyme to the developing chick heart in the absence of cardiac neural crest. *Cell Tissue Res* 1988;252:17–22.
15. Waldo KL, Kumiski D, Kirby ML. Cardiac neural crest is essential for the persistence rather than the formation of an arch artery. *Dev Dyn* 1996;205:281–292.
16. Sater AK, Jacobson AG. The specification of heart mesoderm occurs during gastrulation in Xenopus laevis. *Development* 1989;105:821–830.
17. Farrell MJ, Kirby ML. Unpublished data
18. Farrell MJ, Burch JL, Kumiski D, et al. Pharyngeal endoderm produces a factor that suppresses myocardial calcium transients. Submitted for publication.
19. Farrell MJ, Stadt H, Wallis KT, et al. HIRA, a DiGeorge syndrome candidate gene, is required for cardiac outflow tract septation. *Circ Res* 1999; 84:127–135.

35

Effects of Retinoic Acid and Bis-diamine With Expression of 90-kD Heat Shock Protein and Neurotrophin-3 Genes in Chicks

Hiroshi Sumida, PhD, Tsutomu Kumazaki, PhD, and Harukazu Nakamura, MD

All-trans-retinoic acid (RA) induces cardiac anomalies in chicks.[1] Isolated ventricular septal defect is the most common cardiac anomaly induced by RA in chicks.[2,3] N′N′-bis-(dichloroacetyl)-diamine (BIS), a protein synthesis inhibitor, also induces various cardiac anomalies in chicks.[4,5] Types of cardiac anomalies induced by BIS are different from those induced by RA. BIS induces double outlet right ventricle and persistent truncus arteriosus. Endocardial cushion mesenchymal cells of embryos treated with BIS lose ability of interaction with extracellular matrix.[5,6] Types of anomalies suggest that BIS might disturb the function of neural crest cells. RA might also relate neural crest deficiency.[2] The details of teratogenic mechanisms of both agents are still unknown.

Both RA and BIS possibly induce stress response in embryonic cells. After treatment with RA in maternal mice, 90-kD heat shock protein (HSP90) has been reported to be overexpressed in embryonic target organs of RA.[7] HSP90 is one of the abundant cellular proteins, and

it is believed to act as a molecular shaperonin,[8] though details of the functional feature of HSP90 are still unclear. Level of expression of HSP90 is possibly elevated in embryos treated with RA and BIS by cell damages.

On the other hand, Donovan et al.[9] have reported that neurotrophin-3 (NT-3), a family of neurotrophic factor, deficient results in cardiac insufficiency that might relate to neural crest abnormality in mice. Thus, changes of NT-3 expression in embryos could affect normal functions of neural crest cells.

In our examination concerning expression of HSP90 and NT-3 after treatment of RA or BIS on chick embryos, RA affected embryonic cells very quickly after the treatment (Figs. 1 and 2). Embryos treated with RA overexpressed HSP90 mRNA by 24 hours after treatment (Fig. 1). Western blot analysis indicated an increase of HSP90 level in embryos at 24 hours after treatment of RA, but it returned to the control level until 48 hours after treatment (data not shown). In mammals, HSP90 was classified into two subtypes, HSP90-α and HSP90-β. These two types of HSP90 are consisted in slightly different amino sequences, and may have different functions.[10] It has been reported that RA stimulates expres-

From Clark EB, Nakazawa M, Takao A (eds.): Etiology and Morphogenesis of Congenital Heart Disease: Twenty Years of Progress in Genetics and Developmental Biology. Armonk, NY: Futura Publishing Co., Inc.; © 2000.

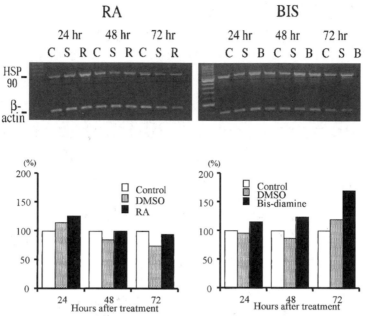

Figure 1. Expression of HSP90 in embryos treated with RA or BIS (see text). C or Control: specimens without treatment; S or DMSO: specimens treated with DMSO; R or RA: specimens treated with RA; B or Bis-diamine: specimens treated with BIS. RA or BIS, 100 μg dissolved in 20 μl dimethyl sulfoxide, was put on the extraembryonic vascular ring of Hi-brown chick embryos incubated for 3 days. To detect expression of HSP90 gene, reverse transcription polymerase chain reaction (RT-PCR) was carried out. Embryos of 24 hours, 48 hours, and 72 hours after treatment were homogenized in the 4.0 M guanidinium isothiocyanate solution. RNA was extracted by a general phenol extraction method. The cDNA solution produced by reverse transcription was reacted with taq polymerase using primers designed with chick HSP90 sequence. The sequence of 5'CCAGAAGATGAAGAAGAGAA3' (5':1661) was used as an upper primer, and 3'TAACCCTTTTGCTCCTAACA5' (3':2660) was used as a lower primer. The PCR product was expected at a size of 1019 bp. Intensity of bands of the PCR products was calibrated by densitometry.

sion of HSP90-α in F9 cells.[11] We preliminarily checked expression of HSP90 by Northern blot using cDNA probes designed for human HSP90-α and -β mRNA (data not shown). The probes are 70% to 75% homologous with chick HSP90 mRNA. At 24 hours and 48 hours after treatment, signals with the HSP90-α probe became more intense than controls. On the other hand, intensity of signals with the HSP90-β probe remained on a similar level with controls. Thus, overexpression of HSP90 by RA seems to be limited within 48 hours after treatment. In contrast, expression of HSP90 in embryos treated with BIS became detectable at 72 hours rather than 24 hours after treatment (Fig. 1). Overexpres-

sion of HSP90 on embryos treated with RA or BIS might indicate embryonic cell damage by these teratogens, although relation between the abnormal heart development and response of HSP90 against RA and BIS has not been clarified yet. The results suggest that RA damaged embryonic cells immediately after treatment and that BIS affects embryonic cells for a longer time. The differences in effective sequence of RA and BIS might relate to differences of types of anomalies induced by each teratogens. Indeed, BIS induces more severe cardiac anomalies than RA. Limited vulnerable period of RA might give chance of recovery from cell damage to embryos.

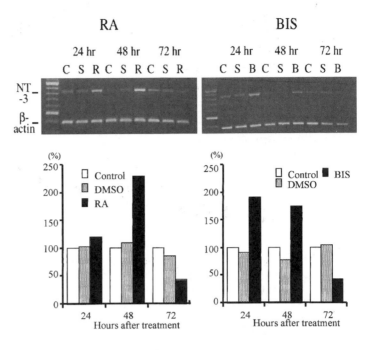

Figure 2. Expression of NT-3 in embryos treated with RA or BIS (see text). C or Control: specimens without treatment; S or DMSO: specimens treated with DMSO; R or RA: specimens treated with RA; B or BIS: specimens treated with BIS; Detection of expression of NT-3 was carried out with the same method for HSP90. For PCR, the sequence of 5'CTTGACTTTCTGTTTCTTTG3' (5':44) was used as an upper primer, and 3'AAATAGGAAGAACATAAATC5' (3':845) was used as a lower primer. The PCR product was expected at a size of 821 bp.

On the other hand, RA and BIS more clearly affected expression of NT-3, which is suggested to be necessary for development of neural crest cells.[12,13] Aspects of expression of NT-3, however, were contrary to our following expectation. We have expected rapid reduction of NT-3 expression after treatment of RA and BIS, because damage of neural crest cells at the early stage of development can easily induce abnormal cardiogenesis.[14,15] NT-3 expression, however, dramatically increased in the embryos from 24 hours to 48 hours after treatment of RA or BIS (Fig. 2). At 72 hours, the expression reduced to less than 50% of that of controls (Fig. 2). Thus, the results raised a new question: Why NT-3 expression was increased at 24 hours after treatment of RA or BIS? It is plausible but we should be cautious in speculating that RA and/or BIS directly induced NT-3 expression. There is another possibility that increasing of expression of NT-3 within 48 hours after treatment was due to a functional compensation of NT-3 production cells against embryonic cell damages. It would be followed by decreasing of expression by reason of consequent cell damage and

probably rebounding against overexpression of NT-3.

There might be a more direct relation between abnormal expression of NT-3 and cardiac anomalies than that of HSP90, because absence of expression of NT-3 results in cardiac anomalies.[9] Because NT-3 possibly regulates proliferation and differentiation of neural crest cells,[12,13] underexpression of NT-3 can cause disintegration of the function of neural crest cells. Cardiac defects by NT-3 deficiency were tetralogy of Fallot, persistent truncus arteriosus and ventricular septal defects,[9] and indeed, these types of anomalies are very similar with those of neural crest deficiency.[16] Furthermore, BIS induces very similar types of cardiac anomalies. And then, abnormal expression of NT-3 in embryos after treatment of BIS might be directly related to the functional insufficiency of neural crest cells and consequent abnormal cardiogenesis. The results of the present study, however, shows another difficulty for explanation of relation between cardiac anomalies induced by RA or BIS and abnormality of neural crest cells. If reduction of NT-3 expression certainly indicates disadvantage to proliferation and differentiation of neural crest cells, our results suggest that RA and BIS disturb functions of neural crest cells. However, at a period of reduction of NT-3 expression, neural crest cells have already migrated into the heart. Thus, we cannot relate dysfunction of neural crest cells on this period with cardiac malformation, unless over-amount of NT-3 damaged neural crest cells at earlier developing stage. We need further information in order to know whether overdose of NT-3 disintegrates function of neural crest cells.

The results of the present study might show that damage of NT-3 producing cells by treatment with RA or BIS results in subsequent dysfunction of neural crest cells. Although our results are very preliminary, we showed a possibility that unusual gene expression induced by teratogens caused abnormal heart development.

References

1. Osmond MK, Butler AJ, Voon FC, et al. The effects of retinoic acid on heart formation in the early chick embryo. *Development* 1991;113:1405–1417.
2. Hart RC, McCue PA, Ragland WL, et al. Avian model for 13-cis-retinoic acid embryopathy: Demonstration of neural crest related defects. *Teratology* 1990;41:463–472.
3. Hart RC, Winn KJ, Unger ER. Avian model for 13-cis-retinoic acid embryopathy: Morphological characterization of ventricular septal defects. *Teratology* 1992;46:533–539.
4. Okishima T, Takamura K, Matsuoka Y, et al. Cardiovascular anomalies in chick embryos produced by bis-diamine in dimethylsulfoxide. *Teratology* 1992;45:155–162.
5. Sumida H, Nakamura H, Matsuo T, et al. Effects of bis-diamine to cardiac mesenchymal cell migration of the chick embryo. *Cong Anom* 1995;35:215–222.
6. Sumida H, Nakamura H, Hisakane M, et al. Reduction of the interaction between vitronectin and cardiac cushion mesenchymal cells of the rat embryo by bisdiamine. *Biomed Res* 1992;13:309–315.
7. Anson J, Laborde JB, Pipkin JL, et al. Target tissue specificity of retinoic acid-induced stress protein and malformations in mice. *Teratology* 1991;44:19–28.
8. Wiech H, Buchner J, Zimmermann R, et al. Hsp90 chaperones protein folding in vitro. *Nature* 1992;358:169–170.
9. Donovan M, Hahn R, Tessarollo L, et al. Identification of an essential nonneuronal function of neurotrophin 3 in mammalian cardiac development. *Nat Genet* 1996;14:210–213.
10. Moore SK, Kozak C, Robinson EA, et al. Murine 86- and 84-kDa heat shock proteins, cDNA sequences, chromosome assignments, and evolutionary origins. *J Biol Chem* 1989;264:5343–5351.
11. Kohda T, Kondo K, Oishi M. Cellular HSP90 (HSP86) mRNA level and in vitro differentiation of mouse embryonal carcinoma (F9) cells. *FEBS Lett* 1991;290:107–110.
12. Pinco O, Carmeli C, Rosenthal A, et al. Neurotrophin-3 affects proliferation and differentiation of distinct neural crest cells and is present in the early neural tube of avian embryos. *J Neurobiol* 1993;24:1626–1641.
13. Kalcheim C, Carmeli C, Rosenthal A. Neurotrophin 3 is a mitogen for cultured neural crest cells. *Proc Natl Acad Sci U S A* 1992;89:1661–1665.
14. Kirby ML, Waldo KL. Neural crest and cardiovascular patterning. *Circ Res* 1995;77:211–215.
15. Nishibatake M, Kirby ML, Van Mierop LH. Pathogenesis of persistent truncus arteriosus and dextroposed aorta in the chick embryo after neural crest ablation. *Circulation* 1987;75:255–264.
16. Kirby ML, Turnage KLd, Hays BM. Characterization of conotruncal malformations following ablation of "cardiac" neural crest. *Anat Rec* 1985;213:87–93.

36

Alterations in RAR and TGF-β Expression in Developing Mouse Hearts Exposed to Retinoic Acid

Sachiko Miyagawa-Tomita, DVM, PhD,
Keiko Komatsu, BSc, Masae Morishima, DVM, PhD,
and Makoto Nakazawa, MD

Introduction

Vitamin A (retinol) and its biologically active derivative retinoic acid (RA) have multiple effects on vertebrate development, cellular differentiation, and homeostasis. The mechanisms by which RA exerts its actions are not fully understood, but several classes of proteins involved in mediating the cellular response to RA have been identified. It is widely accepted that two families of retinoic acid nuclear receptors (RARs and RXRs) act as ligand-dependent transcriptional factors of the RA signal during development.[1] Retinoic acid receptors (RARα, β and γ) are activated by all active forms of retinoic acid, whereas retinoid X receptors (RXRα, β and γ) are activated specifically by 9-cis RA. RXRs cannot only form homodimers with RXRs, but also heterodimers with RARs, thyroid hormone receptors, vitamin D3 receptor, and several orphan receptors.

RA plays an important role in development, especially in cardiogenesis. Exposure of mouse embryos to excess RA induces a high frequency of transposition of the great arteries.[2] Vitamin A deficiency in rat embryos,[3] or mutation of RARs and RXRα[4,5] in mouse embryos are also associated with anomalies of cardiovascular morphology.

Double knock-out of RAR/RAR and RXR/RAR in mice shows several types of congenital heart disease, which are persistent truncus arteriosus, atrioventricular canal defect, aortic arch anomalies, and hypoplastic development of the ventricular myocardium.[4,5] Dysfunction of RA-dependent genes may be a key element in the etiology of congenital heart disease.

Current Research

We examined the expression of RAR-α, RAR-β, and RAR-γ (LGME-U. 184, a gift from Dr. Chambon) in normal and RA-treated mouse embryonic hearts by Northern hybridization, and protein expression by immunohistochemistry (Santa Cruz, Calif). We also looked at transforming growth factor (TGF)-β1,

From Clark EB, Nakazawa M, Takao A (eds.): Etiology and Morphogenesis of Congenital Heart Disease: Twenty Years of Progress in Genetics and Developmental Biology. Armonk, NY: Futura Publishing Co., Inc.; © 2000.

-β2, and -β3 expression (Genentech, Inc., San Francisco, Calif), simultaneously.

All-trans RA dissolved in dimethylsulfoxide was injected, intraperitoneally, into pregnant mice at gestation day 8.5. In RA-treated hearts, the expression of RAR-α, RAR-β, and TGF-βs RNA in the hearts was induced by RA treatment. However, the sensitivity of these gene transcriptions to RA was different in each region when mouse embryonic hearts at gestation day 12.5 were divided to three regions: atria, ventricles, and outflow tract. In the outflow tract of the heart, the expression of RAR-γ and TGF-β3 RNA was upregulated and expression of RAR-β and TGF-β2 was downregulated. In the atrium of the heart, the expression of TGF-β1, TGF-β2, and TGF-β3 was upregulated and expression of RAR-β was downregulated.

An in situ hybridization study showed the expression pattern of RAR transcripts in mouse embryonic heart.[6,7] Detailed expression of the factors was not found. In the immunohistochemistry studies, cardiac muscle expressed three RAR proteins. In the myocardium adjacent to the cushion tissues in the outflow tract and atrioventricular canal regions, the expression of RAR-α and RAR-β proteins was distinctive.

Expression of TGF-β2, TGF-β3, BMP2, and BMP4 transcripts was shown in myocardium of the atrioventricular canal and outflow tract. Expression of TGF-β2 and TGF-β3 transcripts was detected in mesenchymal cells of the atrioventricular canal cushion, and TGF-β1 transcripts in endothelial cells of the atrioventricular canal cushion and outflow tract[8,9,10,11] Expression of TGF-β3 protein was seen weakly and ubiquitously in cushion tissues and myocardium, and TGF-β1 and β2 proteins were expressed in myocardium. It has been thought that RA is capable of indirectly modulating TGF-βs at different levels of their synthesis.[12] Antibody of TGF-β receptor type II blocked activation and migration of cells of the atrioventricular cushion.[13] Although mutation of TGF-β1 or TGF-β3 was seen in mice with a normal heart, TGF-β2 knockout mice showed heart anomalies with a wide range of developmental defects.[14] The TGF-β signaling cascade including the receptors should be clarified in developmental myocardium and epithelial-mesenchymal transformation.[15]

A study of targeted disruptions in the mouse RXRα gene showed hypoplasia of cardiac ventricular muscle, especially compact zone development, and cardiovascular anomalies.[16] It is possible that both RXRα and RARs participate in the mediation of cardiac muscle development.[17] Although downstream genes of RARs and RXRα associated with congenital heart disease have not been found, one of the RXRα downstream targeted genes, cloned G1, has been isolated. Clone G1-encoded protein was involved in intermediary metabolism.[18] Altered intermediary metabolism may contribute to dilated cardiomyopathy in the mice with RXRα mutations. Mice with ventricular cardiomyocytes deficient in RXRα were made with chimeric analysis[19] and a cre/lox recombination strategy,[20] which is a completely different methodology. The mice showed a completely normal phenotype with normal developing hearts. It has been suggested that RXRα functions not in a cardiac myocyte lineage, but in a non-cell-autonomous manner.

In addition to RA nuclear receptors, two cellular cytoplasmic RA binding proteins (CRABPI and CRABPII) have been identified. Both CRABPI and CRABPII transcripts and proteins are expressed in heart muscle and the neural crest in pharyngeal arches during mouse and chick development (Miyagawa-Tomita, et al., unpublished data). However, CRABPI/CRABPII double-mutant mice were essentially normal.[21]

The present results suggest that TGF-β and RAR genes are expressed at appropriate times to influence different aspects of heart development, and each region of the embryonic heart has a different sensitivity to RA. Further detailed studies on RARs and RXRα in cardiogenesis are required.

References

1. Chambon P. A decade of molecular biology of retinoic acid receptors. *FASEB, J* 1996; 10:940–954.
2. Yasui H, Nakazawa M, Morishima M, et al. Morphological observations on the pathogenetic process of transposition of the great arteries induced by retinoic acid in mice.*Circulation* 1995;91:2478–2486.
3. Wilson J, Warkany J. *Am J Anat.* 1949;85: 113–155.
4. Mendelsohn C, Lohnes C, Décimo D, et al. Function of the retinoic acid receptors (RARs) during development (II). Multiple abnormalities at various stages of organogenesis in RAR double mutants. *Development* 1994;120:2749–2771.
5. Lee RY, Luo J, Evans RM, et al. Compartment-selective sensitivity of cardiovascular morphogenesis to combinations of retinoic acid receptor gene mutations. *Circ Res* 1997;80:757–764.
6. Dollé P, Ruberte E, Leroy P, et al. Retinoic acid receptors and cellular retinoid binding proteins. I. A systematic study of their differential pattern of transcription during mouse organogenesis. *Development* 1990; 110:1133–1151.
7. Ruberte E, Dolle P, Chambon P, et al. Retinoic acid receptors and cellular retinoid binding proteins. II. Their differential pattern of transcription during early morphogenesis in mouse embryos. *Development* 1991;111:45–60.
8. Akhurst RJ, Lehnert SA, Faissner A, et al. TGF beta in murine morphogenetic processes: the early embryo and cardiogenesis. *Development* 1990;108:645–656.
9. Millan FA, Denhez F, Kondaiah P, et al. Embryonic gene expression patterns of TGF beta 1, beta 2 and beta 3 suggest different developmental functions in vivo. *Development* 1991;111:131–143.
10. Lyons KM, Pelton RW, Hogan BLM. Organogenesis and pattern formation in the mouse: RNA distribution patterns suggest a role for bone morphogenetic protein-2A (BMP-2A). *Development* 1991;109:833–844.
11. Jones CM, Lyons KM, Hogan BLM. Involvement of Bone Morphogenetic Protein-4 (BMP-4) and Vgr-1 in morphogenesis and neurogenesis in the mouse. *Development* 1991;111:531–542.
12. Mahmood R, Flanders KC, Morriss-Kay GM. The effects of retinoid status on TGF beta expression during mouse embryogenesis. *Anat Embryol* 1995;192: 21–33.
13. Brown CB, Boyer AS, Runyan RB, et al. Antibodies to the Type II TGFbeta receptor block cell activation and migration during atrioventricular cushion transformation in the heart. *Dev Biol* 1996;174: 248–257.
14. Sanford LP, Ormsby I, Gittenberger AC, et al. TGFbeta2 knockout mice have multiple developmental defects that are non-overlapping with other TGFbeta knockout phenotypes. *Development* 1997;124:2659–2670.
15. Brand T, Schneider MD. Transforming growth factor-beta signal transduction. *Circ Res* 1996;78:173–179.
16. Gruber PJ, Kubalak SW, Pexieder T, et al. RXR alpha deficiency confers genetic susceptibility for aortic sac, conotruncal, atrioventricular cushion, and ventricular muscle defects in mice. *J Clin Invest* 1996; 98:1332–1343.
17. Kastner P, Messaddeq N, Mark M, et al. Vitamin A deficiency and mutations of RXRalpha, RXRbeta and RARalpha lead to early differentiation of embryonic ventricular cardiomyocytes. *Development* 1997; 124:4749–4758.
18. Ruiz-Lozano P, Smith SM, Perkins G, et al. Energy deprivation and a deficiency in downstream metabolic target genes during the onset of embryonic heart failure in RXRalpha-/- embryos. *Development* 1998; 125:533–544.
19. Tran CM, Sucov HM. The RXRalpha gene functions in a non-cell-autonomous manner during mouse cardiac morphogenesis. *Development* 1998;125:1951–1956.
20. Chen J, Kubalak SW, Chien KR. Ventricular muscle-restricted targeting of the RXRalpha gene reveals a non-cell-autonomous requirement in cardiac chamber morphogenesis. *Development* 1998;125: 1948–1949.
21. Lampron C, Rochette-Egly C, Gorry P, et al. Mice deficient in cellular retinoic acid binding protein II (CRABPII) or in both CRABPI and CRABPII are essentially normal. *Development* 1995;121:539–548.

37

Essential Role of the Forkhead (Winged Helix) Gene MFH-1 in the Aortic Arch Formation

Naoyuki Miura, MD, PhD, Kiyoshi Iida, MD,
Hideaki Kakinuma, MD, Haruhiko Koseki, MD,
Naoko Kato, MD, Nobuaki Yoshida, MD, PhD,
and Toshihiro Sugiyama, MD

The cardiovascular system undergoes a complex series of morphogenetic events to form a heart and an aorta in fetuses.[1] Formation of the heart and aorta requires migration, differentiation, and precise interactions among multiple cells from several embryonic origins. The aortic arch is formed through an extensive remodeling of arch arteries and dorsal aortas. Neural crest-derived cells are considered to migrate into the pharyngeal arches 3, 4, and 6 and support the endothelium of the aortic arch arteries as the tunica media. In the remodeling of aortic arch, the left fourth arch artery develops to form a part of the aortic arch. The third arch arteries and right fourth artery give rise to the common carotid arteries and the proximal region of the right subclavian artery, respectively. Although anatomic and physiological descriptions of aortic arch anomalies in newborns have existed for half a century,[2-4] the molecular bases underlying the anomalies remain poorly understood.

Winged helix proteins are a family of transcription factors that share an evolutionarily conserved DNA-binding domain.[5,6] Several lines of evidence indicates that the winged helix genes are involved in patterning and morphogenesis during development. We previously isolated the Mesenchyme Fork Head-1 (MFH-1) gene,[7] which is expressed in developing cartilaginous tissues, kidneys, and dorsal aortas.[7,8] Genomic and protein structures of MFH-1 are conserved between human and mouse, and the MFH-1 proteins act as a transactivator.[9]

To examine MFH-1 function during development, we made a knockout mouse of the *MFH-1* gene. Heterozygous mice were indistinguishable from wild-type animals. The homozygotes demonstrated respiratory compromise as evidenced by gasping motions and cyanosis, and died within ten minutes after birth. We found the major anomalies in the aortic arch in the *MFH-1* mutants. The most cases (83%) of homozygous mice displayed type B interruption of the aortic arch where part of the aortic arch between the left common carotid artery and the left subclavian artery did not exist[2] (Fig. 1B). The remaining cases (17%) of mutants showed type C interruption of the aortic arch in which part of the aortic arch

From Clark EB, Nakazawa M, Takao A (eds.): Etiology and Morphogenesis of Congenital Heart Disease: Twenty Years of Progress in Genetics and Developmental Biology. Armonk, NY: Futura Publishing Co., Inc.; © 2000.

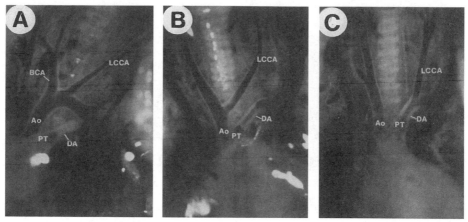

Figure 1. Aortic arch anomalies in *MFH-1*-null mice at day 0 (birth). **A.** Normal aortic arch of wild-type mice. **B** and **C.** Aortic arch anomalies of *MFH-1* (-/-) mice. **B.** Type B interruption of the aortic arch (interrupted between LCCA and LSA). **C.** Type C interruption of the aortic arch (interrupted between BCA and LCCA). Ao, aorta; BCA, brachiocephalic artery; DA, ductus arteriosus Botalli; LCCA, left common carotid artery; LSA, left subclavian artery; RCCA, right common carotid artery; RSA, right subclavian artery; PT, pulmonary truncus.

between the brachiocephalic artery and the left common carotid artery did not exist[2] (Fig. 1C). Aortopulmonary septation was formed normally in all individuals.

Because human patients with type B interruption of the aortic arch also have an associated ventricular septal defect,[2–4] we further examined the intracardiac defects of hearts from newborn homozygotes. Frequently (in 75% of cases), a tiny ventricular septal defect was observed (data not shown). These results indicate that the anomalies in *MFH-1* (–/–) mice are the same as those in humans.

Next, we examined embryos to investigate the pathogenetic process of the anomaly in the aortic arch in *MFH-1*(–/–) mice. The remodeling of the dorsal aorta and arch arteries to generate the aortic arch occurs between 10.5 dpc and 14.5 dpc. Although all embryos younger than 11.5 dpc were alive, dead embryos whose hearts did not beat were found in about half of the embryos older than 13.5 dpc. When we examined embryos at the critical stage around 12.5 dpc (Fig. 2), we found that at 11.5 dpc, the right and left third, fourth, and sixth arch arteries communicated with dorsal aortas in both the wild-type and the mutant fetuses; no dif-

ferences were observed (Fig. 2A, B). At 12.5 dpc, the left fourth arch artery develops to form the isthmus of the aortic arch together with the dorsal aorta. The left third arch artery gives rise to the left common carotid artery. In *MFH-1*(–/–) embryos, the left fourth arch artery disappeared (Fig. 2D) in most cases. We also found that the proximal segment from the left third arch artery was diminished (Fig. 2E) in a small number of cases. The right third and fourth arch arteries were not affected (data not shown). Our results indicate that in mice lacking *MFH-1*, the left fourth arch artery might catastrophically regress during remodeling of the aortic arch around 12.5 dpc.

Then we examined in detail the expression of the *MFH-1* gene in the developing arch arteries by in situ hybridization of sections of embryos from 9.5 dpc to 12.5 dpc in order to clarify the relationship between the phenotype and the expression of the gene. The results indicated that the MFH-1 mRNA was strongly detected in the third, fourth and sixth arch arteries on the right and left sides (data not shown). These results indicate that the area of aortic arch anomalies is more

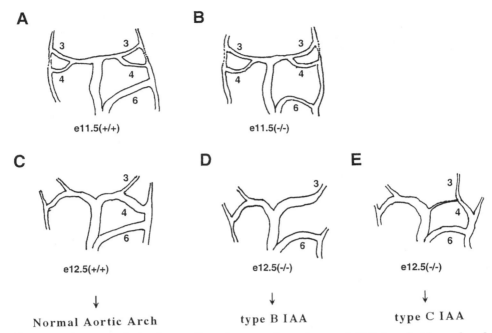

Figure 2. An anomaly in the aortic arch occurs in embryos of 12.5 dpc. **A.** Normal arch arteries in wild-type embryos of 11.5 dpc. **B:** *MFH-1*(−/−) embryos of 11.5 dpc. In **A** and **B**, the third, fourth, and sixth arch arteries communicate with dorsal aortas normally. **C.** Normal arch arteries in wild-type embryos of 12.5 dpc. **D** and **E.** Anomalies in the aortic arch in *MFH-1*(−/−) embryos of 12.5 dpc. In most cases, the left fourth arch artery disappears (**D**), which results in type B interruption of the aortic arch (IAA). In a small number of cases, the segment proximal to the left third arch artery is diminished (**E**), which results in type C IAA. In all cases, the right third and fourth arch arteries are present normally.

restricted than that of *MFH-1* mRNA expression.

Aortic arch development can be divided into two functional phases; first, the generation of the dorsal aorta and arch arteries and subsequently the remodeling of these primary structures. Ablation of the premigratory cardiac neural crest cells in chick embryos results not only in agenesis or hypogenesis of the thymus, thyroid, and parathyroid gland but also in cardiovascular malformations including persistent truncus arteriosus, double-outlet right ventricle, tetralogy of Fallot, and interrupted aortic arch.[10–11] These results imply that accumulation of neural crest-derived cells in prospective arch artery regions is a critical initial process for the subsequent remodeling of the arch arteries. In the mutant mice, the left fourth arch artery was first formed and then dis-

appeared (Fig. 2). Our results indicate that the MFH-1 gene product is not essentially required for the accumulation of neural crest cells and the formation of primary structures, although MFH-1 expression can be seen in the developing arch arteries starting from a very early stage. However, MFH-1 is required for the extensive remodeling of the dorsal aorta and arch arteries to generate the aortic arch, particularly in the derivation of the left fourth arch artery.

DiGeorge syndrome in humans is typically characterized by aplasia or hypoplasia of the thymus, hypoplasia of the parathyroid glands, outflow tract defects of the heart, cleft palate, and mildly dysmorphic facial features.[12,13] Among these criteria, *MFH-1*-deficient mice exhibited type B interruption of the aortic arch with ventricular septal defect, cleft palate, and possibly craniofacial abnormalities, but not defects of the thymus and parathyroid. Thus, phenotypes of *MFH-1*-deficient mice overlapped with those in patients with DiGeorge syndrome. However, the human *MFH-1* gene is located at chromosome 16,[8] not at chromosome 22, which is linked to many cases of DiGeorge syndrome.[12] Therefore, the *MFH-1* gene is unlikely to be the defective gene in DiGeorge syndrome. Rather, an absence or a defect of *MFH-1* positive cells in the prospective aortic arch region might be the cause for interruption of the aortic arch in the DiGeorge syndrome. It is also possible that *MFH-1* gene might be one of the target genes of the DiGeorge gene in subsets of neural crest-derived cells.

MFH-1-deficient mice are useful as a mouse model for interruption of the aortic arch. Molecular analysis of the mutant mice at the stage of remodeling of the aortic arch will open a new era in understanding the gene(s) involved in aortic artery formation.[14]

References

1. Olson EN, Srivastava D. Molecular pathways controlling heart development. *Science* 1996;272:671–676.
2. Celoria GC, Patton RB. Congenital absence of the aortic arch. *Am Heart J* 1959;58:407–413.
3. Moller JH, Edwards JE. Interruption of aortic arch. *Am J Roentgenol* 1965;95:557–572.
4. van Mierop LHS, Kutsche LM. Interruption of the aortic arch and coarctation of the aorta: pathogenetic relations. *Am J Cardiol* 1984;54:829–834.
5. Lai E, Clark KL, Burley SK, et al. Hepatocyte nuclear factor 3/fork head or "winged helix" proteins: a family of transcription factors of diverse biologic function. *Proc Natl Acad Sci U S A* 1993;90:10421–10423.
6. Kaufmann E, Knochel W. Five years on the wings of fork head. *Mech Dev* 1996;57:3–20.
7. Miura N, Wanaka A, Tohyama M, et al. MFH-1, a new member of the fork head domain family, is expressed in developing mesenchyme. *FEBS Lett* 1993;326:171–176.
8. Kaestner KH, Bleckmann SC, Monaghan AP, et al. Clustered arrangement of winged helix genes fkh-6 and MFH-1: possible implications for mesoderm development. *Development* 1996;122:1751–1758.
9. Miura N, Iida K, Kakinuma H, et al. Isolation of the mouse (MFH-1) and human (FKHL 14) mesenchyme fork head-1 genes reveals conservation of their gene and protein structures. *Genomics* 1997;41:489–492.
10. Kirby ML, Waldo KL. Role of neural crest in congenital heart disease. *Circulation* 1990;82:332–340.
11. Kirby ML, Waldo KL. Neural crest and cardiovascular patterning. *Circ Res* 1995;77:211–215.
12. Wilson DI, Burn J, Scambler P, et al. DiGeorge syndrome: part of CATCH 22. *J Med Genet* 1993;30:852–856.
13. Goldmuntz E, Emanuel BS. Genetic disorders of cardiac morphogenesis. The DiGeorge and velocardiofacial syndromes. *Circ Res* 1997;80:437–443.
14. Iida K, Koseki H, Kakinuma H, et al. Essential roles of the winged helix transcription factor MFH-1 in aortic arch patterning and skeletogenesis. *Development* 1997;124:4627–4638.

38

A Dual Pathway to the Heart Links Neural Crest to In- and Outflow Tract Septation and to Differentiation of the Conduction System

Robert E. Poelmann, PhD and
Adriana C. Gittenberger-de Groot, PhD

The embryonic heart is constructed from a number of cells, deriving from various sources during different phases of development. The contractile and conducting cardiomyocytes originate in the cardiogenic plate, and the coronary endothelium and the endocardium arise from various segments of the splanchnic mesoderm. The different echelons of the interstitial, smooth muscle, and fibroblastic cells come from other parts of the splanchnic mesoderm, such as the pro-epicardial organ.[1,2] Finally, an interesting extracardiac subpopulation derives from the rhombencephalon, the dorsal part of which is known as the cardiac neural crest (CNC). It has already been established that the arterial pole of the heart recruits a large number of CNC cells involved in outflow tract septation,[3,4] autonomic innervation[5] and smooth muscle cell[6,7] formation of the pharyngeal arch arteries. We have postulated the possibility that the ventral part of the rhombencephalon may give rise to cells that acquire a position deeper in the heart and that these cells use the dorsal mesocar-

dium at the venous pole as a site of entry.[8] The cells become located in the regions where the conduction system will develop as well as in the atrioventricular cushion mass. The major questions concern the possible role of CNC cells during atrioventricular (AV) and outflow tract septation and in differentiation of the cardiac conduction system. To this aim we used an approach in which cell lineage tracing was combined with differentiation markers.

Cell lineage tracing of neural crest cells was performed using a replication defective spleen necrosis retrovirus harboring the LacZ reporter gene.[9,10] A solution containing 10^6 retroviral particles/mL was applied to the (pre)migratory rhombencephalic neural crest cells at Hamburger Hamilton HH stage 8–12 in chicken embryos. The solution was either flushed onto the neural plate or microinjected into selected parts of the neural tissue. The injections were performed in the ventral part of the neural tissue, or in the dorsal segment. Alternatively, embryos received 1 to 4 microinjections into the migration path of the neural crest cells, i.e., adjacent to the dorsal part of the neural groove. In case of multiple injections the labeled area spanned a length of only one particular somite. In a subset of

From Clark EB, Nakazawa M, Takao A (eds.): Etiology and Morphogenesis of Congenital Heart Disease: Twenty Years of Progress in Genetics and Developmental Biology. Armonk, NY: Futura Publishing Co., Inc.; © 2000.

embryos the dorsal half of the neural tissue was ablated with sharpened tungsten needles,[11] whereas the intact anterior, posterior, or ventral part of the tube was labeled with the retroviral construct. After survival times up to HH stage 38 the labeled cells are visualized using a galactosidase staining procedure.

Immunohistochemical techniques were used to demonstrate the differentiation paths of the CNC and of the cardiac cells. We used the following antibodies: HNK1,[12] to study the migrating neural crest cells and neuronal cells[5]; RMO270, staining neuronal cells (note that both these antibodies stain also the neural crest target areas of the myocardium, albeit in faint way); HHF35, staining actin in both cardiomyocytes and smooth muscle cells; SNAP25, to delineate the conduction system. Using the retroviral labeling many CNC-derived cells have been encountered in the arterial pole (Fig. 1),

including the media of the pharyngeal arch arteries, the vagal innervation, and the mesenchyme of the aortopulmonary septum.[4] In these regions, CNC cells can be found throughout the stages studied. Inside the myocardial sleeve of the heart CNC have been traced into the outflow tract endocardial cushions. After HH 32 the number of crest cells in the cushions decrease dramatically and at HH 36 only a small amount of labeled cells have been encountered in the outflow tract septum.

A hitherto undescribed entrance of rhombencephalic cells to the heart, the venous pole, has been detected with the mentioned approach (Fig. 2). LacZ-positive cells have been encountered in the dorsal mesocardium, the base of the atrium septum, at a dorsal position in the interventricular septum and in a ring encircling the right atrioventricular orifice. These areas are continuous with each other and the pattern of staining strongly

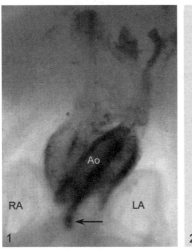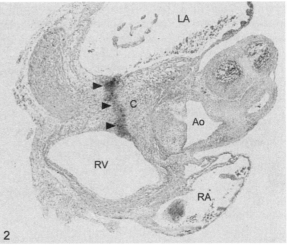

Figure 1. The arterial pole of an HH 35 chick embryo that has been marked with the retrovirus containing LacZ at HH 9. The vessels of the arterial pole show intense staining in the media, indicative of neural crest (NC)-derived smooth muscle cells in this particular embryo. The arrow points toward the NC-derived aortopulmonary septum. Ao, aorta; LA, left atrium; RA, right atrium.

Figure 2. Section through the base of the heart of an HH 30 embryo, treated in a similar way. This particular embryo shows LacZ+, neural crest (NC)-derived cells in both the outflow tract (not presented) and the venous pole. The arrowheads indicate a subpopulation of NC-derived cells that is continuous with both the dorsal mesocardium, including a group of NC cells surrounding the pulmonary veins and the superior cardinal vein, and with the region of the His bundle. C, fused AV cushions; RV, right ventricle.

suggests the venous pole as entrance.[8] As earlier studies using chick-quail chimeras[3,11] did not show targeting to the heart via the venous pole we performed a small set of experiments in which we ablated the posterior rhombencephalon in combination with retroviral marking of either the adjacent anterior, posterior or ventral segments of the neural tissue. The cardiac malformation resulting from the ablation was usually a persistent truncus arteriosus. With concomitant anterior or posterior labeling we were unable to find labeled CNC cells in the heart, partly confirming other's results.[13-15] Ablation combined with labeling of the underlying part of the neural groove, however, gave a substantial number of labeled cells in the both the outflow tract and the inflow part of the heart, in comparable areas as in the non-ablated embryos. This was not found after e.g. DiI 15 labeling. Moreover, retroviral microinjections in the ventral segment of non-ablated embryos resulted in labeled cells in the same areas. These results led us to the conclusion that the dorsal part of the neural groove gives rise to CNC-derived cells in the heart, but the ventral part is also able to give rise to migrating labeled cells. The exact migration route of the ventrally derived cells has yet to be determined. We have the strong impression that these cells use the dorsally located neural crest as site of exit and for the time being we have chosen to include them into the cardiac neural crest. These cells predominantly migrate towards the venous pole. This might explain why chick-quail chimeras in which usually the dorsal part of the chick neural tube has been replaced by a ditto quail heterograft did not show quail cells entering the heart via the venous pole.

The histological observation of apoptotic cells[16-18] prompted us to use the TUNEL approach to determine the areas in which programmed cell death was paramount. These areas coincide with CNC-target areas, even to the extent that many, if not all, LacZ-positive cells showed intense TUNEL-staining. From these observations we concluded that many neural crest cells in the areas of conduction system differentiation and of in- and outflow tract myocardialization are removed by apoptosis. The important question concerns the role of apoptotic CNC cells in these processes. The most straight forward hypothesis is that these cells die because they enter an environment that does not sustain survival, implying no special function other than removal of superfluous cells. However, we propose that the sequel of (1) targeted migration, (2) apoptosis, and (3) final cardiomyocyte differentiation, belong to one specific cascade of events. The myocardial targets of the CNC can be identified by immunohistochemical staining for specific glycoproteins, such as Leu7,[19] HNK1,[12] GlN,[20] and PS-CAM.[21] These very same regions express Msx2,[22] which is known to be involved in signaling for apoptosis in defined segments of the premigratory rhombencephalic neural crest.[23] Apoptosis of CNC that have arrived in the heart may change the microenvironment by, for example, shifting the pH, which is reported to affect the structure of the extracellular matrix and to activate growth factors, like TGFb. Transforming growth factors are present in the heart, but probably in a latent form. We postulate that activated TGFb will be responsible for the myocardialization of the inflow and of the outflow. It is interesting to analyze the heart malformations of the TGFb-2 knock-out mouse,[24] that shows both inflow and outflow malformations. In the human population some clinical features of Down syndrome, i.e., atrioventricular septal defect,[25] can be linked to maldevelopment of this cell population. Other characteristics in Down, such as high incidence of megacolon (Hirschsprung disease) and of diseases of the dental elements are probably also neural crest-related. The other topographical and temporal relationship of apoptotic CNC consists with the final differentiation of the central conduction system. Although it is evident that cardiomyocytes show conductive capacities from very early stages onward, the delineation of specialized conductive cells from the cardiac working myocardium, is only relatively late. We propose that the final differentiation of the AV node (which remains inconspicuous in birds), the bundle of His and the bundle branches is induced by this subpopulation of CNC. As in the chick embryo the neural crest cells take up their position close to the conduction system and become apoptotic in about HH stage 33, we have to contemplate on a function relatively late in differentiation, probably through insulating the conduction system from the surrounding myocardium. It is tempting to speculate what may happen both structurally and functionally with the conduction system after maldevelopment of the neural crest. We suppose that several types of arrhythmia might be related, among which is junctional ectopic tachycardia (JET).

References

1. Vrancken Peeters MPFM, Mentink MMT, Poelmann RE, et al. Cytokeratins as a marker for epicardial formation in the quail embryo. *Anat Embryol* 1995;191:503–508.
2. Gittenberger-de Groot AC, Vrancken Peeters MPFM, Mentink MMT, et al. Epicardial derived cells contribute a novel population to the myocardial wall and the atrioventricular cushions. *Circ Res* 1998;82:1043–1052.
3. Kirby MM, Waldo KL. Role of neural crest in congenital heart disease. *Circulation* 1990;82:332–340.
4. Poelmann RE, Mikawa T, Gittenberger-de Groot AC. Neural crest cells in outflow tract septation of the embryonic chicken heart: Differentiation and apoptosis. *Dev Dyn* 1998;212:373–384.
5. Verberne ME, Gittenberger-de Groot AC, Poelmann RE. Lineage and development of the parasympathetic nervous system of the embryonic chicken heart. *Anat Embryol* 1998;198:171–184.
6. Bergwerff M, DeRuiter MC, Poelmann RE, et al. Onset of elastogenesis and down-regulation of smooth muscle actin as distinguishing phenomena in artery differentiation in the chick embryo. *Anat Embryol* 1996;194:545–557.
7. Bergwerff M, Verberne ME, DeRuiter MC, et al. Neural crest contribution to the developing circulatory system. Implications for vascular morphology? *Circ Res* 1998;82:221–231.
8. Poelmann RE, Gittenberger-de Groot AC. A subpopulation of apoptosis-prone cardiac neural crest cells targets to the venous pole. Multiple functions in heart development? *Dev Biol* 1999;207:271–286.
9. Mikawa T, Fischman DA, Dougherty JP, et al. In vivo analysis of a new LacZ retrovirus for cell lineage marking in avian and other species. *Exp Cell Res* 1991;195:516–523.
10. Noden DM, Poelmann RE, Gittenberger-de Groot AC. Cell origins and tissue boundaries during outflow tract development. *Trends Cardiovasc Med* 1995;5:69–76.
11. Kirby ML. Nodose placode provides ectomesenchyme to the developnig chick heart in the absence of neural crest. *Cell Tissue Res* 1988;252:17–22.
12. Luider TM, Bravenboer N, Meijers C, et al. The distribution and characterization of HNK-1 antigens in the developing avian heart. *Anat Embryol* 1993;188:307–316.
13. Serbedzija GN, Bronner-Fraser M, Fraser SE. Vital dye analysis of cranial neural crest cell migration in the mouse embryo. *Development* 1992;116:297–307.
14. Couly G, Grapin-Botton A, Coltey P, et al. The regeneration of the cephalic neural crest, a problem revisited: The regenerating cells originate from the contralateral or from the anterior and posterior neural fold. *Development* 1996;122:3393–3407.
15. Suzuki HR, Kirby ML. Absence of neural crest regeneration from the postotic neural tube. *Dev Biol* 1997;184:222–233.
16. Pexieder T. Cell death in morphogenesis and teratogenesis of the heart. *Adv Anat Embryol Cell Biol* 1975;51:1–100.
17. Thompson RP, Fitzharris TP. Morphogenesis of the truncus arteriosus of the chick embryo heart: Tissue reorganization during septation. *Am J Anat* 1979;156:251–264.
18. Icardo JM. Distribution of fibronectin during the morphogenesis of the truncus. *Anat Embryol* 1985;171:193–200.
19. Blom NA, Gittenberger-de Groot AC, DeRuiter MC, et al. Development of the cardiac conduction system in human embryos using HNK-1 antigen expression: Possible relevance for understanding of abnormal

atrial automaticity. *Circulation* 1999;99: 800–806.

20. Wessels A, Vermeulen JL, Verbeek FJ, et al. Spatial distribution of "tissue-specific" antigens in the developing human heart and skeletal muscle. III. An immunohisto-chemical analysis of the neural tissue antigen GlN2 in the embryonic heart; implications for the development of the atrioventricular conduction system. *Anat Rec* 1992;232:97–111.

21. Chuck ET, Watanabe M. Differential expression of PSA-CAM and HNK-1 epitopes in the developing cardiac conduction system of the chick. *Dev Dyn* 1997;209:182–195.

22. Chan-Thomas PS, Thompson RP, Robert B, et al. Expression of homeobox genes Msx1 (Hox7) and Msx2 (Hox8) during car-diac development in the chick. *Dev Dyn* 1993;197:203–216.

23. Lumsden A, Graham A. Death in the neural crest: Implications for pattern formation. *Sem Cell Dev Biol* 1996; 7:169–174.

24. Sanford LP, Ormsby I, Gittenberger-de Groot AC, et al. TGFb2 knock out mice have multiple developmental defects that are non-overlapping with other TGFb knock-out phenotypes. *Development* 1997; 124:2659–2670.

25. Marino B. Patterns in congenital heart disease and associated anomalies in children with Down syndrome. In: Marino B, Pueschel SM, eds. *Heart Disease in Persons with Down Syndrome.* Baltimore: Paul H. Brookes Publishing Co.; 1996: 133–140.

39

Molecular Induction of the Cardiac Conduction System

Takashi Mikawa, PhD, Robert G. Gourdie, PhD, Jeanette Hyer, PhD, Yan Wei, PhD, and Kimiko Takebayashi-Suzuki, PhD

A synchronized heart beat is controlled by pacemaking action potentials conducted through Purkinje fibers.[1,2] Dysfunction of this essential tissue is a direct cause of arrhythmias and conduction disturbances, leading to sudden cardiac death. Future therapeutic approaches to repair or regenerate the impulse-conducting tissue after heart injury or congenital disease will benefit from a clear understanding of the mechanisms that regulate its differentiation. We have shown that impulse-conducting Purkinje fibers differentiate from myocytes during embryogenesis,[3] and that the vascular cytokine, endothelin (ET),[4] induces embryonic myocytes to differentiate into Purkinje fibers.[5] Our data indicate that embryonic myocytes have the potential to convert their phenotype into the Purkinje fibers in response to a paracrine signal. In addition to furthering the understanding of the development of specialized myocardial tissues, this study provides a future basis for engineering cardiac pacemaking and impulse-conducting cells.

From Clark EB, Nakazawa M, Takao A (eds.): Etiology and Morphogenesis of Congenital Heart Disease: Twenty Years of Progress in Genetics and Developmental Biology. Armonk, NY: Futura Publishing Co., Inc.; © 2000.

Cardiac Conduction System Development

In the four chambered heart, pacemaking impulse is rhythmically provoked at the sinoatrial node (SA-node)[6] and is conducted as an action potential across the atrial chambers inducing their contraction (Fig. 1A).[7] The pacemaking impulses do not propagate directly to the ventricle. Instead, they first converge on the atrioventricular node (AV-node)[1] and ring (AV-ring), a cellular bundle circumscribing the right and left atrioventricular valves. From the AV-node and ring, the action potential is rapidly propagated along the atrioventricular bundle (AV-bundle)[8] and its branched limbs,[1] finally spreading into the working ventricular muscle via the Purkinje fiber network.[1,9,10]

There was a longstanding debate regarding the ontogeny and developmental process of the cardiac conduction system. Cells of the conduction system can be distinguished from contractile myocytes by their unique expression of genes, which usually appear in neural or skeletal muscle tissues.[11,12] The co-expression of neural and muscle genes has led to the suggestion of two possible origins, myogenic[13,14] and neural crest[11,15] for this specialized tissue. The development of the cardiac conduction system in embryonic

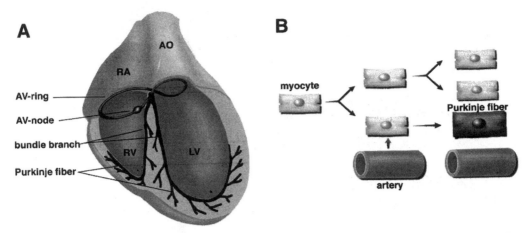

Figure 1. A. Organization of the ventricular conduction system. **B.** Proposed model of induction of Purkinje fibers within the myocyte lineage.

hearts has been studied in a number of species. In all cases, a ringlike structure[16] at the AV-junction has been mapped as the initiation site of conduction system formation. In the chicken embryo, the primary ring can be identified at E2 in the chicken by *Msx-2* expression, which later extends to the proximal conduction system but does not occur in Purkinje fibers.[17] Based on the proximal-distal wave of conduction system development, a model has been proposed wherein a single "primary conduction ring" contains precursor cells that provide progeny that differentiates into the conduction system.[15–18] This hypothesis is based on morphological observations, but until recently lineage relationships within the conduction system remained unsolved.

Myocyte Origin of the Cardiac Conduction System

Without a clear knowledge of the origin and developmental pattern of the conduction system, molecular mechanisms regulating its differentiation could not be established. Using retroviral-mediated approach, single differentiated and contractile myocytes in the tubular heart could be genetically marked.[19] Subsequent inspection of clonal populations (Fig. 1B)[3] have revealed that a subset of clonally related myocytes differentiates into conducting Purkinje fibers, invariably in close spatial association with forming coronary arterial blood vessels. In contrast, infection of cardiac neural crest did not produce β-gal-positive Purkinje fibers. Furthermore, in no case did a clone contain both Purkinje fibers and cells of the central conduction system, such as the AV-bundles or more proximal components. This is the first evidence *in vivo* that Purkinje fibers are locally recruited from myocyte precursors and not from cells of the proximal conduction system. The definitive mapping of Purkinje fiber progenitor cells to a myocyte lineage,[3] and not to neural crest, now allows us to study the mechanisms of Purkinje fiber differentiation by analyzing the process by which heart cells are converted from a contractile to a conductive cell lineage.

Potential Mechanisms for Inducing Purkinje Fibers Within the Myocyte Lineage

The recruitment of Purkinje fibers at periarterial sites within clonally derived populations of differentiated myocytes has led us to hypothesize that embryonic myocytes may be induced to form Purkinje fibers by receiving paracrine signals derived from arterial cells.[20,21] We have tested this hypothesis by checking the inductive activity of several vessel-associated paracrine factors, such as ET, fibroblast growth factor (FGF), and platelet-derived growth factor (PDGF), in culture.[5] Beating myocytes were isolated from embryonic chick ventricles. The conversion of contractile myocytes into conducting cells was monitored by probing for the upregulation of Purkinje fiber-specific genes and the downregulation of cardiac myocyte-specific myofibrillar proteins. Embryonic myocytes could be induced to differentiate into Purkinje cells in response to ET. In contrast, no detectable induction of Purkinje fiber phenotype was obtained following exposure to ET's precursor, big endothelin (big-ET) or by other blood vessel-associated factors, including FGF and PDGF. The response to ET could be neutralized by the addition of selective antagonists to ET-receptors. Thus, induction of Purkinje fibers appeared to be specific to ET. Importantly, the frequency of ET-dependent induction of myocytes into Purkinje fibers declined with progression of embryonic development.

Concluding Remarks

Our results demonstrate for the first time that embryonic myocytes are competent to respond to ET, a paracrine factor prominently secreted from atrial endothelial cells, inducing them to differentiate into Purkinje fibers. The results are consistent with the model illustrated in Fig. 2, where only the subpopulation of myocytes receiving this coronary-derived paracrine signal differentiates into Purkinje fibers, whereas those free from the inductive signal remain as contractile myocytes. Elucidation of how this highly soluble cytokine confines its inductive activity so precisely to just a few cell layers of myocytes will probably have to await a

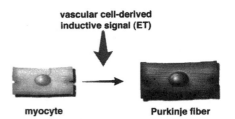

Figure 2. Proposed model of ET-dependent induction of Purkinje fibers.

fuller comprehension of the interaction between the varying temporal sensitivity of myocytes to ET and the spatial distribution of the active ligand in the developing embryonic heart.

Acknowledgement: Supported by NIH (HL54128, HL56987), HFSP, Mathers' Trust, Irma T. Hirschl Trust.

References

1. Tawara S. *Das reizleitungssystem des Säugetierherzens.* Gustav Fischer, Jena;. 1906.
2. Keith A, Flack M. The form and nature of the muscular connections between the primary divisions of the vertebrate heart. *J Anat Physiol* 1907;41:172–189.
3. Gourdie RG, Mima T, Thompson RP, et al. Terminal diversification of the myocyte lineage generates Purkinje fibers of the cardiac conduction system. *Development* 1995;121:1423–1431.
4. Yanagisawa M, Kurihara H, Kimura S, et al. A novel vasoconstrictor peptide produced by vascular endothelial cells. *Nature* 1988;332:411–415.
5. Gourdie RG, Wei Y, Kim D, et al. Endothelin-induced conversion of heart muscle cells into impulse-conducting Purkinje fibers. *Proc Natl Acad Sci U S A* 1998;95:6815–6818.
6. Brooks C McC, Lu H-H. *The Sinoatrial Pacemaker of the Heart.* Springfield, Ill: Charles C Thomas; 1972.
7. Wenckebach KF. Beiträge zur Kenntnis der menschlichen Hetztätigkeit. *Arch Anat Physiol* 1906;2:297–354.
8. His Wm Jr. Die Tätigkeit des embryonalen Herzens und deren Bedeutung für die Lehre von der Herzbewegung beim Erwachsenen. *Arb Med Klin Leipzig* 1893;14.

9. Purkinje J. Mikroskopisch-neurologische Beobachtungen. *Arch Anat Physiol Wiss Med* 1845;12:281–295.

10. Kölliker A. *Gewebeslehre 6 Aufl Lpz;* 1902.

11. Gorza L, Vettore S, Vitadello M. Molecular and cellular diversity of heart conduction system myocytes. *Trends Cardiol Med* 1994;4:153–159.

12. Moorman AFM, de Jong F, Denyn MMFJ, et al. Development of the cardiac conduction system. *Circ Res* 1998;82:629–644.

13. Pattern BM, Kramer TC. The initiation of contraction in the embryonic chick heart. *Am J Anat* 1933;53:349–375.

14. Pattern BM. The development of the sino-ventricular conduction system. *Unv Mich Med Bull* 1956;22:1–21.

15. Gorza L, Schiaffino S, Vitadello M. Heart conduction system: A neural crest derivative. *Brain Res* 1988;457:360–366.

16. Wessels A, Vermeulen JLM, Verbeek FJ, et al. Spatial distribution of "tissue-specific" antigens in the developing human heart. *Anat Rec* 1992;232:97–111.

17. Chan-Thomas PS, Thompson RP, Robert B, et al. Expression of homeobox genes Msx-1 (Hox-7) and Msx-2 (Hox-8) during cardiac development in the chick. *Dev Dyn* 1993;197:203–216.

18. Fishman MC, Chien KR. Fashioning the vertebrate heart: Earliest embryonic decisions. *Development* 1997;124:2099–2117.

19. Mikawa T, Borisov A, Brown AMC, et al. Clonal analysis of cardiac morphogenesis in the chicken embryo using a replication-defective retrovirus: I. Formation of the ventricular myocardium. *Dev Dyn* 1992; 193:11–23.

20. Mikawa T, Hyer J, Itoh N, et al. Retroviral vectors to study cardiovascular development. *Trends Cardiol Med* 1996;6:79–86.

21. Mikawa T, Fischman DA. The polyclonal origin of myocyte lineages. *Ann Rev Physiol* 1996;58:509–521.

40

Adenoviral and Retroviral Gene Targeting of the Cardiac Conduction System

Wanda Litchenberg, PhD, Cheng Gang, MD, PhD,
Sandra C. Klatt, BA, Takashi Mikawa, PhD,
Robert P. Thompson, PhD, and Robert G. Gourdie, PhD

The heterogeneous tissues of the pacemaking and conduction system comprise the "smart components" of the heart, responsible for setting, maintaining and coordinating the rhythmic pumping action of cardiac muscle (Fig. 1A; recent reviews[1,2]). Anomalous development of this essential cardiac system has been implicated in arrhythmogenesis and the emergence of other abnormalities in heart activation in infants and children. In a retroviral lineage tracing study of the developing chick heart, we showed that periarterial Purkinje fibers, the most peripheral cells of the conduction system, share a common myogenic origin with contractive myocytes.[3] Subsequently, it was reported that this recruitment into the peripheral conduction network may occur as a result of instructive cues from coronary arterial tissues.[2,4–7] At present, the cellular origins of other specialized cardiac tissues and the mechanisms giving rise to such tissues remain poorly characterized. Here, complementary adenoviral- and retroviral-based strategies are used to provide evidence that both central and peripheral conduction tissues are largely derived from myocyte progenitors in the embryonic tubular heart. No evidence is found for a direct contribution by neural crest lineages to any part of the conduction system. Replication-defective adenoviral vectors show high-efficiency infection of the early embryonic myocardium, with substantive dilution of lacZ reporter in working myocardial tissues during ensuing development. Interestingly, dramatically higher levels of adenoviral infection are retained in conduction system tissues over the same time course, indicating the utility of these gene vectors in studies targeting the development of specialized myocardial tissues.

Microinjection of replication-defective adenovirus into the pericardial cavity of embryonic day 3 (E3) chick embryos has been reported to result in infection of tissues comprising the tubular heart.[8] In agreement with this, we determined that either of two adenoviral constructs expressing β-Gal (lacZ) under the control of RSV (AdRSVlacZ) or CMV (AdCMVlacZ) promoters, mediated high levels of transgene expression throughout the embryonic heart at E4.5 (Figs. 1B–D). In whole mounts of X-Gal-reacted E4.5 embryos infected by pericardial microinjection the heart was the only organ showing significant levels of β-Gal expression (Fig. 1B).

From Clark EB, Nakazawa M, Takao A (eds.): Etiology and Morphogenesis of Congenital Heart Disease: Twenty Years of Progress in Genetics and Developmental Biology. Armonk, NY: Futura Publishing Co., Inc.; © 2000.

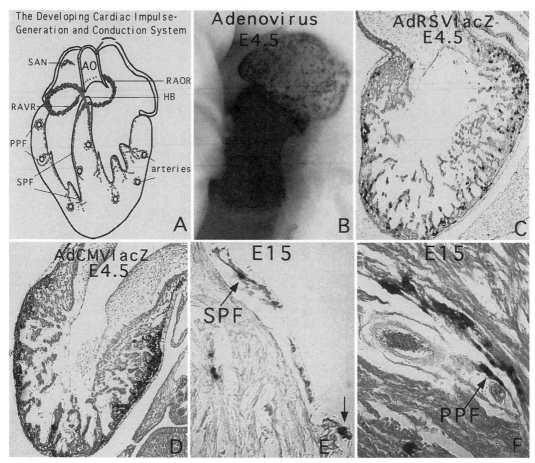

Figure 1. A. Model of the developing chick cardiac conduction system. Dark gray, central conduction system; light gray, proximal His bundle and peripheral conduction system; RAOR, retroaortic ring; RAVR, right atrioventricular ring; HB, His bundle; SAN, sinuatrial node; PPF, periarterial Purkinje fibers; SPF, subendocardial Purkinje fibers; AO, aorta. **B.** X-Gal-reacted embryonic day 4.5 (E4.5) whole-mount chick embryo infected with an adenoviral construct on E3. Replication-defective adenovirus (10^5 pfu) expressing β-galactosidase (β-gal) under control of the RSV or CMV promoter was applied to the external surface of E3 chick hearts in ovo.[8] Hearts were fixed in 2% paraformaldehyde. β-gal expression was detected using the X-Gal reaction. The ventricle shows high levels of uniform infection (as seen by the dark X-Gal signal). Infection in the atria is less uniform. Eosin-stained 10 μm sections of E4.5 hearts infected with AdRSVlacZ (dark nuclear localized signal) **(C)** and AdCMVlacZ (cytoplasmic) at E3 **(D)**. **E.** β-gal+ cells (arrows, and indicated by dark staining nuclei) in an E15 heart infected with AdRSVlacZ at E3 express EAP300, a marker of peripheral Purkinje fibers in chick.[2] **F.** A β-Gal+ periarterial sector (arrows, dark nuclei) containing Purkinje fibers (PPF) in an E15 heart infected with AdRSVlacZ at E3.

No infection was found in neural tissues in embryos targeted thus. Histology of hearts infected by either adenovirus type indicated that β-Gal expression was confined to myocardial cells in the atria, outflow tract, and ventricles (Figs. 1C, D), with no detectable expression in endocardial or epicardial tissues. External inspection of intact hearts sampled over a developmental time course at E4.5, E10, E15 and E19 suggested that the relative abundance of β-Gal expression

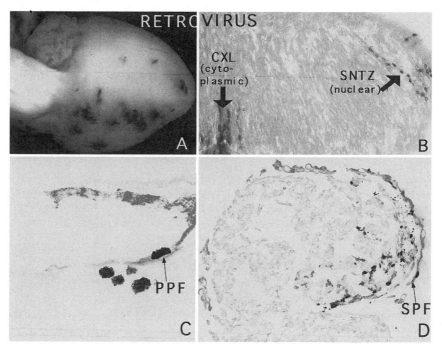

Figure 2. A. X-Gal-reacted hearts from an E14 embryo infected with replication-defective retroviruses on E3. Targeting of the embryonic heart or pre-migratory neural crest with retrovirus, X-Gal reaction, standard histology, and immunohistochemistry are carried out as described in References 3 and 14. **B.** Separate β-Gal-expressing sectors in ventricular myocardium of an E8 heart co-infected with CXL and SNTZ retroviruses. **C.** Double labeling for β-Gal (dark nuclei) and a conduction cell specific marker (light grey, ALD58; see Reference 2) in an E19 heart infected with SNTZ/CXL on E3. A clonal β-Gal+ sector containing a Purkinje fiber (PPF) and working myocytes is seen adjacent to a coronary artery. **D.** Double immunolabeling for β-Gal (dark nuclei) and a conduction cell specific marker (light grey, EAP300; see Reference 2) in an E14 heart infected with SNTZ/CXL on E3. A discrete β-Gal+ clonal sector containing Purkinje fibers (SPF) and working myocytes are seen adjacent to the subendocardium.

in the working myocardial tissues of the atria and ventricles decreased sharply. However, upon dissection of an intact AdRSVlacZ-infected E15 heart following X-Gal reaction, it was noted that there were frequent β-Gal+ cells at the endocardium of the ventricles. Based on histology and immunohistochemistry it was found that this conspicuous population of cells corresponded to subendocardial Purkinje fibers (Fig. 1E). Systematic histological examination of E15 and E19 hearts revealed that ratios of β-Gal-positive to β-Gal-negative cells were dramatically higher in other parts of the atrioventricular conduction system relative to working myocardium (Fig. 1F).

This spatiotemporal pattern of infection was consistent in repetitions of the developmental time course and appeared to be the same for virus-mediated β-Gal expression driven by either RSV or CMV promoters. The episomal genomes of replication-defective adenoviral constructs are thought to be diluted in infected host tissues by cell division.[9] Specialized myocardial tissues are characterized by early withdrawal from proliferation and relatively slow mitosis rates compared to working myocardial tissues.[10,11] Such tissue-specific differences in cell proliferation, between conductive and contractive myocardium, may be an explanation for the time course of adenoviral infection we observe in the developing chick heart.

The spatiotemporal patterns of cardiac infection shown by replication-defective adenoviruses from E3 to E19 are consistent with cells of the mature conduction system being derived from myogenic progenitors present in the tubular heart. However, as only the heart is targeted in this experiment, it cannot be excluded that contributions are not being made from migratory populations such as the cardiac neural crest, as has been suggested by some workers.[12,13] To address this question, replication-defective retroviruses, encoding nuclear (SNTZ) and cytoplasmic (CXL) lacZ (Fig. 2A, B), were specifically targeted by microinjection into either the tubular heart at E3 or the pre-migratory cardiac neural crest (at E2, Hamilton-Hamburges [HH] stages 8–12). The tissue-specific targeting of either myocardial or neural loci used co-infection with CXL and SNTZ viruses to enable discrimination of clones of virally infected cells from polyclones. Following microinjection, embryos were left to develop to between E8 and E18, between which time components of the conduction system become discernible. Only embryos targeted by retroviral microinjection into the tubular heart were found to incorporate β-Gal-expressing cells in the periarterial Purkinje fibers (Fig. 2C), subendocardial Purkinje fibers (Fig. 2D) and components of the central conduction system. These virally tagged cells were of myocardial phenotype and always occurred as part of clonal β-Gal-positive sectors that also incorporated nearby working myocytes. Peripheral conduction cells were never located in clones containing central conduction cells and vice versa. Following viral targeting of cardiac neural crest at E2, β-Gal-expressing cells were detected adjacent to conductive cells and intermingled with contractive myocardial tissues in E10–E14 embryos. However, these neural crest derivatives cells were never later found to be incorporated within definitive central conduction structures.

In summary, our adenoviral and retroviral lineage tracing data suggest that cells of both the central and peripheral conduction system originate largely from myogenic progenitors present in the looped, tubular heart and not from neural crest. Furthermore, retroviral clonal analyses suggest that conductive cells typically share closer lineage relationships with nearby contractive myocytes, than with other, more distally located conductive cells. Finally, the patterns of infection demonstrated by replication-defective adenoviral vectors over cardiac morphogenesis indicate their utility in targeting the development of specialized myocardial tissues.

Acknowledgements: This work was supported by grants to RGG from the NHLBI (HL R01–56728), National Science Foundation (Career Scholarship 9734406) and the March of Dimes Birth Defects Foundation (Basil O'Connor Scholarship FY95 1145, FY96 1139).

References

1. Moorman AFM, Dejong F, Denyn MFJ, et al. Development of the cardiac conduction system. *Circ Res* 1998;82:629–644.
2. Gourdie RG, Kubalak S, Mikawa T. Conducting the embryonic heart: orchestrating development of specialized cardiac tissues.*Trends Cardiovas Med*, 1999;9:18–26.
3. Gourdie RG, Mima T, Thompson RP, et al. Terminal diversification of the myocyte lineage generates Purkinje fibers of the cardiac conduction system. *Development* 1995;121:1423–1431.
4. Gourdie RG, Wei Y, Kim D, et al. Endothelin-induced conversion of embryonic heart muscle cells into impulse-conducting Purkinje fibers. *Proc Natl Acad Sci U S A* 1998;95:6815–6818.
5. Gittenberger deGroot AC, Peeters M, Mentink MMT, et al. Epicardium-derived cells contribute a novel population to the myocardial wall and the atrioventricular cushions. *Circ Res* 1998;82:1043–1052.
6. Hyer J, Johansen M, Prasad A, et al. Induction of Purkinje fiber differentiation by coronary arterialization. *Proc Natl Acad Sci U S A* 1999;96(23):13214–13218.
7. Mikawa T, Gourdie RG, Hyer J, et al., Molecular induction of the cardiac conduc-

tion system. Chapter in Clark EB, Nakazawa M, Takao A (eds.): Etiology and Morphogenesis of Congenital Heart Disease: Twenty Years of Progress in Genetics and Developmental Biology. Armonk, NY: Futura Publishing Co., Inc.

8. Fisher SA, Watanabe M. Expression of exogenous protein and analysis of morphogenesis in the developing chicken heart using an adenoviral vector. *Cardiovasc Res* 1996;31:E86–E95.

9. Mikawa T, Hyer J, Itoh N, et al. Retroviral techniques for studying organogenesis with a focus on heart development. *Trends Cardiovasc Med* 1996;6:79–86.

10. Thompson RP, Kawai T, Germroth PG, et al. Organization and function of early specialized myocardium. In: Clark EB, Markwald RR, Takao A, eds. *Developmental Mechanisms of Congenital Heart Disease*. Armonk, NY: Futura Publishing Co; 1995:269–279.

11. Thompson RP, Soles-Rosenthal P, Cheng G. Origin, and fate of cardiac conduction tissue. In: Clark EB, Takao A, Nakazawa M, eds. Etiology and Morphogenesis of Congenital Heart Disease: Twenty Years of Progress in Genetics and Developmental Biology. Armonk, NY: Futura Publishing Co; 2000.

12. Gorza L, Schiaffino M, Vitadello M. Heart conduction system: a neural crest derivative? *Brain Res* 1988;457:360–366.

13. Vitadello M, Vettore S, Lamar E, et al. Neurofilament M mRNA is expressed in conduction system myocytes of the developing and adult rabbit heart. *J Mol Cell Cardiol* 1998;28:1833–1844.

14. Gourdie RG, Cheng G, Thompson RP, et al. Retroviral cell lineage tracing techniques. In: Twan R, Lo C, eds. *Methods in Molecular Biology. Developmental Biology Protocols*, Vol. 1. In press.

41

EPDC Participate in Formation of Cardiac Valves and Coronary Vascular Wall and Initiate Purkinje Fiber Differentiation

Adriana C. Gittenberger-de Groot, PhD,
Mark-Paul Vrancken Peeters, MD, PhD,
and Robert E. Poelmann, PhD

During development the initially bare myocardial heart tube becomes covered by epicardium that spreads from the pro-epicardial organ, a protrusion from the coelomic wall, originally located on the sinus venosus.[1] The spreading epicardium, as determined by a cytokeratin staining, primarily follows the cardiac transitional zones such as the atrioventricular transition, the primary fold and the outflow tract and only later fills in the open spaces of the free chamber walls. Whether this is the result of differential migration on the basis of special receptors on the myocardium at specific sites, or results from growth differences of the myocardial segments remains to be investigated.[2] Although the epicardium covers the myocardium the subepicardial space is filled by cells that are derived from the epicardial lining.[3,4] These so-called epicardial-derived cells (EPCD) are most probably deposited at this position through an epithelial-mesenchymal transformation process.[4] There are also cells of other extracardiac sources that use the matrix of this subepicardial space to reach the heart. These cells are derived from the neural crest and take part in the autonomous innervation[5,6] and from the sinus venosus and liver endothelium forming the endothelium of the coronary vasculature.[7,8] We have not been able to demonstrate an epithelial-mesenchymal transformation of the surface epicardium to the precursor of the endothelial cells, as others have described this.[3,9] We assume, however, that their tracing technique does not allow determination of exact cell lineages. The question we tried to solve concerns the cell fate of the EPDCs and their role in cardiac differentiation.

The cell lineage of the epicardial cells was studied using the chicken-quail chimera approach, in which we transplanted an embryonic quail pro-epicardial organ (HH15–HH17) into the chicken pericardial cavity of the same developmental stage. The chimeras were harvested between HH25 and HH43. The quail cells, recognized with the anti-quail antibody QCPN, were traced in the host heart and checked for their developmental fate with antibodies demonstrating the differentiation into a number of cell types. These consist of cardiac fibroblasts as detected by pro-collagen staining (antibody M38)

From Clark EB, Nakazawa M, Takao A (eds.): Etiology and Morphogenesis of Congenital Heart Disease: Twenty Years of Progress in Genetics and Developmental Biology. Armonk, NY: Futura Publishing Co., Inc.; © 2000.

and smooth muscle cells (anti-alpha actin HHF35, 1 E12). The transplant also delivered coronary endothelial cells, detected by QH1, as expected from the fact that a piece of liver tissue was included in the transplant. Earlier experiments[7] learned that exclusive transplantation of the pro-epicardial Anlage did not result in coronary endothelial differentiation.

The infestment of the cardiac tube showed a differentiation between the mesenchymal EPDC that contribute to the myocardial wall and subendocardial space and later on to the sulcus tissue and the endocardial cushions, and EPDC that participate in the formation of the media and adventitia of the coronary vasculature. This is both a time and place dependent difference. Initially, the EPDC migrate into the myocardium and through myocardial discontinuities, allowing for intimate contacts between epicardium and endocardium, into the subendocardial region (HH25–HH31). In this developmental period there is no contribution to the atrioventricular cushions or outflow tract cushions. As the coronary endothelial vascular network[8] has not yet connected to the aorta, formation of a coronary vascular media is still absent.

Between HH32 and HH43, with the atrioventricular sulcus separating the atrial and ventricular myocardium, EPDCs have invaded the atrioventricular cushions and sulcus. The presence of EPDCs in the outflow tract cushions could not be evaluated for technical reasons as an overlying quail epicardium was not realized in our experiments.

Interestingly, a close apposition of the coronary endothelial vessels in the periarterial region was seen with the epicardium of the atrioventricular sulcus. The overlying epicardium became cuboidal, subsequently cells detached and seemed to stream towards the future coronary arteries.[8] Staining with smooth muscle cell markers showed that these EPDCs formed the smooth muscle cells of the coronary arterial media that became surrounded by an EPDC-derived population of cardiac fibroblasts constituting the adventitia. The formation of the coronary venous vessel wall takes place much later, immediately before hatching, with cells derived proximally from the myocardium and distally, as in the arteries, from the EPDCs.

The role of the EPDC that invade the myocardium, the subendocardium, the atrioventricular cushions and the atrioventricular sulcus has in part been solved. These cells contribute to the cardiac fibroblast population and to the fibrous heart skeleton. Furthermore, there is a remarkable colocalization between the subpopulation of EPDCs in the periarterial and subendocardial position and the future Purkinje network.[4]

To further scrutinize the function of the EPDCs, we performed two additional sets of experiments. In the first set we inhibited in 15 quail embryos between HH15 and HH18 the epicardial outgrowth, as has been described by Männer[10] for the chick. Our experiments resulted in embryonic death at about HH33 in the quail embryos. One question concerned the capacity of the heart tube to acquire a substitute epicardium inclusive of a coronary vascular network from the coelomic wall at the arterial pole region. We indeed found an outgrowth of a cytokeratin-positive sheath over the myocardium of the outflow tract (Fig. 1), that covered the arterial/myocardial transition at the arterial pole. The endothelial micro-vasculature surrounding the great vessels, most probably the precursor of vasa vasorum, could be detected up to the level of the myocardium and in one case the endothelial cells had formed a lumen contact with the aorta, resembling a coronary artery. There was, however, no connection with the (abnormal) coronary sinusoids that were present at the venous pole of the heart. Obviously, lack of epicardium had impaired proper coronary formation. Besides the lack of formation of a coronary vascular system the heart tube was not well formed. The myocardium showed a thin compact outer layer and the trabeculae were sparse and very thin. The nontrabeculated part of the heart tube showed still the connection of the endocardial outflow tract cushion and

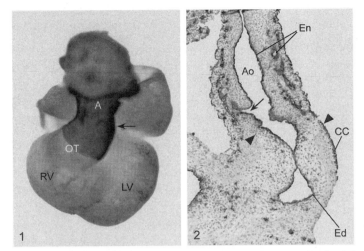

Figure 1. Whole mount of the heart of a HH 29 quail embryo stained with cytokeratin for epicardial formation. The natural outgrowth of the epicardial organ has been inhibited. There is a compensatory outgrowth of coelomic wall from the arterial pole (A) over the outflow tract covering the myocardial (M) vessel wall transition (arrow). LV, left ventricle; RV, right ventricle.

Figure 2. Section through the outflow tract of a quail heart whole mount stained for cytokeratin. The endothelial (En) and endocardial (Ed) cells are stained with an anti-quail endothelial antibody QH1. Along the aortic (Ao) vessel wall endothelial cells are present that at one site make a lumen contact, resembling a coronary artery (arrow). This network is not continuous with a vessel network over the heart that is lacking in this experiment. The arterial pole derived cytokeratin positive coelomic covering (CC) reaches below the mesenchymal/myocardial border (arrow head).

the atrioventricular cushion mass. The cushions showed no signs of myocardialization of the outflow tract or septum formation. A similar lack of septation was seen at the atrioventricular transition. The cushion mass showed a high degree of apoptosis. In general the heart tube persisted in a very immature stage.

The second set of experiments was performed in 8 chicken embryos in which the epicardial formation was similarly delayed by inhibition of the outgrowth as described above for the quail embryo. A quail epicardial organ was added, however, to determine whether a rescue of the embryo and its heart development could be obtained in this case solely by quail epicardium. This proved to be the case. The coronary vasculature, which clearly showed a contribution from both arterial- (chick) and venous- (quail) derived endothelium at the arterial pole, connected to the aorta and a proper network was formed (Fig. 2). These vessels grew into

the myocardium, as did the EPDC subpopulations in the myocardium, subendocardium and the atrioventricular valves. In fact, a rescue of the normal cardiac phenotype with proper myocardial formation and septation was achieved.

In conclusion, we can state that the EPDCs are essential for many aspects of normal cardiac differentiation. It remains to be investigated to what extent the various EPDC populations are involved in both congenital and adult cardiac disease. The most relevant adult disease may be cardiac failure through an improper interstitium. In the neonatal heart, coronary vascular anomalies with myocardial architectural impairment are likely due to EPDC maldevelopment.

References

1. Virágh SZ, Gittenberger-de Groot AC, Poelmann RE, et al. Early development of

quail heart epicardium and associated vascular and glandular structures. *Anat Embryol* 1993;188:381–393.

2. Vrancken Peeters M-PFM, Mentink MMT, Poelmann RE, et al. Cytokeratins as a marker for epicardial formation in the quail embryo. *Anat Embryol* 1995;191: 503–508.

3. Mikawa T, Gourdie RG. Pericardial mesoderm generates a population of coronary smooth muscle cells migrating into the heart along with ingrowth of the epicardial organ. *Dev Biol* 1996;174:221–232.

4. Gittenberger-de Groot AC, Vrancken Peeters M-PFM, Mentink MMT, et al. Epicardial derived cells, EPDC, contribute a novel population to the myocardial wall and the atrioventricular cushions. *Circ Res* 1998;82:1043–1052.

5. Poelmann RE, Mikawa T, Gittenberger-de Groot AC. Neural crest cells in outflow tract septation of the embryonic chicken heart: Differentiation and apoptosis. *Dev Dyn* 1998;212:373–384.

6. Verberne ME, Gittenberger-de Groot AC, Poelmann RE. Lineage and development of the parasympathetic nervous system of the embryonic chicken heart. *Anat Embryol* 1998;198:171–184.

7. Poelmann RE, Gittenberger-de Groot AC, Mentink MMT, et al. Development of the cardiac coronary vascular endothelium, studied with anti-endothelial antibodies, in chicken-quail chimeras. *Circ Res* 1993; 73:559–568.

8. Vrancken Peeters M-PFM, Gittenberger-de Groot AC, Mentink MMT, et al. Smooth muscle cells and fibroblasts of the coronary arteries derive from epithelial-mesenchymal transformation of the epicardium. *Anat Embryol* 1999;199(4):367–378.

9. Dettman RW, Denetclaw W Jr, Ordahl CP, et al. Common epicardial origin of coronary vascular smooth muscle, perivascular fibroblasts, and intermyocardial fibroblasts in the avian heart. *Dev Biol* 1998; 193:169–181.

10. Männer J. Experimental study on the formation of the epicardium in chick embryos. *Anat Embryol* 1993;187:281–289.

42

Origin and Fate of Cardiac Conduction Tissue

Robert P. Thompson, PhD, Patricia Soles-Rosenthal, Med, and Gang Cheng, MD, PhD

Spatial and temporal mapping of cell proliferation in the embryonic chick heart has suggested that early cardiac conduction tissue derives from non- or slowly-dividing populations of inner wall and trabecular myocytes[1,2] that share clonal origin with nearby working myocardium.[3] The possibility that some of these cells might continue slowly dividing, or might disappear through apoptosis,[4] led us to trace conduction tissue kinetics in the embryonic and adult chicken by a complementary method, by label-dilution or "birthdating,"[5] in which a discrete pulse of tritiated-thymidine is followed through lengthy survival. Heavy DNA label is retained only in those cells exiting the cell cycle soon after initial label. As illustrated in Figure 1a, a 24-hour thymidine label from incubation Day 5 (E5-E6) extensively labeled dividing cells in the atrioventricular (AV) cushions and parietal wall (*). Myocytes in the interventricular septum, precursors to central conduction bundles, failed to label between 5 and 6 days, as shown earlier.[1,2] Conversely, in an embryo labeled at E3 and sacrificed at E6 (Fig. 1b), septal trabeculae are heavily labeled, indicating withdrawal of these cells on or soon after E3. Cycling populations (AV cushion and parietal wall, *) show dilution of label in those intervening three days.

In hearts labeled at E1.5, 2, 3, 4, 5, or 6 and allowed to develop through the septation period to E12, 14, 16, 18, or 20, heavy labeling was retained in and only in conduction tissues (Fig. 1c–f), including nonbranching and branching bundles, right atrioventricular ring tissue, left AV junctional tissue, retroaortic ring (arrowheads), and anterior septal branch, seen in more anterior serial sections across the aortic outlet (Ao, d–f), as well as at the sinoatrial junction (not shown). This demonstrates that earliest components of the entire central conduction system terminally differentiate as looping is completed and survive septation with little or no further cell division.

Within the nonbranching His bundle near hatching (Fig. 2a, b, composites from 10–15 sections), core populations remained heavily labeled in embryos labeled at E2; in those labeled at E6, predominately outer layers of this discrete fascicle were heavily labeled. Central conduction tissue cells were rarely labeled after Day 8. This suggests that central conduction fascicles develop by lamellar recruitment of newly quiescent layers of terminally differentiated myocytes throughout the preseptation period, but not thereafter.

Lesser labeling toward peripheral conduction fascicles and earlier clonal marking studies[6] suggested a temporal

From Clark EB, Nakazawa M, Takao A (eds.): Etiology and Morphogenesis of Congenital Heart Disease: Twenty Years of Progress in Genetics and Developmental Biology. Armonk, NY: Futura Publishing Co., Inc.; © 2000.

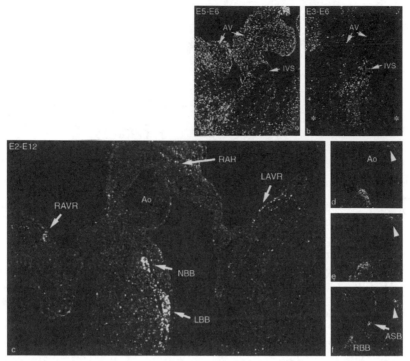

Figure 1. Darkfield autoradiography of thymidine-labeled chick embryo hearts. **a, b.** Hearts at incubatiom Day 6 (E6) after labeling at E5 or E3, as marked. **c–f.** Heart at E12, labeled at E2. ASB, anterior septal branch; AV, atrioventricular cushions; IVS, interventricular septum; LAVR, left AV ring tissue; RAVR, right AV ring tissue; LBB, left bundle branch; RBB, right bundle branch; NBB, nonbranching bundle of His; RAR, retroaortic ring tissue.

gradient of subsequent recruitment of peripheral conduction tissues. This was confirmed in series of embryos labeled on Days 10, 12, 14, 16, or 18, sacrificed on E20, and immunostained for EAP-300[7] before autoradiography (Fig. 2c, d). Note heavily labeled cells terminally differentiated soon after E12 along subendocardial and periarterial Purkinje fibers.

Hearts from hatched chickens 10, 30, 100, or 300 days old, labeled at E2, 3, or 4, retained heavily labeled cells deep in central conduction tissues (Fig. 2e, f). Preliminary counts have suggested gradual decline in such labeled populations, but labeling and immunocytochemistry for bromodeoxyuridine[1] has so far failed to detect quiescent myocytes that reenter the cell cycle; nor have we found apoptosis[4] among long surviving, labeled populations. Although laborious, grain counting may prove a more sensitive method for detecting attrition through slow proliferation, as well as assessing proliferation rates of cycling cell populations in normal and experimentally treated hearts.

In summary, these birthdating studies demonstrate the entire time-course of terminal differentiation and survival of cardiac conduction tissues in the chicken (Fig. 2g); similar to kinetics shown in rodents.[2,8] Earliest quiescent myocytes terminally differentiate from first trabeculae and inner myocardial layers during looping; many of these cells survive into adult life without dividing. Recruitment of newly differentiated myocytes to central conduction fascicles occurs in a lamellar fashion, but only in the pre-septation period, ending by E9. Ramifying recruitment of cells to peripheral Purkinje fiber arborizations continues through the second half of incubation. Proliferation of pa-

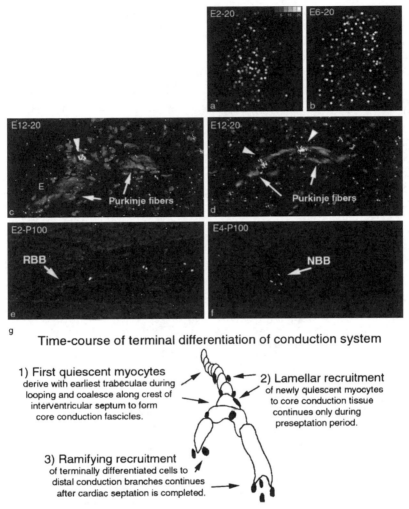

Figure 2. a, b. Locations of labeled cells within nonbranching His bundle of E20 hearts labeled at E2 or E6. Inset: grayscale as grains/nucleus. **c, d.** Heavily labeled nuclei within EAP-300 positive Purkinje fibers in E20 heart labeled at E12. **c:** subendocardial (E); **d.** periarterial. **e, f.** Heavily labeled nuclei in right bundle branch and nonbranching His bundle 100 days posthatching after label at E2 or E4.

rietal wall myocytes continues on into neonatal life.

The current observations of slowly declining label along outflow myocardium and a veil of atrial myocytes along the left, as well as right, AV junction reinforce the idea that AV canal and outlet musculature serve as paired ephemeral sphincters in gating blood flow as valves develop,[9] and may relate to the evolution of conduction tissues, as well as their development. Physically, such a slowly-growing paired-ring structure, similar to early expression of Msx2 in the chick[2,10] and *minK* in the developing mouse,[11] could also serve to deform primary ring tissue[12]during development of definitive conduction tissues. Molecular regulation of conduction tissue differentiation remains to be elucidated. The hypothesis that endothelial signals may mediate such decisions among periarterial and subendocardial Purkinje ramifications[13] might pertain also to early trabeculae as they become intimately associated with endocardium, but inner myocardial layers of AV and outflow myocardium that share cytokinetics with other components of earliest conduction tissues remain well separated from endocardium by intervening cushion matrix throughout preseptation development in vertebrates. Advanced differentiation and organization of inner layers of such intersegmental zones,[9,14] closely correlated with slowed proliferation shown here, may be causally related through greater physical loading and conditioning of such inner myocardial layers and early trabeculae.

Methods

Windowed White Leghorn eggs received a single dose of ^{3}H-methyl-thymidine (80Ci/mmole) upon the air sac membrane and continued incubating at 37.5°C for intervals from hours to months. Dose was normalized with changing embryo DNA content[15] to yield autoradiographic exposures of 1 grain/nucleus/day (Kodak NTB2 emulsion, 5-micron paraffin sections). The dependence of dose upon age was estimated as: dose (uCi) = 0.2 (days of incubation) 2.83 over the first two weeks of incubation. Label increased over the first 36 hours, declining thereafter through depletion of label[5] and dilution of incorporated thymidine (Fig. 1a, b). Labeling density in postmitotic intermediate zone neurons assured uniformity of label. Radiation exposure appears negligible (3 rads/day[16]); early embryos labeled at five times above dose completed septation with no apparent effect. Embryos older than Day 12, and those allowed to survive hatching, were labeled at one-third that dose, with exposure for 60 rather than 20 days.

References

1. Thompson RP, Lindroth JR, Wong YM. Regional differences in DNA-synthetic activity in the preseptation myocardium of the chick. In: Clark E, Takao A, eds. *Developmental Cardiology: Morphogenesis and Function*. Kisko, NY: Futura Press; 1989:219–234.

2. Thompson RP, Kanai T, Germroth PG, et al. Organization, and function of early specialized myocardium. In: Clark EB, Markwald RR, Takao A, eds. *Developmental Mechanisms of Congenital Heart Disease*. Armonk, NY: Futura Publishing Co; 1995: 269–279.

3. Litchenberg W, Cheng G, Klatt SC, et al. Adenoviral, and retroviral gene targeting of the cardiac conduction system. In: Clark EB, Nakazawa M, Takoa A (eds). *Etiology and Morphogenesis of Congenital Heart Disease: Twenty Years of Progress in Genetics and Developmental Biology*. Futura Publishing Company, Inc. Armonk, NY, 2000.

4. Cheng G, Wessels A, Gourdie RG, et al. Spatiotemporal distribution of apoptosis in embryonic chicken heart. *Anat Rec* (in press).

5. Yurkewicz L, Lauder JM, Marchi M, et al. ^{3}H-thymidine long survival autoradiography as a method for dating the time of neuronal origin in the chick embryo: The locus coeruleus and cerebellar Purkinje cells. *J Comp Neurol* 1981;203:257–267.

6. Gourdie RG, Mima T, Thompson RP, et al. Terminal diversification of the myocyte lineage generates Purkinje fibers of the cardiac conducting system. *Development* 1995;121:1423–1431.

7. McCabe CF, Gourdie RG, Thompson RP, et al. The developmentally regulated protein EAP-300 is expressed by myocardium and cardiac neural crest during chick embryogenesis. *Dev Dyn* 1995;203:51–60.

8. Thompson RP, Lindroth JR, Alles A, et al. Cell differentiation birthdates in the embryonic rat heart. *Proc NY Acad Sci* 1990; 588:446–448.

9. Ya J, Schilham MW, Clevers H, et al. Animal models of congenital defects in the ventriculoarterial connection of the heart. *J Mol Med* 1997;75:551–566.

10. Chan-Thomas PS, Thompson RP, Robert B, et al. Expression of homeobox genes Msx-1 (Hox-7) and Msx-2 (Hox-8) during cardiac development in the chick. *Dev Dyn* 1993;197:203–216.

11. Kupershmidt S, Yang T, Anderson ME, et al. Replacement by homologous recombination of the *minK* gene with *lacZ* reveals restriction of *minK* expression to the

mouse cardiac conduction system. *Circ Res* 1999;84:146–152.

12. Wessels A, Vermeulen JL, Verbeek FJ, et al. Spatial distribution of "tissue-specific" antigens in the developing human heart and skeletal muscle. III. An immunohistochemical analysis of the distribution of the neural tissue antigen G1N2 in the embryonic heart; implications for the development of the atrioventricular conduction system. *Anat Rec* 1992;232:97–111.

13. Gourdie RG, Kubalak S, Mikawa T. Conducting the embryonic heart: Orchestrating development of specialized cardiac tissues. *Trends Cardiovasc Med* 1999;9:18–26.

14. Wenink ACG, Spliet WGM, Mansoer JR. Entwicklung der Šumlichen Anordnung des Myokardiums. *Wien Klin Woch* 1988;24:805–811.

15. Romanoff A. *Biochemistry of the Avian Embryo.* New York: John Wiley & Sons; 1967:24.

16. Dewey WC, Sedita BA, Humphrey RM. Chromosomal aberrations induced by tritiated thymidine during the S and G2 phases of Chinese hamster cells. *Int J Radiat Biol* 1967;12:597–600.

43

The Form and Function of the Developing Cardiac Conduction System

Michiko Watanabe, PhD, David S. Rosenbaum, MD, Imad Libbus, MD, and Emil Thomas Chuck, PhD

Introduction

The excitation and contraction sequences of the mature four-chambered heart are coordinated by the specialized cardiomyocytes of the His-Purkinje system (HPS). Abnormal development or disease of the HPS may result in life-threatening reentrant arrhythmias and heart block. The development of this critical system has been a challenge to study because it is difficult to distinguish these special cardiomyocytes from the neighboring working cardiomyocytes until the system is well on its way to maturity.[1] The recognition that this system expresses a different set of genes, proteins, and carbohydrates from the rest of the myocardium (reviewed[2]) has been valuable in tracking this tissue during the less mature stages. The deployment of contemporary molecular biology techniques[3] supports a cardiomyocyte origin of these specialized cells. Despite these advances, many basic questions still remain unresolved. During early cardiogenesis, the tubular heart begins to contract without a specialized ventricular conduction system[5] by slow homogeneous cell-cell propagation through the muscular atrioventricular junction (AVJ). The aim of our

studies has been to determine when this immature heart eventually acquires an HPS and achieves its mature pattern of electrical conduction.

Methods and Results

Our studies provide evidence that when the chicken heart becomes a four-chambered structure around embryonic stage 30 (incubation day 6.5)[5] the characteristic wishbone-shaped form of the HPS is delineated by markers[6,7] simultaneously with the appearance of an apex-to-base activation sequence in the left ventricle characteristic of HPS conduction.[8] The two markers, identified using monoclonal antibodies to the polysialylated neural cell adhesion molecule (PSA-NCAM) and the HNK-1 sulfated carbohydrate epitope, label the HPS in a complementary rather than an overlapping pattern. The PSA-NCAM is detected in the distal HPS structures such as the right and left bundle branches and the Purkinje fibers adjacent to the endocardium lining the ventricular lumen, whereas the HNK-1 marks the more central HPS structures connected to a dorsal atrioventricular (AV) node-comparable region. At approximately the same stages, extracellular electrodes placed on the left ventricle allowed detection of a transition in the pattern of activation from the immature

From Clark EB, Nakazawa M, Takao A (eds.): Etiology and Morphogenesis of Congenital Heart Disease: Twenty Years of Progress in Genetics and Developmental Biology. Armonk, NY: Futura Publishing Co., Inc.; © 2000.

base-to-apex pattern to that of the mature apex-to-base pattern. Additionally, an apparently intermediate pattern of simultaneous apex and base activation was transiently detected. The apex-to-base pattern is associated with conduction through the HPS. These results indicate that the period around stage 30 is a critical time in maturation of cardiac conduction which warrants further detailed analysis.

The technique of two-dimensional optical mapping using voltage-sensitive dyes has been used to study the electrophysiology of tissues such as the adult guinea pig heart.[9] Voltage-sensitive dyes avidly bind the plasma membrane of nearly all excitable cells and change their fluorescence intensity linearly with changes in the transmembrane potential of the cells. The changes in fluorescence intensity can be detected using an array of 256 photodetectors and analyzed to obtain a two-dimensional map of electrical activity with high spatial and temporal resolution. A similar system in conjunction with a fluorescence microscope has been used to record the action potentials from tubular chicken embryo hearts at stages when the embryonic tissue is transparent.[10] We now have the capability to record from older chicken embryo hearts that are not transparent by using an epifluorescence imaging microscope using a different dye di-4-ANEPPS. Our system can record at temporal resolutions as high as 0.29 msec and with a spatial resolution of 1.0 mm to 0.027 mm. With this level of resolution, it will be possible to record transmembrane potentials in cardiac tissue at the single cell level.

Preliminary results indicate that our fluorescence microscope-based optical mapping system allows collection of high fidelity action potentials from the adult guinea pig heart preparation that are comparable to that obtained from the standard previously validated optical mapping system.[11] Action potentials from stage 28–35 chicken embryo hearts in the normal sinus rhythm have also been obtained using our current system (Fig. 1).

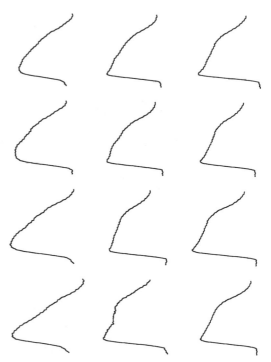

Figure 1. Action potentials recordings from a chicken embryo heart. White Leghorn chicken (*Gallus gallus*) eggs were incubated in humidified air at 37.5°C. All animals were handled in accordance with the *Guide for the Care and Use of Laboratory Animals* (NIH publication 85–23, revised 1985). Stage 28 chicken embryo hearts were excised, placed in warmed tissue bath with oxygenated (95% O_2, 5% CO_2) Tyrode's solution (35+/–2°C, pH 7.6), superfused with the voltage sensitive dye di-4-ANEPPS (15 μm) and DAM (diacetyl monoxime; 10 mM) for 10 minutes in warmed Tyrode's buffer before recording from a photodiode array connected to an epifluorescence microscope (Nikon Eclipse E400) with fluorescence objectives and filter cubes. Recordings were collected from the dorsal surface of the ventricles using a 10× objective. Each action potential represents 250 msec.

Discussion

Stage 30, the stage at which we detect the emergence of both the form and function of the HPS, is a critical period in the morphogenesis of the heart. Other events occurring at approximately the same time are the completion of septation of the cardiac outflow tract and the ventricular chambers[12] and the apparent displacement of the muscular atrioventricular connection by connective tissue[13] except at the site where the HPS traverses. There is evidence from other studies that the HPS components may be present and functioning before the transition period at stage 30. Studies using extracellular recordings indicate that there is a preferential pathway of faster conduction along the ventricular trabeculae as early as stage 23.[14] There are also indications from intracellular microelectrode recordings[15] that components of the central HPS, the AV node and upper bundle, become functionally distinct from surrounding myocardium at 5.5 to 6 days (comparable to stage 28), which is just before the transition that we have detected at stage 30. These findings considered with ours suggest the possibility that the transition in the overall left ventricular activation pattern occurs at stage 30 not only because the individual HPS components finally become functional at that time but also because the other avenue for ventricular activation, the AVJ myocardium, disappears (Fig. 2).

Listed below are potential explanations for our observations at the HPS transition period.

1. The HPS system appears at stage 30 and finally provides an avenue to connect the AV node-equivalent tissue to the apical myocardium of the ventricle.
2. The HPS system is present before stage 30 but not functionally mature until stage 30.
   A. The HPS was not endogenously mature. It had the wrong ion channel properties or the HPS cardiomyocytes were not connected to each other in the proper way.
   B. The central HPS was not properly disconnected/insulated from the surrounding working cardiomyocytes.
3. The HPS system was present and functioning in a mature fashion but the ventricular myocardium was preferentially responding to the activation

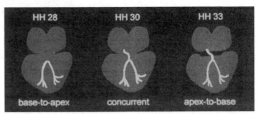

Figure 2. Model to explain the transition in pattern of ventricular conduction. The HPS is immature before stage 30 (HH 28) and a base-to-apex ventricular conduction is driven by the AVJ myocardium. When both the HPS and the AVJ myocardium connection are in place, concurrent conduction is detected at stage 30 (HH 30). When the HPS is in place and the AVJ myocardium breaks elsewhere, the only avenue of conduction is through the HPS which conducts the impulse to the apical myocardium by passing the base resulting in the mature apex-to-base conduction sequence (HH 33).

through the AVJ until this avenue of activation was deleted.

The method of optical mapping could help us to test these possibilities by providing the two-dimensional pattern of activation over the surface of the developing heart and the conduction velocity in any direction. These two parameters could reveal the functional maturity of the HPS and the relationship of this specialized tissue to the surrounding myocardium during development of the heart.

The appearance of the markers PSA-NCAM and HNK-1 on putative HPS cardiomyocytes around the time of appearance of the HPS-like conduction may have significance for the cellular events occurring during HPS development. These two carbohydrate components are both implicated in regulating cell interactions in the nervous system[16,17] and may be serving similar functions on the myocardium. Their role in regulating cardiomyocyte interactions is unknown. It is intriguing that the proximal region of the common or His bundle can be distinguished from the distal region by immunostaining properties. Is the HNK-1-positive region comparable to the penetrating bundle that is it spared the fate of the rest of the cardiomyocytes at the atrioventricular junction?

We have determined that stage 30 is an important transition time for the HPS both in its form and function. Our current more challenging aim is to determine why and by what mechanism this transition occurs at this particular stage. Answering these questions will require a detailed understanding of the changes in cardiomyocyte interactions not only within the HPS but also at the AVJ and in the cardiomyocytes adjacent to the HPS simultaneously. This information can be provided by using traditional histological techniques in combination with the two-dimensional optical mapping technique at the microscopic level.

Acknowledgements: These studies were supported by NIH grant HL38172 (M.W.), the fellowship in Cardiac Pacing and Electrophysiology from the North American Society of Pacing and Electrophysiology (E.T.C.), the Medical Research Service of the Department of Veterans Affairs, NIH grant HL54807, and the National American Heart Association Grant-in-Aid (D.S.R.).

References

1. Vassall-Adams PR. The development of the atrioventricular bundle and its branches in the avian heart. *J Anat* 1982; 134:169–183.
2. Moorman AFM, de Jong F, Denyn MMFJ, et al. Development of the cardiac conduction system. *Circ Res* 1998;82:629–644.
3. Gourdie RG, Mima T, Thompson RP, et al. Terminal diversification of the myocyte lineage generates Purkinje fibers of the cardiac conduction system. *Development* 1995;121:1423–1431.
4. Patten BM. The development of the sinoventricular conduction system. *Univ Mich Med Bull* 1956;22:1-21.
5. Hamburger V, Hamilton JL. A series of normal stages in the development of the chick embryo. *J Morphol* 1951;88:49.
6. Watanabe M, Timm M, Fallah-Najmabadi H. Cardiac expression of polysialylated NCAM in the chicken embryo: Correlation with the ventricular conduction system. *Dev Dyn* 1992;194:128–141.
7. Chuck ET, Watanabe M. Differential expression of PSA-NCAM and HNK-1 epitopes in the developing cardiac conduction system of the chick. *Dev Dyn* 1997; 209:182–195.
8. Chuck ET, Freeman DM, Watanabe M, et al. Changing activation sequence in the embryonic chick heart. Implications for the development of the His-Purkinje system. *Circ Res* 1997;81:470–476.
9. Laurita KR, Girouard SD, Rosenbaum DS. Modulation of ventricular repolarization by a premature stimulus. Role of epicardial dispersion of repolarization kinetics demonstrated by optical mapping of the intact guinea pig heart. *Circ Res* 1996;79: 493–503.
10. Kamino K. Colon adenocarcinomas in European hamsters after application of N-nitroso-bis 2-oxypropyl-amine. *Physiol Rev* 1991;71:53–58.
11. Girouard SD, Laurita KR, Rosenbaum DS. Unique properties of cardiac action potentials recorded with voltage-sensitive dyes. *J Cardiovasc Electrophysiol* 1996;7:1024–1038.
12. Ben-Shachar G, Arcilla RA, Lucas RV, et al. Ventricular trabeculations in the chick embryo heart and their contribution to ventricular and muscular septal development. *Circ Res* 1985;57:759–766.
13. Arrechedera H, Strauss M, Argüello C, et al. Ultrastructural study of the myocardial wall of the atrio-ventricular canal during the development of the embryonic chick heart. *J Mol Cell Cardiol* 1984;16: 885–895.
14. de Jong F, Opthof T, Wilde AA, et al. Persisting zones of slow impulse conduction in developing chicken hearts. *Circ Res* 1992; 71:240–250.
15. Argüello C, Alanís J, Valenzuela B. The early development of the atrioventricular node and bundle of His in the embryonic chick heart. An electrophysiological and morphological study. *Development* 1988; 102:623.
16. Rutishauser U, Landmesser LT. Polysialic acid in the vertebrate nervous system: a promoter of plasticity in cell-cell interactions. *Trends Neurosci* 1996;19:422–427.
17. Schachner M, Martini R, Hall H, et al. In: Yu ACH, et al., eds. *Gene Expression in the Central Nervous System.* New York: Elsevier Science; 1995:183.

44

Accelerated Maturation of the Ductus Arteriosus With Retinoic Acid in the Fetal Rat

Kazuo Momma, MD

Patent ductus arteriosus (PDA) is a frequent complication in premature infants.[1] It has been established both clinically[2] and in experimental animals[3] that maturation of the fetal DA is associated with increased constriction in response to maternally administered indomethacin (Ind). Ind has been widely used to close the PDA in premature infants.[4,5] Recent study with the transgenic mouse has shown that "endogenous retinoic acid (RA) signaling colocalizes with advanced expression of the adult smooth muscle myosin heavy chain isoform during development of DA,"[6,7] suggesting an important role of retinoic acid in DA maturation. We studied the effects of retinoic acid on DA maturation in fetal rats.

Indomethacin-Induced DA Constriction With and Without RA Pretreatment

In total, 8 studies were performed. In all protocols, DA/pulmonary artery (PA) inner diameter ratio was studied at 1:00 PM hours of the 21st day, with or without administration of 1 mg/kg of

Ind at 9:00 AM of the same day. In comparison to the moderate DA constriction with Ind without pretreatment with retinoic acid (DA/PA = 0.54), stronger constriction occurred with Ind after two days' administration of RA (10 mg/kg) on Days 19 and 20 (late fetal stage), with DA/PA decreased to 0.31 (Figs.1 and 2).[8] RA administered in the early fetal stage (Days 15–17) had different effects. No accelerated maturation was noticed with RA doses of 1 or 10 mg/kg.

Mechanism of RA

The importance of vitamin A in the development of the cardiovascular system and DA was first demonstrated by Wilson and Warkany.[9,10] They showed that fetuses from mother rats with vitamin A deficiency developed anomalies of the aortic arch, its branches, and DA. Later studies showed teratogenic effects of large doses of vitamin A.[11] RA is an active form of retinol, vitamin A. In the last 10 years, it has been clearly shown that RA and RA receptors are important in regulation of development, especially regulation of maturation of a variety of organs[12] including the cardiovascular system.[13] Recently Colbert et al.[6] have shown in transgenic mice that "endogenous retinoic acid signaling colocalizes with advanced expression of the adult smooth muscle my-

From Clark EB, Nakazawa M, Takao A (eds.): Etiology and Morphogenesis of Congenital Heart Disease: Twenty Years of Progress in Genetics and Developmental Biology. Armonk, NY: Futura Publishing Co., Inc.; © 2000.

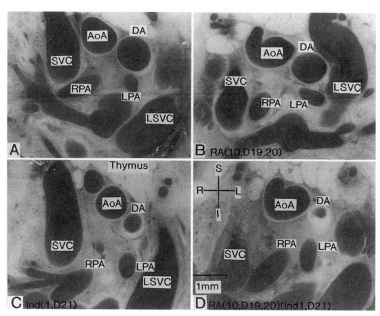

Figure 1. A. The ductus arteriosus of the fetus was widely patent on the 21st day in those fetuses without administration of indomethacin. Frontal cut of the dilated ductus arteriosus (**A–D**). **B.** The ductus arteriosus of the fetus was widely patent on 21st day in those fetuses with treatment of retinoic acid (10 mg/kg of retinoic acid on the 19th and 20th days) and without administration of indomethacin. **C.** Constricted ductus arteriosus 4 hours after administration of indomethacin,1 mg/kg through orogastric tube, on 21st day. **D.** Severely constricted ductus arteriosus following intramuscular injection of 10 mg/kg of retinoic acid on 19th and 20th days and 4 hours after orogastric administration of indomethacin on the 21st day in near term fetus. AoA, aortic arch; DA, ductus arteriosus; LA, left atrium; LPA, left pulmonary artery; RPA, right pulmonary artery; SVC, superior vena cava. Methods: *Animals*: Thirty virgin Wistar rats (pregnancy period 21.5 days) were mated overnight from 5:00 PM to 9:00 AM. *Retinoic acid administration*. All-*trans*-retinoic acid (Sigma Chemical Co., St. Louis, Mo) was used. Retinoic acid was dissolved in safflower seed oil just before injection to a concentration of 1 mg/mL for injection of 1 mg/kg and 10 mg/mL for injection of 10 mg/kg, and injected into the dorsum of pregnant rats intramuscularly at 9:00 AM. *Measurements*. To study in situ morphology of the fetal ductus arteriosus, a rapid whole-body freezing method was used as described in an earlier study.[4,7–10] Constriction of the ductus arteriosus was studied on the 21st day (near-term fetus). Indomethacin (1 mg/kg) was administered through an orogastric tube to the pregnant rat at 9:00 AM on the 21st day. Four hours later, fetuses were delivered by caesarean section, and frozen immediately in acetone cooled to –80°C by dry ice. Frozen thorax was cut on a freezing microtome in the frontal plane, and the cut surface was photographed with binocular stereoscopic microscope and color film.

osin heavy chain isoform during development of ductus arteriosus." In the mouse, expression of the retinoic acid receptor begins at 13.5 days in the mesenchyme surrounding the ductus, becomes very intense by 15.5 days on the DA, and is present on the smooth muscle layers of the tunica media of the ductus by the 17.5th day. The developmental stages of the cardiovascular system in the rat embryo is delayed by one to two days compared to those of the mouse, and developmental stage of the 17.5th day in the mouse fetus corresponds approximately to the 19th day in the rat fetus.

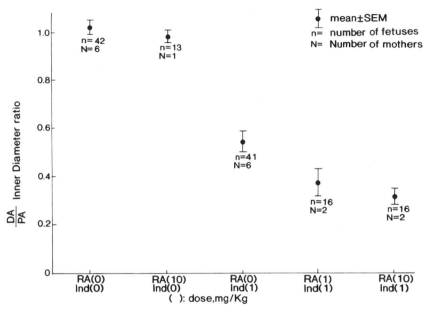

Figure 2. Constriction of DA on the 21st day in fetal rats treated with RA on the 19th and 20th days. The vertical axis shows fetal inner diameter ratio of DA to main PA. In horizontal axis, five experimental groups are shown. Without administration of RA and Ind (RA(0) Ind(0)), the inner diameter ratio of the DA to the main PA (DA/PA) was 1.0. DA/PA was 1.0 following administration of RA (10 mg/kg) on the 19th and 20th days. Moderate ductal constriction (DA/PA = 0.56) was induced by Ind (1mg/kg) 4 hours after orogastric administration without pretreatment by RA. Severe ductal constriction was induced by Ind (1 mg/kg) with pretreatment by RA (1 mg/kg and 10 mg/kg on the 19th and 20th days), and DA/PA was 0.38 and 0.31. Methods: Frozen thorax was cut on a freezing microtome in the frontal plane, and the inner diameters of the main PA and the DA were measured every 100 um in 10 to 15 planes with a microscope and a micrometer. Constriction of the ductus was not uniform, but most severe at the aortic end.[9] The narrowest DA diameter was used to get the inner diameter ratio of DA to main PA (DA/PA).

Vitamin A and Fetal Development

Studies in human infants have shown that neonates have little reserve of vitamin A,[14,15] and some neonates, especially premature infants, show deficient plasma levels of RA and vitamin A.[16] Developmental changes in endogenous retinoids during pregnancy and embryogenesis were studied in the mouse[17] and rat.[18] Maternal plasma vitamin A levels decrease profoundly at mid-gestation. Retinol level of the embryo and fetus increase during organogenesis and fetal development. Large amounts of vitamin A are demanded in embryonic and fetal life.

RA and Endothelial Factors

Other possible mechanisms of acceleration of fetal maturation of the DA include endothelial factors. In addition to prostaglandins, endothelium-derived nitric oxide is important in maintaining fetal patency of the DA.[19] Nitric oxide synthase is controlled by interleukin beta and cyclic adenosine monophosphate.[20] Endothelin is a potent vasoconstrictor and constricts the DA postnatally.[21] Possibly the effects of retinoids on production of nitric oxide or endothelin and its effects on ductal constriction would be a more likely target for the action of exogenous vitamin A.

Acknowledgments: Editorial help of Leonard M Linde, MD, Professor of Pediatric Cardiology, University of Southern California School of Medicine, is highly appreciated.

References

1. Neal WA. Patent ductus arteriosus. In: Moller JH, Neal WA, eds. *Fetal, Neonatal, and Infant Cardiac Disease*. Norwalk, Conn: Appleton & Lange; 1990:391–400.
2. Moise KJ. Effect of advancing gestational age on the frequency of fetal ductal constriction in association with maternal indomethacin use. *Am J Obstet Gynecol* 1993;168:1350–1353.
3. Momma K, Takao A. In vivo constriction of the ductus arteriosus by nonsteroidal antiinflammatory drugs in near-term and pre-term fetal rats. *Pediat Res* 1987;22:567–572.
4. Heymann MA. Patent ductus arteriosus. In Adams FH, Emmanouilides GC, eds. *Moss' Heart Disease in Infants, Children, and Adolescents*. 3rd ed. Baltimore, Md: Williams & Wilkins; 1983:158–171.
5. Olley PM. The ductus arteriosus, its persistence and its patency. In Anderson RH, Macartney FJ, Shinebourne EA, et al., eds. *Paediatric Cardiology*. Edinburgh: Churchill Livingstone; 1987:931–958.
6. Colbert MC, Kirby ML, Robbins J. Endogenous retinoic acid signaling colocalizes with advanced expression of the adult smooth muscle myosin heavy chain isoform during development of the ductus arteriosus. *Circ Res* 1996;78:790–798.
7. Momma K, Takao A. Right ventricular concentric hypertrophy and left ventricular dilatation by ductal constriction in fetal rats. *Circ Res* 1989;64:1137–1146.
8. Momma K, Konishi T, Hagiwara H. Characteristic morphology of the constricted fetal ductus arteriosus following maternal administration of indomethacin. *Pediat Res* 1985;19:483–500.
9. Wallenstein S, Zucker CL, Fleiss JL. Some statistical methods used in circulation research. *Circ Res* 1980;47:1–9.
10. Wilson JG, Warkany J. Aortic-arch and cardiac anomalies in the offspring of vitamin A deficient rats. *Am J Anat* 1949;85:113–155.
11. Lammer EJ, Chen DT, Hoar RM, et al. Retinoic acid embryopathy. *N Engl J Med* 1985;313:837–841.
12. Hofmann C, Eichele G. Retinoids in development. In: Sporn MB, Roberts AB, Goodman DS, eds. *The Retinoids: Biology Chemistry, and Medicine*. 2nd ed. New York: Raven Press; 1994:387–435.
13. Mably JD, Liew C-C. Factors involved in cardiogenesis and the regulation of cardiac-specific gene expression. *Circ Res* 1996;79:4–13.
14. Underwood BA. Maternal vitamin A status and its importance in infancy and early childhood. *Am J Clin Nutr* 1994;59(suppl):517S–524S.
15. Godal JC, Basu TK, Pabst HF, et al. Perinatal vitamin A (Retinol) status of northern Canadian mothers and their infants. *Biol Neonat* 1996;69:133–139.
16. Woodruff CW, Latham CB, James EP, et al. Vitamin A status of premature infants: The influence of feeding and vitamin supplements. *Am J Clin Nutr* 1986;44:384–389.
17. Satre MA, Ugen KE, Kochhar DM. Developmental changes in endogenous retinoids during pregnancy and embryogenesis in the mouse. *Biol Reprod* 1992;46:802–810.
18. Willingford JC, Underwood BA. Vitamin A status needed to maintain vitamin A concentrations in nonhepatic tissues of the pregnant rats. *J Nutr* 1987;117:1410–1415.
19. Coceani F, Kelsey L, Seidlitz E. Occurrence of endothelium-derived relaxing factor-nitric oxide in the lamb ductus arteriosus. *Can J Physiol Pharmacol* 1993;72:82–88.
20. Hirokawa K, O'Shaughnessy K, Moore K, et al. Induction of nitric oxide synthase in cultured vascular smooth muscle cells: The role of cyclic AMP. *Br J Pharmacol* 1994;112:396–402.
21. Coceani F, Kelsey L, Seidlitz E. Evidence for an effecter role of endothelin in closure of the ductus arteriosus at birth. *Can J Physiol Pharmacol* 1992;70:1061–1064.

45

Increased SM2 Myosin Heavy-Chain mRNA Expression Just Before Birth and Induction of Apoptosis After Birth Are Observed in Longitudinally Oriented Smooth Muscle Cells in the Inner Media of the Ductus Arteriosus

*Shin-ichiro Imamura, DVM, PhD, Toshio Nishikawa, MD,
Eriko Hiratsuka, BSc, Atsuyoshi Takao, MD,
and Rumiko Matsuoka, MD, PhD*

The ductus arteriosus (DA) is a unique blood vessel that changes dramatically, from patency of the vessel during fetal life to closure at birth. Hyperoxygen tension induces contraction of the DA,[1-3] and its closure is attributed to contraction of the smooth muscle cells (SMCs). Increased intracellular Ca^{2+} concentration also causes contraction of the DA.[4] However, detailed mechanisms of ductal closure and ligament formation are still unclear, as are the mechanisms of patency.

To understand better the mechanisms of ductal closure and remodeling of the DA after birth, we examined when and where smooth muscle-2 (SM2) myosin heavy-chain (MHC) mRNA expression, which is associated with the contraction of smooth muscle,[5-7] and apoptosis

From Clark EB, Nakazawa M, Takao A (eds.): Etiology and Morphogenesis of Congenital Heart Disease: Twenty Years of Progress in Genetics and Developmental Biology. Armonk, NY: Futura Publishing Co., Inc.; © 2000.

are detectable in the DA. In a preliminary study, we found that apoptotic cell death was clearly detected in the SMCs of the DA after birth. Apoptosis may play a role in vascular remodeling of the DA.[8]

Localization in situ of the SM2 MHC mRNA was performed using T-T dimerized SM2 MHC cDNA probe[9] (Fig. 1). In situ hybridization revealed that SM2 MHC mRNA expression was strongly positive in the longitudinally oriented SMCs and in the inner layer of the circularly oriented SMCs of the DA just before birth (Fig. 1A). However, in the outer layer of the circularly oriented SMCs of the DA and in the pulmonary artery (PA) and aortic artery (Ao), the SM2 MHC mRNA expression was weak. These observations suggest that the inner media of the DA may play an important role in ductal closure, because the SM2 MHC isoform is thought to be associated with the contractile phenotype of smooth muscle cell.[5-7]

Apoptotic features were detected using in situ detection of DNA strand

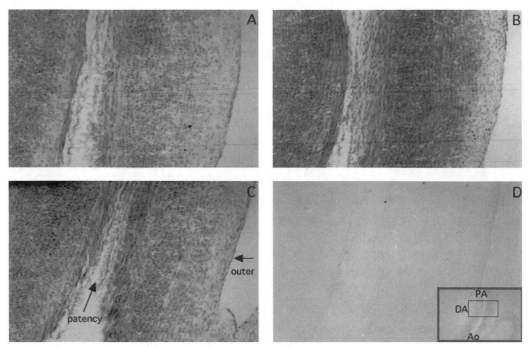

Figure 1. In situ hybridizations using the SM2 antisense oligo-DNA probe (**A**) and the SM1 and SM2 antisense oligo-DNA probe (**B**), and the complementary 28S rRNA probe (**C**) as a positive control and the nonirradiated complementary 28S rRNA probe (**D**) as a negative control were performed (×200). The SM2 MHC mRNA expression was strongly positive in the longitudinally oriented smooth muscle cells and in the inner layer of the circularly oriented smooth muscle cells (**A**). DA, ductus arteriosus; PA, pulmonary artery; Ao, aortic artery.

breaks (TUNEL method), transmission electron microscopical analysis and electrophoretic analysis of total DNA. Apoptotic cells were detected in the SMCs of the DA from 1 day after birth. Interestingly, significant numbers of TUNEL-positive nuclei were detected in the longitudinally oriented SMCs and in the inner layer of the circularly oriented SMCs. Very few nuclei of the outer layer of the circularly oriented SMCs were stained by TUNEL. Transmission electron micrographs (Figs. 2A–D) revealed that the cells had become smaller and nuclear chromatin condensation and nuclear shrinkage could be seen, but the integrity of the plasma membrane had been retained in the SMCs of the DA. Electrophoretic analysis (Figs. 2E–G) showed that a faint but visible ladder was observable from 1 day after birth. However, in the PA and Ao, no ladder formation could be detected. Apoptotic cells were not de-

tected in the PA and Ao. Masson's stained sections showed that the TUNEL-positive area in the DA was replaced by connective tissue from 1 day after birth. At 9 days after birth, the DA had become thin, the number of TUNEL-positive nuclei had decreased in the inner layer and the amount of connective tissue had increased. However, the SMCs in the media were still alive. These results indicate that apoptotic cell death observed in the SMCs of the DA may play an important role in the remodeling of the DA after birth and ligament formation starts at the inner media of the DA.

From these results, we conclude that increased SM2 smooth muscle MHC mRNA expression and induction of apoptosis are observed at the same position in the media of the DA, indicating their important role in ductal closure and remodeling of the vessel wall.

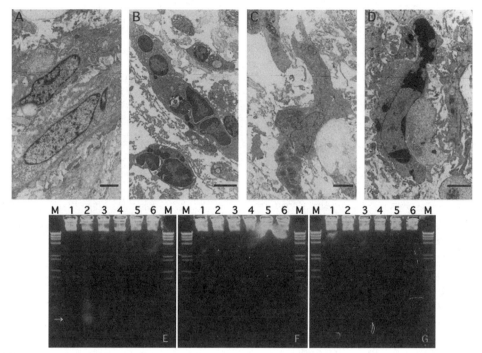

Figure 2. Transmission electron microscopic photographs of smooth muscle cells of the ductus arteriosus on gestational day 29 (**A**), and at 1 (**B**), 3 (**C**), and 7 (**D**) days after birth. Characteristic features of the apoptotic process were observed from 1 day after birth. Bar indicates 2 μm. Electrophoretic gel for detection of DNA strand breaks of smooth muscle cells of the ductus arteriosus (**E**), pulmonary artery (**F**), and aortic artery (**G**). In the ductus arteriosus, a faint but visible ladder is observable from 1 day after birth (**E**). Arrow indicates mononucleosome (180 bp). Lane 1, gestational day 29; lane 2, day 1; lane 3, day 3; lane 4, day 5; lane 5, day 7; lane 6, day 9; M, molecular markers

Materials and Methods

Animals

Japanese White rabbits on gestational day 29, and at 1, 3, 5, 7, and 9 days after birth were used. Briefly, the DA was excised from the animal with or without the PA and Ao.

In Situ Hybridization

The probe (antisense oligo-DNA with auxiliary ATT repeats at both 3′ and 5′ ends) was designed from the 39 nucleotides from rabbit SM2 smooth muscle cDNA, which were inserted in SM1, and it is not homologous with SM1.[5] This probe was irradiated with ultraviolet light at a dose of approximately 10 kJ/m^2 to form thymine-thymine (T-T) dimers.[9] A 34-nucleotide sequence complementary to part of the 28S rRNA[10] was also used as a positive control probe, and the SM2 sense oligo-DNA and nonirradiated complementary 28S rRNA probes were used as negative control probes.

The procedures, sensitivity, and reliability of in situ hybridization using the T-T dimerized oligo-DNA probe have been described previously in detail.[9,11]

In Situ Detection of DNA Strand Breaks

To identify nuclei with DNA strand breaks at the cellular level, TUNEL was performed using an ApopTag Plus kit (Oncor).

Hematoxylin-eosin (H-E) and Masson's staining was also performed for control and detection of connective tissue, respectively.

Electrophoretic Analysis of Extracted DNA

Frozen samples were minced and 5 to 10 μL of the samples were used. Forty microliters of lysis buffer [50 mM Tris-HCl (pH 7.8), 10 mM EDTA, 0.5% w/v N-lauroylsarcosine sodium salt (Nacalai Tesque Inc., Osaka, Japan)] were added and mixed well. Then, 4 μL of proteinase K (10 mg/mL) were added and mixed well, and the samples were incubated at 50°C for 90 minutes. Next, 2 μl of RNase A (10 mg/mL, Sigma) were added and mixed well, and the samples were incubated at 50°C for 30 minutes. These samples were then run on 2% agarose gel (1 g of agarose/50 mL, 40 mM Trizma Base, 5 mM glacial acetic acid, 2 mM EDTA) and stained with ethidium bromide.

References

1. Kovalcik V. The response of the isolated ductus arteriosus to oxygen and anoxia. *J Physiol* 1962;169:185–197.
2. Fay FS. Guinea pig ductus arteriosus. I. Cellular and metabolic basis for oxygen sensitivity. *Am J Physiol* 1971;221:470–479.
3. Roulet MJ, Coburn RF. Oxygen-induced contraction in the guinea pig neonatal ductus arteriosus. *Circ Res* 1981;49:997–1002.
4. Nakanishi T, Gu H, Hagiwara N, et al. Mechanisms of oxygen-induced contraction of ductus arteriosus isolated from the fetal rabbit. *Circ Res* 1993;72:1218–1228.
5. Sakurai H, Matsuoka R, Furutani Y, et al. Expression of four myosin heavy chain genes in developing blood vessels and other smooth muscle organs in rabbits. *Eur J Cell Biol* 1996;69:166–172.
6. Imamura S, Sakurai H, Takao A, et al. Changes in myosin heavy chain gene expression of cultured aortic smooth muscle cells induced by cyclic mechanical stretching. *Circulation* 1992;86(suppl 1):830.
7. Kim H-S, Aikawa M, Kimusa K, et al. Ductus arteriosus: Advanced differentiation of smooth muscle cells demonstrated by myosin heavy chain isoform expression in rabbits. *Circulation* 1993;88(part 1):1804–1810.
8. Slomp J, Gittenberger-de Groot A, Glukhwa WA, et al. Differentiation, dedifferentiation, and apoptosis of smooth muscle cells during the development of the human ductus arteriosus. *Arterioscler Thromb Vasc Biol* 1997;17:1003–1009.
9. Koji T, Nakane PK. Localization *in situ* of specific mRNA using thymine-thymine dimerized DNA probes: Sensitive and reliable non-radioactive in situ hybridization. *Acta Pathol Jpn* 1990;40:793–807.
10. Koji T, Nakane PK. Recent advances in molecular histochemical techniques: *In situ* hybridization and southwestern histochemistry. *J Electron Microsc* 1996;45:119–127.
11. Koji T, Chedid W, Rubin JJ, et al. Progesterone-dependent expression of keratinocyte growth factor mRNA in stromal cells of the primate endometrium: Keratinocyte growth factor as a progestomedin. *J Cell Biol* 1994;125:393–401.

Section VI

46

Overview: Function, Biomechanics, and Control of Developing Cardiovascular Systems

Bradley B. Keller, MD

Overview

Throughout life, cardiovascular (CV) structure and function interact dynamically in all species.[1] The developing CV system has been the focus of both scientists and clinicians for centuries in a broad search for the mechanisms responsible for normal CV morphogenesis and the etiologies of congenital CV anomalies. Definition of CV morphogenesis using light and electron microscopic techniques has provided detailed information on this complex process in numerous species.[2–5] Recent application of molecular biologic and immunohistochemical techniques have dramatically expanded our understanding of cell fates in the developing CV system.[6] Recent reviews have summarized the functional maturation of the embryonic CV system.[7,8]

Function of Developing CV Systems

The embryonic CV system generates forward blood flow and blood pressure to support the metabolic demands of the rapidly growing embryo.[9–11] Embryonic CV function is defined using quantitative measures of venous return, atrial function,[12] ventricular performance,[7,13] and arterial load.[14] These functional indices include individual measures (heart rate, blood pressure and flow, mean vascular resistance) and integrated measures (end-diastolic volume vs stroke volume relations and pressure-volume relations,[15] stress-strain relations, and arterial impedance.)[16] Embryonic CV function has been investigated in a broad range of species, including chick,[9,17] rat,[18] mouse,[15] *Xenopus,*[19] and zebrafish.[20] These developing CV systems can adjust CV function acutely to compensate for changes in chamber filling or vascular tone.[21] Despite limited myofiber maturation, the embryonic myocardium contains a positive force-length relationship and can adjust Ca^{2+} flux to compensate for changes in pacing interval (Keller, unpublished).

Embryonic arterial load is a critical, dynamic determinant of global CV performance. As in the mature arterial circulation, embryonic arterial impedance is defined using simultaneous blood pressure and velocity data.[16,22] The embryonic vasculature acutely adjusts vascular impedance to compensate for changes in cardiac function.[16] Diffusible mediators of altered embryonic vascular tone include atrial

From Clark EB, Nakazawa M, Takao A (eds.): Etiology and Morphogenesis of Congenital Heart Disease: Twenty Years of Progress in Genetics and Developmental Biology. Armonk, NY: Futura Publishing Co., Inc.; © 2000.

natriuretic peptide[23] and nitric oxide,[24] though there are likely many additional regulators of global and regional vascular tone and permeability. As in the mature heart, stroke volume is more sensitive to changes in peripheral vascular resistance than to acute changes in intrinsic myocardial contractility. Prior to autonomic innervation, these acute adjustments in myocardial and vascular function likely occur via local regulatory mechanisms. Of note, there are important species differences in the function and regulation of embryonic CV systems.[8] One obvious and important aspect of mammalian CV development is the coupling of the embryonic CV system to the placental circulation and thus to the maternal circulation.[25,26]

Chronic changes in embryonic CV function occur via modified contractile mass and performance and may also occur via altered myofiber maturation, vasoregulation, and/or neurohumoral control. Chronically increased ventricular afterload produced by conotruncal banding in the chick embryo results in acutely increased developed pressure and myocardial hyperplasia.[27] This translation of changes in CV function to changes in structure likely occurs via the transduction of altered force and deformation within the developing myocardium.[5,28] These forces may affect endothelial cells via fluid shear as well as myocardial cells and nonmyocytes via wall strain and/or stress.

The rapid development of genetically targeted animals with cardiac phenotypes has required the application of techniques developed to define cardiovascular physiology in the chick to the mouse embryo.[8] In addition, novel technologies including optical coherence tomography[29] and high-frequency ultrasound[30] show promise for increased spatial and temporal resolution of the beating embryonic heart in situ. Each of these methods will require careful validation to determine their sensitivity and specificity for defining normal and altered embryonic cardiovascular function.

Biomechanics of Developing Cardiovascular Systems

Biomechanics approaches can now define the passive and active properties of the developing myocardium as well as the impact of altered morphogenesis on muscle performance.[31] We can tag the embryonic epicardium and determine acute and chronic, regional epicardial strains.[32] Using simple geometric models, simultaneous ventricular pressure and strain data are used to define stress-strain relations. As in the mature heart, embryonic end-systolic stress-strain relations are linear, load-independent, and correlate with acute changes in embryonic myocardial contractility (K. Tobita, personal communication). We can also suspend isolated embryonic myocardial specimens in a force-length chamber to determine in vitro myocardial viscoelastic[33] and contractile properties.[8] The functionally immature embryonic myocardium has a positive postsystolic and postextrasystolic force augmentation consistent with modest intracellular Ca^{2+} storage but develops reduced active force in response to shortened pacing interval, consistent with limited Ca^{2+} transport. The measurement of isotonic force during constant shortening velocity allows the calculation of actin-myosin cross-bridge kinetics in the embryonic myocardium (E. Schroder, personal communication). These quantitative measures are also crucial in the mathematical modeling of CV functional and structural development.

Control of Developing Cardiovascular Systems

Unfortunately, we know too little about the "control" systems that regulate embryonic CV performance acutely and that coordinate the adaptation of the developing CV system. In the absence of obvious environmental or metabolic stimuli, embryonic arterial tone varies in a nonrandom fashion, likely related to both tissue level and circulating regulatory mechanisms. We know that the embryonic myocardium responds to adrenergic and purinergic stimulation prior to functional autonomic innervation suggesting that these pathways may have regulatory roles. Likewise, both sodium nitroprusside and 1-arginine acutely reduce embryonic vascular tone, consistent with a nitric oxide mediated mechanism. An additional, critical level of embryonic CV regulation occurs in mammalian embryos due to transplacental maternal-embryonic coupling.[25,34] At the present time, we know very little about the dynamic coupling between the maternal and embryonic circulations during the period of primary cardiac morphogenesis.[15,26]

Thus, the past 25 years have resulted in dramatic progress in the investigation of embryonic CV function and links between changes in function and morphogenesis in several species.[1,18,27,35] The experimental paradigms for investigation of CV development include a wide range of species and teratogenic, surgical, and molecular interventions.[8,36,37] The final CV phenotype represents a complex balance of morphological and functional mechanisms that dynamically interact throughout development.[8] Quantitative measures of performance and biomechanics in the developing myocardium and vasculature can provide insights into the mechanisms that link morphogenesis and function in this complex system.

References

1. Keller BB. Embryonic cardiovascular function, coupling, and maturation: A species view. In: Burggren W, Keller BB, eds. *Development of Cardiovascular Systems: Molecules to Organisms.* Cambridge Univ Press; New York: 1997:65–87.
2. Pexieder T, Christen Y, Vuillemin M, et al. Comparative morphometric analysis of cardiac organogenesis in chick, mouse, and dog embryos. In: Nora JJ, Takao A, eds. *Congenital Heart Disease: Causes and Processes.* Mount Kisco, New York: Futura Publishing Co; 1984:423–438.
3. Vuillemin M, Pexieder T. Normal stages of cardiac organogenesis in the mouse, I: De-velopment of the external shape of the heart. *Am J Anat* 1989;184:101–113.
4. Vuillemin M, Pexieder T. Normal stages of cardiac organogenesis in the mouse, II: Development of the internal relief of the heart. *Am J Anat* 1989;184:114–128.
5. Sedmera D, Pexieder T, Hu N, et al. Developmental changes in the myocardial architecture of the chick. *Anat Rec* 1997;248:421–432.
6. Gittenberger de-Groot AC, Vrancken Peeters MP, Mentink MM, et al. Epicardium-derived cells contribute a novel population to the myocardial wall and the atrioventricular cushions. *Circ Res* 1998;82:1043–1052.
7. Keller BB, Hu N, Tinney JP. Embryonic ventricular diastolic and systolic pressure-volume relation. *Cardiology Young* 1994;4:19–27.
8. Keller BB. Methods to detect cardiovascular phenotypic changes during development. In: Hoit BD, Walsh RA, eds. *Cardiovascular Physiology in the Genetically Engineered Mouse.* New York: Kluwer Academic Publishers; 1998:260–275.
9. Clark EB, Hu N. Developmental hemodynamic changes in the chick embryo from stages 18 to 27. *Circ Res* 1982;51:810–815.
10. Hu N, Clark EB. Hemodynamics of the stage 12 to stage 29 chick embryo. *Circ Res* 1989;65:1665–1670.
11. Keller BB. Functional maturation and coupling of the embryonic cardiovascular system. In: Clark EB, Markwald RR, Takao A, eds. *Developmental Mechanisms of Heart Disease.* Mount Kisco, New York: Futura Publishing; 1995:367–386.
12. Hu N, Keller BB. Relationship of simultaneous atrial and ventricular pressures in the stage 16 to 27 chick embryo. *Am J Physiol* 1995;269:H1359–H1362.
13. Casillas CB, Tinney JP, Keller BB. Influence of acute alterations in cycle length on ventricular function in the chick embryo. *Am J Physiol* 1994;267:H905–911.
14. Yoshigi M, Hu N, Keller BB. Dorsal aortic impedance in the stage 24 chick embryo following acute changes in circulating blood volume. *Am J Physiol* 1996;270:H1597–1606.
15. Keller BB, MacLennan MJ, Tinney JP, et al. In vivo assessment of embryonic cardiovascular dimensions and function in day 10.5 to 14.5 mouse embryos. *Circ Res* 1996;79:247–255.
16. Yoshigi M, Keller BB. Characterization of the embryonic aortic impedance with

lumped parameter models. *Am J Physiol* 1997;273:H19–H27.

17. Keller BB, Hu N, Clark EB. Correlation of ventricular area, perimeter, and conotruncal diameter with mass and function in the stage 12 to 24 chick embryo. *Circ Res* 1990;66:109–114.

18. Nakazawa M, Miyagawa S, Ohno T, et al. Developmental hemodynamic changes in rat embryos at 11 to 15 days of gestation: Normal data of blood pressure and the effect of caffeine compared to data from chick embryo. *Pediatr Res* 1988;23:200–205.

19. Fritsche R, Burggren WW. Development of cardiovascular responses to hypoxia in larvae of the frog *Xenopus laevis*. *Am J Physiol* 1996;271:R912–917.

20. Stainier DY, Fouquet B, Chen JN, et al. Mutations affecting the formation and function of the cardiovascular system in the zebrafish embryo. *Development* 1996; 123:285–292.

21. Keller BB, Yoshigi M, Tinney JP. Ventricular-vascular uncoupling by acute conotruncal occlusion in the stage 21 chick embryo. *Am J Physiol* 1997;273: H2861–H2866.

22. Zahka KG, Hu N, Brin KP, et al. Aortic impedance and hydraulic power in the chick embryo from stages 18 to 29. *Circ Res* 1989;64:1091–1095.

23. Hu N, Hansen AL, Clark EB, et al. Atrial natriuretic peptide reduces diastolic filling in the stage 21 chick embryo. *Pediatr Res* 1995;37:465–468.

24. Bowers PN, Tinney JP, Keller BB. Nitroprusside selectively reduces ventricular preload in the stage 21 chick embryo. *Cardiovasc Res* 1996;31:E132–E138.

25. Ursem NTC, Brinkman HJF, Struijk PC, et al. Umbilical artery waveform analysis based on maximum, mean, and mode velocity in early human pregnancy. *Ultrasound Med Biol* 1998;24:1–7.

26. MacLennan MJ, Keller BB. Umbilical arterial bloodflow during development and following acutely increased heart rate. *Ultrasound Med Biol* 1998 25:361–370 1999.

27. Clark EB, Hu N, Frommelt P, et al. Effect of increased ventricular pressure on heart growth in chick embryo. *Am J Physiol* 1989;257:H55–H61.

28. Sedmera D, Pexieder T, Hu N, et al. A quantitative study of the ventricular myoarchitecture in the stage 21–29 chick embryo following decreased loading. *Eur J Morphol* 1998;36:105–119.

29. Boppart SA, Bouma BE, Pitris G, et al. In vitro cellular optical coherence tomotraphic imaging. *Nature Medicine* 1998; 4:861–865.

30. Srinivasan S, Baldwin HS, Aristizabal O, et al. Noninvasive, in utero imaging of mouse embryonic heart development with 40-MHz echocardiography. *Circulation* 1998; 98:912–918.

31. Taber LA. Mechanical aspects of cardiac development. *Prog Biophys Mol Biol* 1998; 69:237–255.

32. Taber LA, Sun H, Cartmell JS, et al. Epicardial strains in the stage 16–24 embryonic chick ventricle. *Circ Res* 1994;75: 896–903.

33. Miller CE, Vanni MA, Taber LA, et al. Passive stress-strain measurements in the stage 16 and stage 18 embryonic chick heart. *J Biomech Eng JBME* 1997;119: 445–451.

34. Furukawa S, MacLennan MJ, Keller BB. Hemodynamic response to anesthesia in pregnant and nonpregnant ICR mice. *Lab Animal Sci* 1998;48:357–363.

35. Pexieder T, Janecek P. Organogenesis of the human embryonic and early fetal heart as studied by microdissection and SEM. In: Nora JJ, Takao A, eds. *Congenital Heart Disease: Causes and Processes*. Mount Kisco, New York: Futura Publishing Co; 1984:401–421.

36. Dyson E, Sucov HM, Kubalak SW, et al. Atrial-like phenotype is associated with embryonic ventricular failure in retinoid X receptor I −/− mice. *Proc Natl Acad Sci U S A* 1995;92:7386–7390.

37. Gui YH, Linask KK, Khowsathit P, et al. Doppler echocardiography of normal and abnormal embryonic mouse heart. *Pediatr Res* 1996;40:633–642.

47

MRI and Analysis of the Embryonic and Fetal Heart

Bradley R. Smith, PhD

Introduction

Magnetic resonance microscopy (MRM) is a fast and nondestructive, three-dimensional imaging technique that is effective for analyzing cardiovascular development. Technologies for the analysis of genetically-altered animal models have not kept pace with the very rapid increase in the production of animals with mutant phenotypes.[1] Storage, interpretation and distribution of data concerning these new animal models present an important challenge. Careful classification and characterization of phenotypes is essential for ultimately mapping the genes responsible for normal and abnormal development.[2] The researchers who are well trained in generating animals with altered gene expression are frequently not well trained or equipped to assess the results of their specialized work. Here we show the utility of MRM for qualitative and quantitative analysis of normal and abnormal cardiovascular development.

Findings

MRM adapts the noninvasive techniques of clinical magnetic resonance imaging (MRI) for small specimens. These

adaptations include the use of stronger magnetic fields (2–14 Tesla), stronger gradient coils to perturb the magnetic field, specialized imaging coils to accommodate small specimen sizes, and pulse sequences designed to maximize signal-to-noise ratios from very small sample sizes. MRM has been used successfully to investigate fixed embryo specimens[3–7] as well as live embryos.[8,9] It can currently produce three-dimensional data sets with 20 μm resolution in all dimensions in fixed embryo specimens and approximately 190 μm for live in utero imaging of embryos. It has several distinct strengths when compared to other imaging techniques used to investigate cardiovascular development: (1) it is fast, (2) it acquires three-dimensional data, (3) it can produce multiple "stains" of each specimen, and (4) it is nondestructive.

MRM generates nondistorted three-dimensional data that can be manipulated interactively in a fraction of the time required by traditional optical image reconstruction techniques. A three-dimensional data set (128 × 256 × 256 voxels) can be produced from a fixed embryo specimen in 1.75 hours and then processed and loaded into visualization software for real-time manipulation in another 15 minutes.

The three-dimensional nature of MRM data allows the creation of visual models that can be manipulated for fast and easy interpretation. This is accomplished by: (1) digitally slicing the image data in any ori-

From Clark EB, Nakazawa M, Takao A (eds.): Etiology and Morphogenesis of Congenital Heart Disease: Twenty Years of Progress in Genetics and Developmental Biology. Armonk, NY: Futura Publishing Co., Inc.; © 2000.

entation including arbitrary cutting planes (Fig. 1), (2) volume rendering multiple stacked image slices with control over the opacity (alpha-channel) of voxels based on their signal intensity (Fig. 2b), (3) segmentation (isolation) of structures based on seeding, connectivity and threshold levels (Fig. 2), and (4) creation of animations to emphasize spatial relationships between structures that are not apparent in static two-dimensional images.

In addition to the qualitative capabilities mentioned above, MRM permits quantitative assessment of three-dimensional structures. Accurate calculation of cardiac function depends on reliable volumetric measurement of the cardiac chambers. Although videomicro-

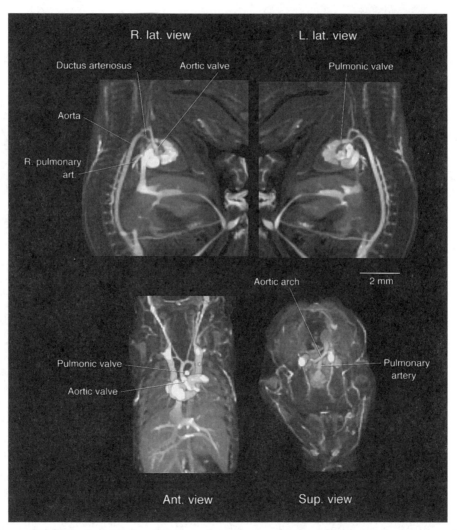

Figure 1. MRM of a 14.5-day mouse embryo thorax demonstrates major cardiovascular anatomical landmarks in this fixed specimen over-expressing the gap junction gene connexin 43. Three-dimensional data arrays permit image displays in multiple sectioning planes and with selectable section thickness, all from the same specimen. The top row shows right and left lateral views with a slice thickness of approximately 0.5 mm. The bottom row shows an anterior view and a superior view (dorsal to the top of the page, embryos left to the right of the page) with a slice thickness of about 2 mm. The data are from a collaboration with Cecilia Lo at the University of Pennsylvania.[7]

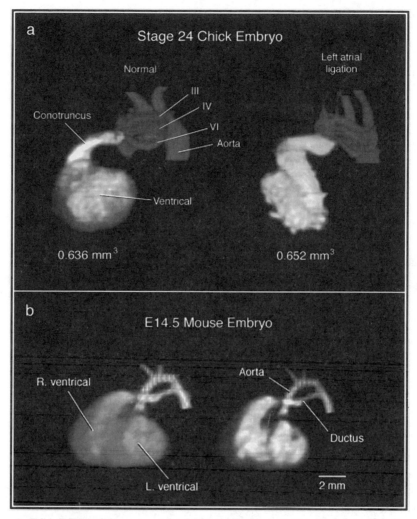

Figure 2. BSA-DTPA-Gd contrast highlights the ventricular and vascular lumens in these chick and mouse embryos. Isolation of the ventricles and conotruncus is achieved with seeding and thresholding of the three-dimensional data. This digital model of the heart and major vessels can be rotated for observation and measured for quantitative analysis. **a.** Normal and surgically manipulated chick embryo hearts are compared. The data are from a collaboration with Brad Keller and Norman Hu. **b.** Changing the alpha-channel (image opacity) renders the myocardium transparent and reveals the ventricular lumen in this normal mouse embryo.

graphy can be used to *calculate* ventricular volume in live embryonic hearts,[10] MRM can produce direct volume measurements in the hearts of sacrificed embryos (Fig. 2a). This ability to generate measurements of lengths, areas, and volumes in three-dimensions is important because the assessment of cardiac phenotypes in genetically altered animals is moving from a simple diagnosis of normal versus abnormal to the more informative quantification of phenotypic variation.[2]

MRM also provides the means to investigate a specimen with multiple pulse sequences to obtain a series of images with different tissue to tissue contrasts. Intrinsic properties of tissues can be exploited to produce various light-to-dark contrasts between structures by the selection of different imaging pulse sequences during image acquisition (similar to using several optical stains in histology) (Fig. 3a). Additionally, contrast agents can be added in order to increase or decrease the MR signal in regions of interest that do not have sufficient intrinsic contrast (Fig. 3b).

The nondestructive nature of MRM makes it suitable for investigating live embryos. Data on the development of mammalian embryos are typically collected from observations of many embryos sacrificed at various stages of growth because direct observation of the live embryo is very difficult in mammals. The ability to make repeated observations of a single live embryo as it grows reduces the number of animals needed to achieve statistically reliable evidence for the mechanisms being studied. Live rat embryos have been followed with repeated MRM in utero imaging at embryonic days 13, 16, and 20.[9] Although in utero MRM imaging is not yet ready to evaluate details of cardiovascular development, it does provide adequate image contrast and resolution to readily identify major anatomical features including the placenta, amniotic fluid, umbilical stalk, limb buds, neural tube, telencephalic and mesencephalic vesicles, cardinal veins, heart chambers, aorta, and sinus venosus (Fig. 4).

Discussion

The nondestructive and high-resolution capability of MRM to generate three-dimensional images in live and fixed embryos permits the study of phenomena that are of great interest to investigators of cardiovascular development. However, limited resolution with respect to optical techniques and low contrast levels at very high resolution are challenges currently facing MRM in fixed embryos. For in utero imaging, motion within the mother, motion of the embryo, motion within the embryo, and even the diffusion of water through the embryo constrain image resolution and contrast. Pulse sequences are being developed that can be triggered by physiological events in the mother and that can acquire data very rapidly to accommodate the motion that is inherent in live embryo imaging. Techniques that can target MRI contrast agents to specific gene products are in great demand but have yet to be identified or constructed. Such contrast agents could act as markers to illuminate the temporal and spatial expression of selected genes in whole embryos.

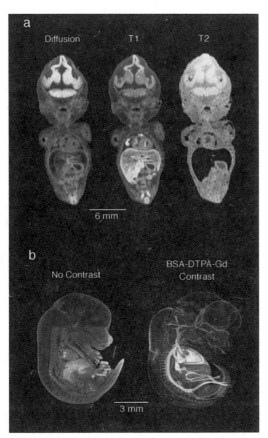

Figure 3. a. Diffusion-weighted, T1-weighted, and T2-weighted images from a Carnegie stage 22 human embryo demonstrate the variation in image contrasts that can be obtained from a single specimen. **b.** BSA-DTPA-Gd contrast reveals in a day 12 mouse embryo cardiovascular structures that are not apparent in a contrast-free specimen.

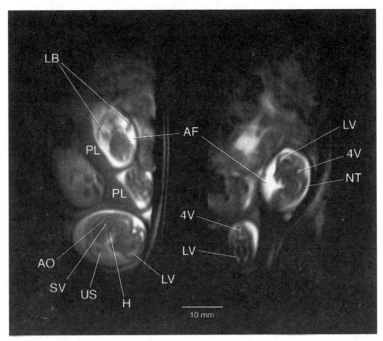

Figure 4. In utero images of live day 16 rat embryos. 4V, fourth ventricle of brain; AF, amniotic fluid; AO, aorta; H, heart; LB, limb buds; LV, lateral ventricle of brain; NT, neural tube; PL, placenta; SV, sinus venosus; US, umbilical stalk.

Acknowledgements: The author wishes to thank Cecilia Lo for including MRM as a part of her investigations of connexin gap junction genes and their role in cardiac development, Bradley Keller and Norman Hu for their collaboration with the left atrial ligation studies in chick embryos, and Dr. G. Allan Johnson and the staff of the Center for In Vivo Microscopy for their expertise which has made the imaging of embryos possible. This work was supported by the following grants: P41 RR05959 NIH (G. Allan Johnson), and N01-HD-6-3257 NIH (Bradley Smith).

References

1. Nagy A, Rossant J. Targeted mutagenesis: analysis of phenotype without germ line transmission. *J Clin Invest* 1996;97:1360–1365.
2. Chien K. Genes and physiology: molecular physiology in genetically engineered animals. *J Clin Invest* 1996;97:901–909.
3. Kornguth S, Bersu E, Anderson M, et al. Correlation of increased levels of class I MHC H-2Kk in the placenta of murine trisomy 16 conceptuses with structural abnormalities revealed by magnetic resonance microscopy. *Teratology* 1992;45:383–391.
4. Smith BR, Effmann EL, Johnson GA. MR microscopy of chick embryo vasculature. *J Magn Reson Imaging* 1992;2:237–240.
5. Smith BR, Johnson GA, Groman EV, et al. Magnetic resonance microscopy of mouse embryos. *Proc Natl Acad Sci U S A* 1994; 91:3530–3533.
6. Smith B. Magnetic resonance microscope *Trends Cardiovasc Med* 1996;6:247–254.
7. Huang G, Wessels A, Smith BR, et al. Alteration in connexin 43 gap junction gene dosage impairs conotruncal heart development. *Dev Biol* 1998;198:32–44.
8. Jacobs RE, Fraser SE. Magnetic resonance microscopy of embryonic cell lineages and movements. *Science* 1994;256: 681–684.
9. Smith BR, Shattuck MD, Hedlund LW, et al. Time-course imaging of rat embryos in utero with magnetic resonance microscopy. *Magn Reson Med* 1998;39(4):673–677.
10. Tanaka N, Mao L, DeLano FA, et al. Left ventricular volumes and function in the embryonic mouse heart. *Am J Physiol* 1997;273:H1368–H1376.

48

The Similarity of Ventricular Function and Morphology of the Embryonic Heart of ET-1 Knockout and Retinoic Acid-Treated Mice

Makoto Nakazawa, MD, Hiroshi Yasui, MD,
Masae Morishima, DVM, PhD,
Sachiko M. Tomita, DVM, PhD, Yukiko Kurihara, MD,
Hiroki Kurihara, MD, and Naohito Yamasaki, MD

Endothelin-1 (ET-1) is also one of the essential factors in morphogenesis, especially of the cardiac outflow tract. Kurihara et al. first reported that ET-1 knockout homozygous mice had an anomaly complex similar to 22q11.2 partial deletion syndrome.[1,2] We have been interested in hemodynamics and cardiac function of mouse embryos, and we analyzed the heart of ET-1 knockout mice during embryonic days 10 to 12. During the study, we noticed that the morphology of the embryonic heart was somewhat different from what we had expected from the final morphology which was originally reported, and more interestingly that it was very similar to that of embryos which were produced by treatment of dams with all trans retinoic acid at embryonic day (ED) 8.5.[3,4]

As we have previously reported, all hearts of retinoic acid treated embryos showed a hypoplasia and dysplasia of the proximal outflow cushion as a common

finding, which was associated with a spectrum of cardiac outflow tract morphology when observed at ED 12. The one end was that the aorta shifted to the right and overrode on the interventricular septum, which we called dextroposed aorta, but the pulmonary artery still connected to the right ventricle. And, the other extreme, which was seen in approximately 80% of embryos, was complete transposition of the great arteries, in which the aorta arose completely from the right ventricle and the pulmonary artery arose completely from the left ventricle. In this retinoic acid treated model, transposition was much more frequent than hearts with dextroposed aorta.

We were able to examine 10 embryos of ET-1 knockout mouse. The hypoplasia and dysplasia of the outflow cushion was a little mild compared to the retinoic acid treated embryo, but the outflow tract morphology showed the similar spectrum from dextroposed aorta to complete transposition of the great arteries. The only difference was that complete transposition was less frequent and seen in only 2 out of 10 of the ET-1 knockout embryos and there were 2 embryos with com-

From Clark EB, Nakazawa M, Takao A (eds.): Etiology and Morphogenesis of Congenital Heart Disease: Twenty Years of Progress in Genetics and Developmental Biology. Armonk, NY: Futura Publishing Co., Inc.; © 2000.

pletely normal great arteries. The other six showed the dextroposed aorta. Thus, two models showed very similar outflow tract morphology during relatively early stages of cardiac development (Fig. 1) although the incidence of each morphology was different among these two models.

The morphological findings seen in the ET-1 knockout mouse was first surprising since this peptide is well known as a potent vasoactive as well as inotropic and chronotropic substance,[5,6] and it has been recently clarified also as an important factor in the myocardial hypertrophy.[7] On the other hand, retinoic acid was first recognized as a teratogene, and the

late Pexieder and his associates have disclosed that retinoic acid given during early development causes abnormal myocardial function in the chick embryo.[8] In addition, it was also reported that knockout of the retinoic acid X receptor (RXR) resulted in the very thin compact layer of the ventricular wall and depression of pump function of the ventricles.[9] These studies have indicated that retinoic acid should also play an important role in myogenesis and cardiac function beside the well known role in morphogenesis. Thus, it would be questioned that cardiac function and cardiac myogenesis may be affected in the lack of endothelin-1 and the excess of retinoic acid, both of which

ET-1 knockout embryo

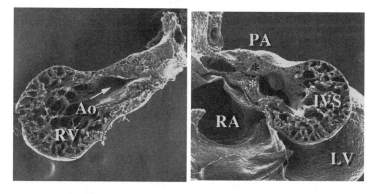

Retinoic acid treated embryo

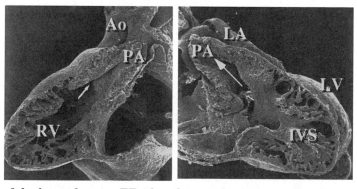

Figure 1. SEM of the heart from an ET-1 knockout embryo (upper photos) and from a retinoic acid treated embryo (lower photos). The inside view of the right ventricular free wall is shown on the left, and the left side half of the heart is on the right. Both hearts showed a typical morphology of complete aortopulmonary transposition. Ao, aorta; PA, pulmonary artery; RV, right ventricle; LV, left ventricle; IVS, interventricular septum.

cause a common outflow tract morphology as described above.

A new technology which we have developed enables us to observe embryonic heart of the mammalian in situ, and thus to evaluate physiology of early developmental stages of the cardiovascular system.[10] Using our bathing system, we have analyzed characteristics of ventricular size and pump function in embryos of both ET-1 knockout and retinoic acid treated mouse at ED 12. The findings in these two models was almost identical in many aspects (Fig. 2). Firstly, the primitive right ventricle (RV) was almost equal in size to the primitive left ventricle (LV) in both models. This is abnormal because the RV being larger than the LV is a specific finding in the control mouse of the strain that we used, that was the ICR mouse. Pump function, evaluated with ejection fraction as in the mature subject, of the RV was depressed and that of the LV was rather augmented in both endothelin-1 knockout and retinoic acid treated embryos. The ratio of the RV/LV of size and ejection fraction was very similar in both groups and this finding was only subtle (statistically not significant) at ED 11 (data not shown), but became obvious at ED 12 as presented in Figure 2. Another finding was that the atrium and sinus venosus were enlarged in retinoic acid treated embryos and they were even larger in endothelin-1 knockout embryos, which were, however, unable to be quantitated be-

cause a large part of them was hidden behind the ventricles.

The data showed that, in both ET-1 knockout and retinoic acid treatment, morphological abnormality was confined at the outflow tract of the heart, and this abnormal morphology may have resulted in the dysfunction of the RV. Pump function of the LV was normal or it looked even somewhat augmented, and gross structure of trabeculation and free wall of the LV was completely normal (data not shown), indicating that both intervention have nothing to do with organogenesis of the LV. Thus, it should be speculated that these two interventions may utilize a common molecular and genetical pathway of morphogenesis which is confined only at the outflow tract. One possible explanation may be a role of the neural crest cell. Kurihara et al. first indicated that the morphology of ET-1 knockout mouse could be a result of abnormality in neural crest cell function, and they have later implied that ET-1 may a key factor in cell differentiation at the target tissues of neural crest cells.[11] It is also recently shown that the neural crest cell migrates into the outflow tract of the developing heart.[12] These facts suggest that abnormal morphology seen in this study have resulted from abnormal neural crest cell function. This may not, however, explain why the whole RV was small and its function was depressed. In this symposium, Dr. Kirby has suggested that cardiac neu-

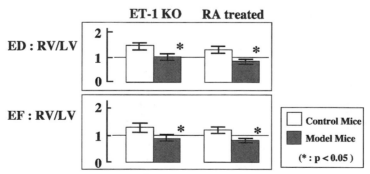

Figure 2. The ratio of end-diastolic size between the right and left ventricles (ED: RV/LV) was larger than 1.0 in both ET-1 knockout and retinoic acid treated embryos, which was significantly larger than that of controls. The ratio of ejection fraction (EF: RV/LV) was similar.

ral crest cells affect myocardial development via a fibroblast growth factor (FGF)-like signal,[13] which would be a hypothesis supportive of our findings. Retinoic acid is also an important factor in the cardiovascular morphogenesis especially in relation to the neural crest cell. Several studies have revealed that the anomaly complex produced by neural crest deprivation was identical, or nearly identical if not completely, to that seen in mice of double knockout of retinoic acid receptors (RARs) such as RARα/RARβ, RARα/RARγ, RXRα/RARγ, or RXRα/RARα.[14,15] Thus, it may be speculated that the two models which we showed in the present study utilize a common molecular and genetical pathway which would be strongly related to the neural crest cell. It is very unlikely that the lack of ET-1 or overdose of retinoic acid acts directly on development of the whole heart, since left ventricular shape and function were not affected at all.

References

1. Kurihara Y, Kurihara H, Suzuki H, et al. Elevated blood pressure and craniofacial abnormalities in mice deficient in endothelin-1. *Nature* 1994;368:703–710.
2. Kurihara Y, Kurihara H, Oda H, et al. Aortic arch malformations and ventricular septal defect in mice deficient in endothelin-1. *J Clin Invest* 1995;96:293–300.
3. Yasui H, Nakazawa M, Morishima M, et al. Morphological observations on the pathogenetic process of transposition of the great arteries induced by retinoic acid in mice. *Circulation* 1995;91:2478–2486.
4. Yasui H, Nakazawa M, Morishima M, et al. Cardiac outflow tract septation process in the mouse model of transposition of the great arteries. *Teratology* 1997;55:353–363.
5. Masaki T. Possible role of endothelin in endothelial regulation of vascular tone. *Ann Rev Pharmacol Toxicol* 1995;35:235–255.
6. Concas V, Laurent S, Brisac AM, et al. Endothelin has potent direct inotropic and chronotropic effects in cultured heart cells. *J Hypertens.* 1989;7(suppl):S96–S97

7. Ponicke K, Heinroth-Hoffmann I, Becker K, et al. Trophic effect of angiotensin II in neonatal rat cardiomyocytes: Role of endothelin-1 and non-myocyte cells. *Br J Pharmacol* 1997;121:118–124.
8. Pexieder T, Blanc O, Pelouch V, et al. Late fetal development of retinoic acid-induced transposition of great arteries: Morphology, physiology, and biochemistry. In: Clark EB, Markwald RR, Takao A, eds. *Developmental Mechanisms of Heart Disease.* Armonk, NY: Futura Publishing Co; 1995:297–307.
9. Dyson E, Sucov HM, Kubalak SW, et al. Atrial-like phenotype is associated with embryonic ventricular failure in retinoid X receptor alpha −/− mice. *Proc Natl Acad Sci U S A* 1995;92:7386–7390.
10. Nakazawa M, Morishima M, Tomita H, et al. Hemodynamics and ventricular function in the day-12 rat embryo: Basic characteristics and the responses to cardiovascular drugs. *Pediatr Res* 1995;37:117–123.
11. Kurihara H. Endothelin-1 as a regulator of cardiac neural crest development. Presented at the Fifth International Symposium on Etiology and Morphogenesis of Congenital Heart Disease: Twenty Years' Progress, December 7–9, 1998, Tokyo, Japan.
12. Karen W, Tomita S-M, Kumiski D, et al. Cardiac neural crest cells provide new insight into septation of the cardiac outflow tract: Aortic sac to ventricular septal closure. *Dev Biol* 1998;196:129–144.
13. Kirby ML, Farrell M, Karen W, et al. Novel mechanisms used by cardiac neural crest cells in supporting structural and functional heart development. In: Clark EB, Nakazawa M, Takao A, eds. *Etiology and Morphogenesis of Congenital Heart Disease: Twenty Years of Progress in Genetics and Developmental Biology.* Armonk, NY: Futura Publishing Co., 2000.
14. Dyson E, Sucov HM, Kuralak SW, et al. Atrial-like phenotype is associated with embryonic ventricular failure in retinoid X receptor a −/− mice. *Proc Natl Acad Sci U S A* 1995;92:7386–7390.
15. Lee RY, Luo J, Evans RM, et al. Compartment-selective sensitivity of cardiovascular morphologenesis to combinations of retinoic acid receptor gene mutations. *Circ Res* 1997;80:757–764.

49

In Utero High-Frequency (40 MHz) Echocardiographic Analysis of Murine Embryonic Heart Development

Michael Artman, MD, Shardha Srinivasan, MD,
Colin Phoon, MD, Orlando Aristizabal, PhD,
and Daniel H. Turnbull, PhD

The increasing number of genetically engineered murine models with potential abnormalities in cardiovascular development[1] has resulted in a need for noninvasive techniques of serially analyzing cardiovascular structure and function in live embryonic mice. Presently available methods of studying embryonic and fetal murine development include standard histological analysis of fixed specimens, scanning electron microscopy,[2,3] and magnetic resonance microscopy.[4] Real-time imaging has been achieved using high-speed video microscopy,[5,6] but this technique requires surgical exposure of the embryos and is therefore not suited to serial measurements. High-frequency (40–50 MHz) ultrasound imaging has been used to provide high-resolution imaging of live mouse embryos in utero.[7] We therefore applied this technique to study cardiovascular development in live mouse embryos from gestational age 8.5 to 13.5 days (E8.5–E13.5).

Images obtained by 40 MHz echocardiography in the present study differ in some ways from those obtained by lower frequency clinical ultrasound. At this high frequency, the blood pool is echogenic so that the heart is identified as a bright, highly echogenic structure and flow in the vasculature exhibits a speckled pattern. Cardiac contractions could be identified in some E8.5 embryos and the common atrium and ventricle could be reliably observed by E9.5. The progressive development of the ventricles, outflow tract and chamber growth were tracked from E9.5 to E13.5. A total of 234 embryos were imaged over the course of this project. In order to confirm the feasibility of serial studies, four litters were repeatedly imaged on three consecutive days from E11.5 to E13.5. The following day, the anesthetized mother was killed and the embryos were examined under a dissecting microscope. In all embryos in these four litters (n = 31) the ultrasound images and gross morphology were normal.

Planimetry of the epicardial surfaces was used as a measure of chamber growth and measurements recorded in end-systole and end-diastole were used as an index of contractile function. The combined end-diastolic ventricular area increased from 1.47 ± 0.33 at E10.5 to 2.02 ± 0.21 mm^2 at E11.5. The presumptive right and left ventricles could be distinguished after E11.5, so separate mea-

From Clark EB, Nakazawa M, Takao A (eds.): Etiology and Morphogenesis of Congenital Heart Disease: Twenty Years of Progress in Genetics and Developmental Biology. Armonk, NY: Futura Publishing Co., Inc.; © 2000.

surements were performed at E12.5 and E13.5. No significant difference was observed between the ventricles at these stages, although progressive growth was noted [right ventricular (RV) end-diastolic area = 1.21 ± 0.17 at E12.5 and 1.47 ± 0.20 mm² at E13.5; left ventricular (LV) end-diastolic area = 1.22 ± 0.18 at E12.5 and 1.51 ± 0.24 mm² at E13.5]. RV and LV fractional area changes were approximately 34% ± 6% at E12.5 and E13.5.

The present system is somewhat limited by the relatively slow frame rate (8 images/second). If the embryonic heart rate is near 200 bpm, then each cardiac cycle will be completed in only 2 to 4 frames. We attempted to minimize the potential error by averaging 4 separate measurements of apparent end-diastole and end-systole. The inherent limitations of the frame rate combined with the maternal respirations made it difficult to accurately assess embryonic heart rate visually from the 2-dimensional images. Using a prototype of a new ultrasound-guided Doppler system being developed in our laboratory, we found the embryonic heart rate to be quite sensitive to maternal temperature and level of anesthesia. However, further studies are necessary to non-invasively characterize embryonic heart rate, blood flow velocities, and ventricular function at various stages of development.

We conclude that high-frequency ultrasound can be used to identify key elements of normal murine embryonic cardiovascular development. The developmental stages studied correspond to approximately 3–6 weeks of gestation in humans and are the earliest to be studied in utero in the developing mouse. This technique should be useful for the non-invasive evaluation of cardiac structural and functional development in a variety of murine models of cardiovascular pathology.

Methods

Developing hearts of mouse embryos in utero were studied from gestational age 8.5 to 13.5 days (E8.5 to E13.5) using 40 MHz ultrasound. Timed-pregnant CD1 mice were anesthetized (sodium pentobarbital 5mg/100gm and magnesium sulfate 10mg/100gm body weight) and the abdominal area was shaved. A small water bath was fitted to the skin to provide a coupling medium for the transducer. Transabdominal scans were performed using a focused 40-MHz transducer with measured lateral resolution of 90 μm, axial resolution of 30 μm and depth of penetration of 7 to 10 mm. The transducer is coupled to a mechanical scanning system, which produces real time images at 8 frames/second. This system was developed and constructed in our laboratory and the details have been previously described.[8,9]

Imaging was started from one flank and embryos were sequentially imaged across the lower abdomen. Sequential linear scans were obtained at increments of 20 or 100 μm, depending on the size of the embryo and the region of interest. The consistent orientation of normal mouse embryos with the placenta and tail to the right of the embryo was used as a landmark to help identify proper orientation of cardiac structures. Atrial and ventricular contractions and changes in cardiac morphology were recorded from E9.5 to E13.5. Hyperechoic streaming patterns revealed flow through the umbilical, vitelline and other vessels. Doppler recordings were obtained from the major blood vessels and across the cardiac inflow and outflow tracts. Planimetry of the epicardial borders was used to measure ventricular growth and the change in ventricular area during systole and diastole was used as an index of contractile function.[9] Several pregnant mice were studied repeatedly to confirm the utility of this approach for serial analyses within the same litter.

References

1. Rossant J. Mouse mutants and cardiac development: new molecular insights into cardiogenesis. *Circ Res* 1996;78:349–353.

2. Vuillemin M, Pexieder T. Normal stages of cardiac organogenesis in the mouse: I. Development of the external shape of the heart. *Am J Anat* 1989;184:101–113.

3. Vuillemin M, Pexieder T. Normal stages of cardiac organogenesis in the mouse: II. Development of the internal relief of the heart. *Am J Anat* 1989;184:114–128.

4. Smith BR, Johnson GA, Groman EV, et al. Magnetic resonance microscopy of mouse embryos. *Proc Natl Acad Sci U S A* 1994; 91:3530–3533.

5. Dyson E, Sucov HM, Kubalak SW, et al. Atrial-like phenotype is associated with embryonic ventricular failure in retinoid X receptor alpha −/− mice. *Proc Natl Acad Sci U S A* 1995;92:7386–7390.

6. Yasui H, Nakazawa M, Morishima M, et al. Cardiac outflow tract septation process in the mouse model of transposition of the great arteries. *Teratology* 1997;55:353–363.

7. Turnbull DH, Bloomfield TS, Baldwin HS, et al. Ultrasound backscatter microscope analysis of early mouse embryonic brain development. *Proc Natl Acad Sci U S A* 1995;92:2239–2243.

8. Turnbull DH, Starkoski BG, Harasiewicz KA, et al. A 40–100 MHz B-scan ultrasound backscatter microscope for skin imaging. *Ultrasound Med Biol* 1995;21:79–88.

9. Srinivasan S, Baldwin HS, Aristizabal O, et al. Noninvasive, in utero imaging of mouse embryonic heart development with 40-MHz echocardiography. *Circulation* 1998;98:912–918.

50

Calcium Regulation in the Developing Heart

Michael Artman, MD, Peter S. Haddock, PhD, and William A. Coetzee, DSc

The sarcoplasmic reticulum (SR) and T-tubule (TT) networks of adult mammalian ventricular myocytes are coupled by diadic junctions, linking depolarization-induced Ca^{2+} entry to a spatially homogeneous release of SR Ca^{2+} stores.[1,2] In view of the central role of TT-SR junctions in facilitating SR Ca^{2+} release, we hypothesized that immature cardiac myocytes, which lack T-tubules and have altered expression of key proteins involved in excitation-contraction coupling may exhibit subcellular Ca^{2+} gradients during normal contraction and relaxation. To test this hypothesis, we compared the excitation-contraction coupling phenotype of newborn (1–5 days of age) rabbit ventricular myocytes with adult ventricular myocytes. Using confocal microscopy, we measured fluo-3 Ca^{2+} transients in the sub-sarcolemmal space (SS) and cell center (CC) of field-stimulated (0.5 Hz) myocytes from each age group. In adults, line-scan images revealed spatially and temporally uniform changes in $[Ca^{2+}]_i$ across the entire width of the cell. Peak systolic $[Ca^{2+}]_i$ was similar in the SS (940 ± 76 nM) and CC (1002 ± 70 nM, n = 9) and subsequently declined with similar time constants (τ_{relax} SS: 154 ±

13; CC: 148 ± 17 msec; n = 5). These data are consistent with an excitation-contraction coupling phenotype in which mature T-tubule and SR networks facilitate the triggered homogeneous release of SR Ca.

Newborn myocytes were smaller and had a greater surface area-to-volume ratio compared to adult cells.[3] Composite line-scan images in newborn myocytes revealed striking regional and temporal differences in $[Ca^{2+}]_i$ during steady-state stimulation. During the initial phase of each transient, Ca^{2+} increased significantly in the sub-sarcolemmal space prior to a smaller rise in the cell center. Local Ca^{2+} transients obtained at the sub-sarcolemmal space also had a more rapid upstroke than at the cell center. Furthermore, peak systolic Ca^{2+} was significantly higher in the subsarcolemmal space compared to the cell center (SS: 1128 ± 65; CC: 549 ± 23 nM, n = 13), and declined more rapidly during relaxation (τ_{relax} SS: 307 ± 16; CC: 515 ± 26 msec; n = 6).

We next assessed the contribution of SR Ca^{2+} stores to the Ca^{2+} transients and patterns of subcellular Ca^{2+} distribution by comparing Ca^{2+} gradients in field-stimulated myocytes that were either untreated or exposed to thapsigargin (TG, 10 μM) to deplete SR Ca^{2+} (confirmed by rapid application of 10 mM caffeine). As shown in Figure 1, TG treatment of adult

From Clark EB, Nakazawa M, Takao A (eds.): Etiology and Morphogenesis of Congenital Heart Disease: Twenty Years of Progress in Genetics and Developmental Biology. Armonk, NY: Futura Publishing Co., Inc.; © 2000.

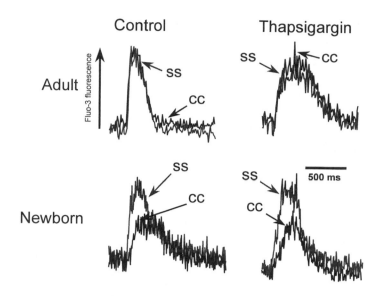

Figure 1. Ca^{2+} transients recorded from the subsarcolemmal space (SS) and cell center (CC) in the absence and presence of thapsigargin to deplete SR Ca^{2+} stores. Thapsigargin prolonged the transients in adult cells, but had no effect on either the time course of the transient or the spatial inhomogeneity in newborn myocytes.

myocytes prolonged the time course of the $[Ca^{2+}]_i$ transient to a similar degree at both the sub-sarcolemmal space and cell center (τ_{relax} SS: 432 ± 28; CC: 446 ± 28 msec; n = 6). However, the homogeneous spatial distribution of the Ca^{2+} transient remained. In contrast, TG did not affect the time course or spatial inhomogeneity of $[Ca^{2+}]_i$ transients in newborn myocytes (τ_{relax} SS: 274 ± 19; CC: 473 ± 17 msec; n = 5–6). These results indicate that the SR participates minimally during normal contraction and relaxation in myocytes from newborn rabbits.

To further define postnatal changes in the excitation-contraction coupling phenotype, we investigated the spatial relationship between key proteins involved in Ca^{2+} transport. We used confocal imaging of myocytes co-immunolabeled with antibodies against the cardiac isoforms of the Na-Ca exchanger (NCX1; the dominant pathway for sarcolemmal Ca^{2+} fluxes at birth) and the ryanodine receptor (RyR2; the Ca^{2+} release channel in the junctional SR). In newborn ventricular myocytes, NCX1 labeling was observed exclusively at the sarcolemma. RyR2 expression was confined solely to the cell interior such that no NCX1-RyR2 co-localization was observed. These data indicate a spatial separation of the sarco-

lemma and SR at birth, consistent with diminished utilization of SR Ca^{2+} during excitation-contraction coupling. In myocytes from 10–14 day old rabbits, a narrow sub-sarcolemmal band of antigen co-localization appeared, suggesting the presence of peripheral sarcolemmal-SR couplings. This may be an important intermediate stage in the transition to an SR-dependent phenotype. In contrast to immature myocytes, NCX1 and RyR2 co-localized at each Z-line in adult myocytes consistent with maturation of the T-tubule system and close approximation of the sarcolemma with the SR Ca^{2+} release sites.

Our results indicate that the absence of T-tubules and lack of tight spatial coupling between the sarcolemma and SR appears to functionally isolate the SR from effective participation in excitation-contraction coupling in the newborn rabbit heart. Consequently, the immature heart utilizes transsarcolemmal Ca entry to evoke contractions consistent with an SR-independent excitation-contraction coupling phenotype. The transition to an adult SR-dependent pattern of excitation-contraction coupling is dependent upon the coordinated acquisition of an extensive T-tubule network and formation of diadic junctions with the SR.

Methods

Confocal T-tubule and Ca Imaging

In all experiments, newborn (1–5 day), juvenile (10–14 day), and adult ventricular myocytes were isolated from the hearts of New Zealand White rabbits.[3] Myocytes were incubated in di-8-ANEPPS (5 μM; 5 minutes at 22°C), a plasma membrane-selective fluorescent dye, to fluorescent-label the sarcolemma and allow identification of the T-tubule network.[4] The dye was excited with the 488-nm line of an argon laser and emitted fluorescence > 510 nm recorded in image-scan mode.

To observe spatial and temporal changes in $[Ca^{2+}]_i$ myocytes were loaded (newborn: 10 minutes; adult: 30 minutes; 22°C) with the Ca^{2+} fluorophore, fluo-3 (1 μM). Myocytes were electrically stimulated (22°C, 0.5 Hz) and calcium transients recorded in line-scan mode. In all experiments, the confocal plane in the z-dimension was set in the cell center. Intracellular calcium was calibrated according to the formula $[Ca^{2+}]_i = K_d * R/((K_d/[Ca]_{rest})-R + 1)$,[5] where R is the normalized fluorescence (F/F_{rest}) and K_d is the dissociation constant of the Ca^{2+}-fluo-3 complex. We used a minimum estimate of the K_d in the cytoplasmic environment of muscle cells of 1.1 μM[6], and age-appropriate values for $[Ca]_{rest}$ of 244 and 160 nM determined in field-stimulated (0.5 Hz), indo-1 loaded, newborn and adult myocytes, respectively.

Immunofluorescence Analysis

Myocytes were fixed and permeabilized in 3.7% paraformaldehyde/0.2% Triton-X100 and were co-immunolabeled with antibodies raised against cardiac isoforms of the NCX1 and RyR2.[7] Appropriate FITC and Texas Red-conjugated secondary antibodies revealed spatial patterns of antigen expression and co-localization in confocal optical sections obtained at the mid z-plane of each cell.

References

1. Callewaert G. Excitation-contraction coupling in mammalian cardiac cells. *Cardiovasc Res* 1992;26:923–932.
2. Wier WG, Egan TM, Lopez-Lopez JR, et al. Local control of excitation-contraction coupling in rat heart cells. *J Physiol* 1994;474: 463–471.
3. Haddock PS, Coetzee WA, Artman M. Na^+/Ca^{2+} exchange current and contractions measured under $Cl(^-)$-free conditions in developing rabbit hearts. *Am J Physiol* 1997;273:H837–H846.
4. Huser J, Lipsius SL, Blatter LA. Calcium gradients during excitation-contraction coupling in cat atrial myocytes. *J Physiol* 1996;494:641–651.
5. Cannell MB, Cheng H, Lederer WJ. Spatial non-uniformities in $[Ca^{2+}]_i$ during excitation-contraction coupling in cardiac myocytes. *Biophys J* 1994;67:1942–1956.
6. Harkins AB, Kurebayashi N, Baylor SM. Resting myoplasmic free calcium in frog skeletal muscle fibers estimated with fluo-3. *Biophys J* 1993;65:865–881.
7. Kieval RS, Bloch RJ, Lindenmayer GE, et al. Immunofluorescence localization of the Na-Ca exchanger in heart cells. *Am J Physiol* 1992;263:C545–C550.

51

Ca^{2+}-Induced Ca^{2+} Release in Developing Rabbit Heart

Glenn T. Wetzel, MD, PhD, Michael J. Bransby, BS, Fuhua Chen, MD, and Joshua I. Goldhaber, MD

In mature mammalian ventricular heart cells, Ca^{2+} influx across the cell membrane serves as a trigger to stimulate the release of intracellular Ca^{2+} stores, resulting in cell contraction.[1] In contrast, cells from immature hearts exhibit little reliance on intracellular Ca^{2+} stores.[2–5] The paucity of such Ca^{2+}-induced Ca^{2+} release (CICR) in immature heart is apparently not the result of a primary defect in the Ca^{2+} storage or release systems.[2,3] We have examined the time course and intracellular localization of the rise in intracellular Ca^{2+} concentration associated with cell contraction in immature heart. Here we show that the expression of a mature pattern of CICR develops rapidly in cultured neonatal rabbit myocytes. Furthermore, during cell contraction, acutely isolated neonatal rabbit myocytes exhibit waves of increased intracellular Ca^{2+} concentration which originate near the cell membrane and travel rapidly toward the center of the cell. These observations suggest that the primary defect in Ca^{2+}-induced Ca^{2+} release in developing heart is an inability to couple Ca^{2+} entry to Ca^{2+} release in an efficient fashion.

Immature myocytes lack a well-developed T-tubule system and generally appear to be more dependent on transsarcolemmal Ca^{2+} influx for tension generation than their adult counterparts.[2–5] The age-related increase in expression of CICR in the heart is associated with an increase in the abundance of several sarcoplasmic reticulum (SR) proteins related to the release of intracelluar Ca^{2+} stores (the Ca^{2+} release channel [ryanodine receptor], the Ca^{2+} pump [SERCA], calsequestrin, and junctin).[6–10] However, variations in these results between preparations and species have been reported.[9–11] Furthermore, immunofluorescence microscopy using probes specific for the ryanodine receptor or SERCA has demonstrated that these proteins are present and well organized within the sarcomere in immature heart.[12] These proteins are likely incorporated into a corbular form of SR, prior to the formation of junctional SR later in development. We also found that the SR in immature heart is able to store physiologically significant quantities of Ca^{2+} and that the ryanodine receptors are capable of releasing these intracellular Ca^{2+} stores.[2,3] Thus, the decreased reliance of immature myocytes on CICR may not follow directly from the decreased abundance of SR proteins in those cells.

In order to study the factors that mediate these developmental changes in excitation-contraction coupling in a controlled environment, a cell culture model for rabbit myocyte development has been established. (Single, Ca^{2+}-stable, cardiac ventricular myocytes are isolated from neonatal rabbit hearts as previously described.[13] Experiments are performed at 37°C. Cells are superfused with Tyrode's solution: 136 mM NaCl, 5.4 mM KCl, 0.3 mM NaH_2PO_4, 1 mM $MgCl$, 10 mM HEPES, 4 mM D-mannitol, 0.6 mM thiamin HCl, 10 mM glucose, 2 mM pyruvic acid, 1.8 mM $CaCl_2$, pH 7.4. Isolated myocytes from 2-day-old rabbits are cultured in minimum essential media with Earle's salts, 25 mM Na-HEPES, pH 7.4, 2 mM glutamine, 500 U/mL penicillin G, 500 (g/mL streptomycin, 0.1 μM Ara-C, 10% fetal bovine serum, and triiodothyronine. The cells are maintained at 37°C in a humidified atmosphere of 95% air–5% CO_2.[14]) Interestingly, after only 2 days in culture, myocytes from a 2-day-old rabbit respond to reloading of the SR Ca^{2+} stores in a fashion similar to that of mature myocytes (Fig. 1). Unlike acutely isolated neonatal myocytes, in mature myocytes and cultured neonatal myocytes restoration of SR Ca^{2+} stores results in a shortening of the time to peak intracellular $[Ca^{2+}]$ and an increase in peak $[Ca^{2+}]$. (Isolated myocytes are loaded with the Ca^{2+} sensitive fluorescent dye, Indo-1 AM, (0.1–1 (M) for 10 minutes at 37°C. The time course of the $[Ca^{2+}]$ transient is reflected by the ratio of the fluorescence

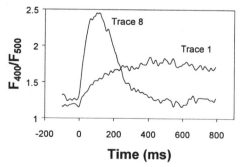

Figure 1. Ca^{2+} transients in a cultured neonatal myocyte. SR Ca^{2+} stores were depleted by a 1-second application of 10 mM caffeine and subsequently replenished by 8 field-stimulation induced contractions. The figure shows Ca^{2+} transients (reflected by the F400/F500 ratio) for the 1st and 8th contractions after SR depletion (Traces 1 and 8, respectively).

emitted at 400 nm and 500 nm (F400/F500) after nonspecific fluorescence is subtracted (exitation wavelength = 350 nm). This finding suggests that the maturation of excitation-contraction coupling is accelerated under standard cell culture conditions. Our preliminary experiments indicate that neonatal myocytes do not exhibit significant T-tubule development during the 2 days in culture. Thus, the ômatureö pattern of CICR occurs without the close coupling of the Ca^{2+} channels and Ca^{2+} release channels found in the junctional SR of mature heart.[15]

Additional experiments have been performed to evaluate the spatial distribution of the rise in intracellular $[Ca^{2+}]$, the $[Ca^{2+}]_i$ transient, during contractions in immature heart. $[Ca^{2+}]_i$ transients were recorded during field-stimulation induced contractions using a Noran laser scanning confocal microscope. ($[Ca^{2+}]_i$ transient subcellular localization is determined using the Noran Odyssey XL confocal system. Isolated myocytes are loaded with Fluo-3. Probe fluorescence is excited by a 100 mW krypton-argon laser (488 nm wavelength) and emitted light (515 nm) recorded using a Zeiss Axiovert 100 TV fluorescence microscope with a Zeiss C-apochromat 40× water immersion objective lens.) Two-dimensional images demonstrate that depolarization-induced $[Ca^{2+}]_i$ transients originate in the subsarcolemmal space. A line scan recording of a $[Ca^{2+}]_i$ transient is depicted in Figure 2. The cell nucleus is seen as a consistently bright fluorescent image in the middle of the cell. A wave of increased $[Ca^{2+}]_i$ can be seen to originate near the sarcolemmal membrane. The rate of propagation of the $[Ca^{2+}]_i$ transient toward the center of the cell is indicated by the slope of the thick white line (220 (m/sec). This is considerably faster than that reported for propagated Ca^{2+} waves in mature ventricular myocytes (50–120 (m/sec) and may reflect differences in cell ultrastructure or intracellular Ca^{2+} buffering.[16]

In addition to the depolarization-induced contractions described above, some cells exhibited spontaneous, local-

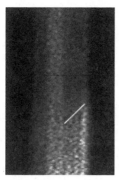

Figure 2. Linescan of a depolarization-induced Ca^{2+} transient in a neonatal rabbit ventricular myocyte. In linescan mode, the cell is repeatedly scanned across the short axis of the cell (depicted on the horizontal axis) and sequentially repeated measurements of [Ca^{2+}]$_i$ are stacked as a function of time from the top of the image to the bottom.

ized [Ca^{2+}]$_i$ transients. These transients typically originate near the sarcolemmal membrane and spread toward the cell interior. These localized [Ca^{2+}]$_i$ transients terminate spontaneously and resemble the Ca^{2+} "sparks" observed in mature myocardium.[1,17,18] Other [Ca^{2+}]$_i$ transients develop into waves of increased intracellular Ca^{2+} that propagate throughout the myocyte. Transients that originate proximal to the ends of the cell can propagate in both directions. These findings demonstrate that acutely isolated neonatal myocytes can exhibit CICR. However, as we have previously shown, such CICR does not play a significant role in contraction of immature rabbit myocytes.[2,3,19]

The rapid development of CICR expression under cell culture conditions demonstrates that a T-tubule system is not required for CICR expression. Furthermore, neonatal myocytes can express CICR as propogated [Ca^{2+}]$_i$ transients similar to Ca^{2+} sparks and waves reported in mature myocardium. In contrast, physiological contractions progress rapidly from the cell edge toward the cell center. These results suggest that CICR does not play a physiologically significant role in tension generation in immatue

heart due to an inability to efficiently couple Ca^{2+} entry to Ca^{2+} release.

References

1. Cheng H, Lederer MR, Xiao RP, et al. Excitation-contraction coupling in heart: new insights from Ca^{2+} sparks. *Cell Calcium* 1996;20:129–140.
2. Miller MS, Friedman WF, Wetzel GT. Caffeine-induced contractions in developing rabbit heart. *Pediatr Res* 1997;42:287.
3. Balaguru D, Haddock PS, Puglisi JL, et al. Role of the sarcoplasmic reticulum in contraction and relaxation of immature rabbit ventricular myocytes. *J Mol Cell Cardiol* 1997;29:2747–2757.
4. Bransby M, Chen F, Wetzel GT. *Pediatr Res* 1998;43(part 2):18A.
5. Chin TK, Christiansen GA, Caldwell JG, et al. Contribution of the sodium-calcium exchanger to contractions in immature rabbit ventricular myocytes. *Pediatr Res* 1997;41(4 Pt 1):480–485.
6. Komazaki S, Hiruma T. Development of mechanisms regulating intracellular Ca^{2+} concentration in cardiac muscle cells of early chick embryos. *Dev Biol* 1997;186:177–184.
7. Brillantes AM, Bezprozvannaya S, Marks AR. Developmental and tissue-specific regulation of rabbit skeletal and cardiac muscle calcium channels involved in excitation-contraction coupling. *Circ Res* 1994;75:503–510.
8. Arai M, Otsu K, MacLennan DH, et al. Regulation of sarcoplasmic reticulum gene expression during cardiac and skeletal muscle development. *Am J Physiol* 1992;262:C614–620.
9. Lompre AM, Lambert F, Lakatta EG, et al. Expression of sarcoplasmic reticulum Ca^{2+}-ATPase and calsequestrin genes in rat heart during ontogenic development and aging. *Circ Res* 1991;69:1380–1388.
10. Ding S, Chen F, Wetzel GT. *Pediatr Res* 1998;43(part 2):20A.
11. Moorman AF, Vermeulen JL, Koban MU, et al. Patterns of expression of sarcoplasmic reticulum Ca^{2+}-ATPase and phospholamban mRNAs during rat heart development. *Circ Res* 1995;76:616–625.
12. Chen F, Mottino G, Klitzner TS, et al. Distribution of the Na$^+$/Ca^{2+} exchange protein in developing rabbit myocytes. *Am J Physiol* 1995;268:C1126–1132.

13. Wetzel GT, Chen F, Klitzner TS. Ca^{2+} channel kinetics in acutely isolated fetal, neonatal, and adult rabbit cardiac myocytes. *Circ Res* 1993;72:1065–1074.

14. Shannon KM, Klitzner TS, Chen F, et al. Effects of triiodothyronine on retention of beta-adrenergic responsiveness of voltage-gated transmembrane calcium current during culture of ventricular myocytes from neonatal rabbits. *Pediatr Res* 1995;37:277–282.

15. Adachi-Akahane S, Cleemann L, Morad M. Cross-signaling between L-type Ca^{2+} channels and ryanodine receptors in rat ventricular myocytes. *J Gen Physiol* 1996; 108:435–454.

16. Niggli E, Lipp P. Subcellular features of calcium signalling in heart muscle: what do we learn? *Cardiovasc Res* 1995;29:441–448.

17. Wier WG, ter Keurs HE, Marban E, et al. Ca^{2+} 'sparks' and waves in intact ventricular muscle resolved by confocal imaging. *Circ Res* 1997;81:462–469.

18. Tanaka H, Sekine T, Kawanishi T, et al. Intrasarcomere [Ca^{2+}] gradients and their spatio-temporal relation to Ca^{2+} sparks in rat cardiomyocytes. *J Physiol* (Lond) 1998; 508:145–152.

19. Wetzel GT, Chen F, Klitzner TS. Na^+/Ca^{2+} exchange and cell contraction in isolated neonatal and adult rabbit cardiac myocytes. *Am J Physiol* 1995;268:H1723–733.

52

Developmental Changes in Contractile System of the Vascular Smooth Muscle Cells and the Effect of Acidosis

Toshio Nakanishi, MD and Hong Gu, PhD

In the vascular smooth muscle cells, Ca enters into the cell via Ca channel and possibly via Na-Ca exchange, and additional Ca is released from endoplasmic reticulum. Stimulation of (-adrenoreceptor increases Ca influx across the sarcolemma and Ca release from intracellular Ca store sites. Membrane depolarization also opens Ca channel and increases Ca influx across the sarcolemma.[1,2] The increased Ca influx may further induce Ca release from intracellular Ca store sites and the increased $[Ca]_i$ results in vascular contraction. Little is known about developmental changes in Ca channels and Na-Ca exchange of the smooth muscle cells. We review recent data regarding developmental changes in the sarcoplasmic reticulum.

Several studies have shown that both respiratory and metabolic acidosis cause vasodilation of aorta, coronary artery, cerebral artery, and pulmonary artery.[3–11] Although the mechanisms for the vasodilation remain unclear, regulation of $[Ca]_i$ may be altered during acidosis.[12,13] We will also review our recent data regarding Ca metabolism during acidosis in the vascular smooth muscle.

Kullama et al.[14] showed in the rat aorta that the vasorelaxant effect of diltiazem on contraction in the newborn was less than in the adult. In contrast, Karaki et al.[15] and Seguchi et al.,[16] using the rabbit aorta, showed that the effect of verapamil and diltiazem on KCl^- or norepinephrine-induced contraction in the newborn was similar to or greater than that in the adult. Seguchi et al.[16] also showed that caffeine-induced contraction of the aorta in the newborn was less than in the adult, suggesting that contraction of the aorta in the newborn depends more on Ca influx across the sarcolemma and less on intracellular Ca pool than in the adult.

Contractile system of vascular smooth muscle cells in the small arteries may be different from that in the aorta. The size of the intracellular Ca pool was examined using caffeine and noradrenaline. These drugs release Ca from intracellular store sites.[17–19] Clauvin et al.[17] showed that norepinephrine-induced contraction in the absence of extracellular Ca decreased from proximal to distal arteries, suggesting that the amount of intracellular Ca pool is less in the more distal arteries. Small arteries are physiologically important because they regulate resistance of the circulation.

Membrane depolarization activates slow Ca channels and induces Ca release from the intracellular Ca store sites. In

From Clark EB, Nakazawa M, Takao A (eds.): Etiology and Morphogenesis of Congenital Heart Disease: Twenty Years of Progress in Genetics and Developmental Biology. Armonk, NY: Futura Publishing Co., Inc.; © 2000.

order to estimate the role of Ca channels in the vascular contraction, the effect of the Ca antagonist was examined in the mesenteric small artery. 10^{-7} M diltiazem caused a small increase in developed tension in the fetus (to 116% ± 5%), but not in the newborn rabbit. This concentration of diltiazem significantly decreased developed tension in the adult rabbit. Diltiazem higher than 10^{-7} M caused vasorelaxation in all age groups and the vasorelaxant effect in the fetus and newborn was significantly less than in the adult. The study showed that the vasorelaxant effect of diltiazem in the fetus and newborn was less than in the adult. The result suggested that the Ca channels in the immature small artery were less sensitive to blockade by diltiazem than in the mature small artery and Ca channels might change qualitatively with development.

The size of intracellular Ca pool was estimated using caffeine and noradrenaline in the mesenteric small artery.[20] The caffeine-induced and noradrenaline-induced contraction in the Ca and Na-free solution in the newborn and fetus was similar and it was significantly greater than in the adult. The data suggested that the size of intracellular Ca pool was greater in the premature vessels than in the adult.

The tension-$[Ca]_i$ relationship was determined in the skinned smooth muscle fibers of the mesenteric artery in order to estimate sensitivity of myofibrils to Ca in three age groups. At pCa 6.0, the relative degree of activation in the adult was greater than in the newborn and fetus.[20] The result suggests that Ca concentration required by the myofibrils in the mature artery is lower than that in the premature artery and there is developmental change in the quality of contractile proteins.

The ultrastructural study also showed a greater amount of the endoplasmic reticulum in the premature vessels than in the mature vessels.[20] Because the endoplasmic reticulum is an important organelle regulating intracellular Ca, the ultrastructural study seems to be in agreement with the results using caffeine and noradrenaline.

Although the precise mechanisms for the regulation of vascular tone during acidosis are not yet clear, previous studies have shown that vascular contraction during acidosis is mainly regulated by $[Ca]_i$ and the sensitivity of contractile apparatus to Ca.

We previously studied the effect of respiratory acidosis on norepinephrine-induced contraction in the aorta.[21] In vessels precontracted by either norepinephrine or high KCl, the acidosis-induced decrease in developed tension in the newborn was significantly greater than that in the adult.

In the mesenteric artery, respiratory acidosis caused a transient vasoconstriction in the adult,[22] but only a small vasorelaxation in the newborn. The contraction induced by noradrenaline increased to 135% ± 2% of control during acidosis in the adult and decreased to 83% ± 5% of control in the newborn.

Upon induction of respiratory acidosis, pH_i fell rapidly, and the depression of pH_i was similar in the two age groups. Upon induction of acidosis, the fura-2 fluorescence ratio increased transiently and the net change of the ratio was similar in the two age groups.[22] Because the change in $[Ca]_i$ during acidosis was similar in the two age groups, the age-related difference in the effect of acidosis on vascular tone cannot be explained by $[Ca]_i$.

The decrease in pH_i during acidosis may reduce the sensitivity of myofibrils to Ca and induce vasorelaxation. If the sensitivity of myofibrils to low pH is different in the two age groups, this could result in different degrees of vasorelaxation for the same degree of changes in pH_i and $[Ca]_i$ during acidosis. The tension-$[Ca]i$ relationship was determined in the skinned smooth muscle fibers of the mesenteric small artery in order to estimate sensitivity of myofibrils to Ca in the two age groups. In the adult, the tension-[Ca] relationship at pH 7.1 was not significantly different from that at pH 6.8.[22] In contrast, the tension-[Ca] relationship curve at pH 6.8 was shifted to the right compared to that at pH 7.1 in the newborn. Therefore, the depression of contractile force observed in the newborn might be due to decreased sensitivity of myofibrils to Ca.

Solaro et al.[23,24] showed previously that myofibrillar ATPase activity of the premature myocardium (dog and rat) was insensitive to changes in pH. They attributed the decreased pH sensitivity of the premature myocardium to the age-related transition of troponin isoforms. In the vascular smooth muscle, sensitivity of myofibrils to Ca is, at least in part, regulated by the degree of myosin light chain phosphorylation,[25] which in turn is dependent on myosin light chain kinase and phosphatase activities. Whether an age-related difference in the sensitivity of these enzymes to pH exists or not is unknown. Vascular smooth muscle contraction is activated by calcium which is bound to calmodulin. Whether or not the calmodulin-calcium interaction is sensitive to pH in the newborn is also unknown and the mechanisms for the age-related difference in the sensitivity of myofibrils to pH remain to be studied.

We studied developmental changes in the contractile system of the pulmonary resistance arteries using small arteries of the rabbit with the diameter of between 100 to 300 um. The effect of diltiazem in the adult was greater than in the newborn and fetus, suggesting that the premature pulmonary arteries are less dependent on Ca influx from extracellular space.[26]

The caffeine-induced contraction in the fetus was greater than in the newborn and adult rabbit. However, the caffeine induced contraction in the newborn was still twice as much as that in the adult. These data suggest that intracellular Ca pool is greater in the newborn and fetus than in the adult.[26] We conclude that in the small pulmonary artery, in the small mesenteric artery, intracellular Ca pool is well developed, and it decreases with development.

In the pulmonary artery, we used acidosis as a tool to induce Ca release from SR under pathological conditions. Phorbol

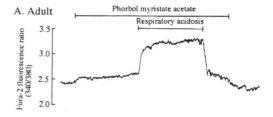

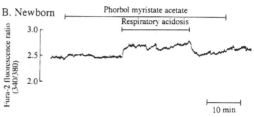

Figure 1. Effect of respiratory acidosis on the fura-2 fluorescence ratio in the rabbit small pulmonary artery. Phorbol ester was given initially and then acidosis was induced. In the pulmonary artery pretreated by phorbol ester, acidosis caused big increase in contraction in the adult, but not in the newborn.

ester was given initially and then acidosis was induced. In the pulmonary artery pretreated by phorbol ester, acidosis caused a big increase in contraction in the adult, but not in the newborn. Ca increased significantly in the newborn and adult, and the increase in the adult was greater than in the newborn (Fig. 1).

From these data, we conclude that in the small pulmonary artery, in which an intracellular Ca pool is activated by phorbol ester, the amount of Ca released by acidosis is greater in the adult than in the newborn. Whether Ca pool studied by caffeine is different from that studied by acidosis remain to be investigated. It is possible that there is a Ca pool which is different from SR and that Ca in the adult is greater than in the newborn.

Acknowledgements: This study was supported by a grant-in-aid from the Japan Research Promotion Society for Cardiovascular Diseases.

References

1. Karaki H, Weiss GB. Calcium release in smooth muscle. *Life Sci* 1988;42:111–122.

2. Nelson MT. Ca-activated potassium channels and ATP-sensitive potassium channels as modulators of vascular tone. *Trends Cardiovasc Med* 1993;3:54–60.

3. Aalkjaer C. Regulation of intracellular pH and its role in vascular smooth muscle function. *J Hypertens* 1990;8:197–206.

4. Jensen PE, Hughes A, Boonen HCM, et al. Force, membrane potential, and [Ca]i during activation of rat mesenteric small arteries with norepinephrine, potassium, aluminum, fluoride, and phorbol ester. *Circ Res* 1993;73:314–324.

5. Loutzenhiser R, Matsumoto Y, Okawa W, et al. H+-induced vasodilation of rat aorta is mediated by alterations in intracellular calcium sequestration. *Circ Res* 1990;67: 426–439.

6. Rinaldi GJ, Gattaneo A, Gingolani HE. Interaction between calcium and hydrogen ions in canine coronary arteries. *J Mol Cell Cardiol* 1987;19:773–784.

7. Kontos HA. Regulation of the cerebral circulation. *Annu Rev Physiol* 1981;43: 397–407.

8. Krampetz IK, Rhoades RA. Intracellular pH: Effect on pulmonary arterial smooth muscle. *Am J Physiol* 1991;260:L516–L521.

9. Furtado MR. Effect of NH4Cl on the contractility of isolated vascular smooth muscle. *Life Sci* 1987;41:95–102.

10. Nielsen H, Aalkjaer C, Mulvany MJ. Differential contractile effects of changes in carbon dioxide tension on rat mesenteric resistance arteries precontracted with noradrenaline. *Pflugers Arch* 1991;419: 51–56.

11. Aalkjaer C, Mulvany MJ. Effect of changes in intracellular pH on the contractility of rat resistance vessels. *Prog Biochem Pharmacol* 1988;23:150–158.

12. Irisawa H, Sato R. Intra- and extracellular actions of protons on the calcium current of isolated guinea pig ventricular cells. *Circ Res* 1986;59:348–365.

13. Wray S. Smooth muscle intracellular pH: Measurement, regulation, and function. *Am J Physiol* 1988;254:C213–C225.

14. Kullama LK, Balaraman V, Claybaugh JR, et al. Differential ontogeny of in vitro vascular responses to three categories of calcium channel antagonists in rats. *Pediatr Res* 1991;29:278–281.

15. Karaki H, Nakagawa H, Urakawa N. Age-related changes in the sensitivity to verapamil and sodium nitroprusside of vascular smooth muscle of rabbit aorta. *Br J Pharmacol* 1985;85:223–228.

16. Seguchi M, Nakazawa M, Nakanishi T, et al. Developmental change of vascular smooth muscle contraction in the rabbit thoracic aorta. *Circulation* 1990;82:491.

17. Cauvin C, Saida K, van Breemen C. Extracellular Ca dependence and diltiazem inhibition of contraction in rabbit conduit arteries and mesenteric resistance vessels. *Blood Vessels* 1984;21:23–31.

18. Kanaide H, Kobayashi S, Nishimura J, et al. Quin2 microfluorometry and effects of verapamil and diltiazem on calcium release from rat aorta smooth muscle cells in primary culture. *Circ Res* 1988;63:16–26.

19. Cauvin C, Lukeman S, Cameron J, et al. Differences in norepinephrine activation and diltiazem inhibition of calcium channels in isolated rabbit aorta and mesenteric resistance vessels. *Circ Res* 1985;56: 822–828.

20. Nakanishi T, Gu H, Abe K, et al. Developmental changes in the contractile system of the mesenteric small artery of rabbit. *Pediatr Res* 1997;41:65–71.

21. Nakanishi T, Gu H, Momma K. Effect of acidosis on contraction, intracellular pH, and calcium in the newborn and adult rabbit aorta. *Heart Vessels* 1997;12:207–215.

22. Nakanishi T, Gu H, Momma K. Developmental changes in the effect of acidosis on contraction, intracellular pH, and calcium in the rabbit mesenteric small artery. *Pediatr Res* 1997;42:750–757.

23. Solaro RJ, Kumar P, Blanchard EM, et al. Differential effects of pH on calcium activation of myofilaments of adult and perinatal dog hearts. *Circ Res* 1986;58:721–729.

24. Dieckman LJ, Solaro RJ. Effect of thyroid status on thin-filament Ca regulation and expression of troponin I in perinatal and adult rat hearts. *Circ Res* 1990;67:344–351.

25. Kitazawa T, Gaylinn BD, Denney GH, et al. G-protein mediated Ca sensitization of smooth muscle contraction through myosin light chain phosphorylation. *J Biol Chem* 1991;266:1708–1715.

26. Nakanishi T, Gu H, Seguchi M. Developmental changes in contractile sytem of rabbit arterial smooth muscle. In: Clark EB, Markwald RR, Takao A, eds. Developmental *Mechanisms of Heart Disease*. New York: Futura; 1995:1994:449–458.

53

Mechanisms of HERG Gating in the Heart

Gail A. Robertson, PhD, Jinling Wang, MS, and Matthew C. Trudeau, PhD

The *human ether-a-go-go-related gene* (*HERG*) encodes a subunit of the ion channels underlying cardiac I_{Kr},[1,2] a potassium current that contributes to the terminal repolarization of the ventricular action potential.[3] When I_{Kr} is disrupted by mutations in the *HERG* gene or blocked by drugs, life-threatening arrhythmias known as torsades de pointe can result. The HERG polypeptide is structurally similar to members of the S4-containing superfamily of ion channels[4] and its behavior can be described by typical gating properties such as a sigmoidal time course of activation[2] and C-type inactivation.[5–7] Despite these similarities, HERG currents differ from other K^+ currents because of the temporal relationships among these gating transitions: at positive voltages, channels inactivate quickly, spending little time in the open state; at repolarizing voltages, deactivation is slow, resulting in relatively greater occupancy of the open state as channels recover from inactivation.[1,2,8] A simple scheme can be written as:

$$C_1 \underset{}{\overset{depolarization}{\rightleftarrows}} C_2 \rightleftarrows \ldots \rightleftarrows C_n \underset{slow}{\overset{fast}{\rightleftarrows}} O \underset{repolarization}{\rightleftarrows} I$$

where C represents the closed states, O is the open state, and I the inactivated state. As a consequence of the fast inactivation and slow deactivation, the corresponding macroscopic currents reach their maximum amplitude not at positive voltages like most voltage-gated channels, but instead at more negative voltages during a subsequent repolarizing step. The resulting profile of I_{Kr} during the cardiac action potential, inferred from expression studies of HERG in heterologous systems[9] and modeled for native tissues,[10] is a resurgent current that is suppressed at the peak of the action potential but rebounds during repolarization. The timing and amplitude of this resurgent current are thus determined by the rate of recovery from inactivation and the subsequent rate of deactivation during the repolarization phase of the cardiac action potential.

Previous studies have demonstrated that the rate of deactivation in HERG channels is dramatically increased when the N terminus is deleted.[6,11] Isoforms with truncated or alternative, short N termini and correspondingly fast deactivation rates are encoded by splice variants of Merg1, the mouse ortholog to HERG.[12,13] The same splice variants arise from the HERG locus.[14] Thus, the N terminus regulates deactivation gating and represents a mechanism by which functional diversity is generated in HERG and related channels.

We are interested in the gating mechanisms that specialize HERG for its physiological role in the heart. In our most recent study, we explored the mechanism

From Clark EB, Nakazawa M, Takao A (eds.): Etiology and Morphogenesis of Congenital Heart Disease: Twenty Years of Progress in Genetics and Developmental Biology. Armonk, NY: Futura Publishing Co., Inc.; © 2000.

A.

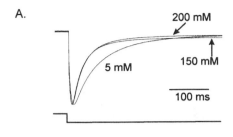

B. Deactivation Time Constant

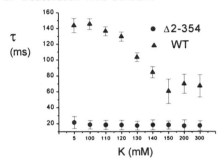

C. Fractional Change in Deactivation Rate

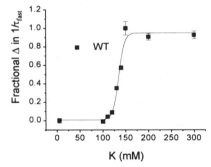

by which the N terminus slows deactivation and thus allows the HERG current to rebound during repolarization.[14] Using two approaches, we demonstrated that the N terminus action involves the internal mouth of the pore. First, elevating external K^+ concentration increased the rate of deactivation, as if the permeating K^+ ions destabilize the binding of the N terminus to the mouth of the pore (Fig. 1). Second, NEM modification of an aphenotypic cysteine at the putative internal mouth of the pore (S4-S5 linker) phenocopied the N terminal deletion as if sterically hindering the N terminus from reaching its site of interaction there (Fig. 2).

The N terminus also has the effect of promoting C-type inactivation, and channels with an N terminal deletion inactivate more slowly and less completely. Two lines of investigation indicate that deactivation and inactivation are regulated by functionally and structurally independent N terminus mechanisms. First, the slowing of deactivation by the N terminus was equally effective whether in a wild type background or when C-type inactivation was disabled by mutation. This rules out the possibility that the slowing of deactivation is a secondary consequence of the lowering of the free energy of the inactivated state by the N

Figure 1. Deactivation rate in HERG channels increases with elevated external K^+. **A.** Scaled tail currents from WT channels in 5 mM, 150 mM, and 200 mM external K^+. Currents were evoked at -100 mV subsequent to a 3-sec step to 60 mV. **B.** Deactivation time constants at various external K^+ concentrations for both WT ($n = 6$) and $\Delta2$–354 channels ($n = 5$) for tail currents evoked as described in **A.** Tail currents were fit with a single exponential function in this case because at -100 mV the fast component accounts for over 90% of the current. **C.** The change in deactivation rate ($1/\tau$) with increasing external K^+ exhibits a saturating dose-response behavior with a Hill coefficient of 5.36 ± 0.69. At -100 mV, the forward (activation) rate is negligible and most of the deactivating current is described by the fast deactivation tau so the deactivation

rate $\cong 1/\tau_{fast}$. As shown, deactivation rate increased in a dose-dependent manner with increased external K^+ ions. These data were fitted with the Hill equation: $ln[(1-S')/S'] = -n(lnK-lnL)$ where $S' = S/S_o$ is the fraction of sites occupied by the ligand; S is the number of sites occupied; S_o is the total number of sites available; K is the dissociation constant of the ligand; L is the ligand concentration; and n is the Hill coefficient. We determine S' using the formula $(k - k_5)/(k_{300} - k_5)$, where k is the deactivation rate ($1/\tau$ at -100 mV) at any given external potassium concentration, k_5 is the rate at 5 mM [K]o and k_{300} the rate at 300mM $[K]_o$. The S' values at different $[K]_o$ (i.e., L) were plotted as fractional increase of deactivation rate in Fig.1C. The resulting sigmoidal dose response curve was then fitted with the Hill equation indicated above to obtain the Hill coefficient.

A. Deactivation Currents

B. Deactivation Time Constants

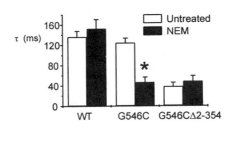

Figure 2. NEM modification of the S4-S5 linker mimics the N terminus deletion. **A.** Families of tail currents from G546C channels before and after NEM modification. **B.** Summary of effects of NEM modification on WT, G546C and G546CΔ2–354 channels. Time constants were determined by fitting tail currents to a single exponential function because at −100 mV the fast component accounts for over 90% of the current. The first pair of bars indicates that NEM modification does not significantly affect deactivation time constants for wild type channels. The second set of bars shows marked effect of NEM modification on G546C mutant. The third set of bars shows that modification of G546CΔ2–354 does not further accelerate the deactivation rate, indicating that NEM and deletion of the N terminus disrupt the same process ($n = 6$ for each construct).

terminus. Second, a small deletion of the first 16 amino acids caused rapid deactivation characteristic of the complete N terminus deletion but had no effect on inactivation. Thus, inactivation is regulated by a physically separate domain. However, effects of the N terminus on deactivation and inactivation were both disrupted by modification of the S4-S5 linker, indicating that both mechanisms may depend on the docking of the N terminus near the internal mouth of the pore.

In summary, I_{Kr} is produced at least in part by the assembly of HERG subunits, the specific gating properties of which create an outward, resurgent K^+ current that contributes to the terminal repolarization of the ventricular action potential. C-type inactivation is responsible for suppressing the current during the initial depolarization, and the N terminus stabilizes the open state to allow the development of a large current during repolarization. Isoforms with altered gating may be produced by alternative splicing of the N terminus, but in which tissues or at what developmental stage such regulation takes place remains to be determined. Also unknown are the structural details of the various conformations of the

channel, although through continued structure-function studies we expect to discover more about the residues involved and their points of interaction within the channel complex.

References

1. Sanguinetti MC, Jiang C, Curran ME, et al. A mechanistic link between an inherited and an acquired cardiac arrhythmia: HERG encodes the IKr potassium channel. *Cell* 1995;81:299–307.
2. Trudeau MC, Warmke JW, Ganetzky B, et al. HERG, a human inward rectifier in the voltage-gated potassium channel family. *Science* 1995;269:92–95.
3. Sanguinetti MC, Jurkiewicz NK. Two components of cardiac delayed rectifier K+ current. Differential sensitivity to block by class III antiarrhythmic agents. *J Gen Physiol* 1990;96:195–215.
4. Warmke JW, Ganetzky B. A family of potassium channel genes related to eag in Drosophila and mammals. *Proc Natl Acad Sci U S A* 1994;91:3438–3442.
5. Smith PL, Baukrowitz T, Yellen G. The inward rectification mechanism of the HERG cardiac potassium channel. [see comments]. *Nature* 1996;379:833–836.

6. Schonherr R, Heinemann SH. Molecular determinants for activation and inactivation of HERG, a human inward rectifier potassium channel. *J Physiol Lond* 1996; 493:635–642.

7. Herzberg IM, Trudeau MC, Robertson GA. Transfer of rapid inactivation and E-4031 sensitivity from HERG to M-EAG channels. *J Physiol (Lond)* 1998;511:3–14.

8. Shibasaki T. Conductance and kinetics of delayed rectifier potassium channels in nodal cells of the rabbit heart. *J Physiol (Lond)* 1987;387:227–250.

9. Zhou Z, Gong Q, Ye B, et al. Properties of HERG channels stably expressed in HEK 293 cells studied at physiological temperature. *Biophys J* 1998;74:230–241.

10. Zeng J, Laurita KR, Rosenbaum DS, et al. Two components of the delayed rectifier K+ current in ventricular myocytes of the guinea pig type. Theoretical formulation and their role in repolarization. *Circ Res* 1995;77:140–152.

11. Spector PS, Curran ME, Zou A, et al. Fast inactivation causes rectification of the IKr channel. *J Gen Physiol* 1996;107: 611–619.

12. Lees-Miller JP, Kondo C, Wang L, et al. Electrophysiological characterization of an alternatively processed ERG K+ channel in mouse and human hearts. *Circ Res* 1997;81:719–726.

13. London B, Trudeau MC, Newton KP, et al. Two isoforms of the mouse ether-a-go-go-related gene coassemble to form channels with properties similar to the rapidly activating component of the cardiac delayed rectifier K+ current. *Circ Res* 1997;81:870–878.

14. Wang J, Trudeau MC, Zappia AM, et al. Regulation of deactivation by an amino terminal domain in HERG potassium channels. *J Gen Physiol* 1998;112: 637–647.

54

Hypoxic Induction of Adrenomedullin in Human Umbilical Vein Endothelial Cells

Teruhiko Ogita, MD, PhD, Takashi Nakaoka, MD, PhD,
Yuji Kira, MD, PhD, Rumiko Matsuoka, MD, PhD,
and Toshiro Fujita, MD, PhD

Several well-known biological responses occur to compensate for hypoxic stress. Pulmonary vessels respond to local hypoxia by vasoconstricting, thereby shunting blood to better oxygenated areas of the lung, whereas blood vessels in other parts of the body vasodilate to deliver more oxygen-carrying blood to hypoxic tissues.[1,2] Over the past few years, hypoxia has been shown to induce increased expression of several mammalian genes, including erythropoietin, platelet-derived growth factor B chain, endothelin, IL-1α, IL-8, vascular endothelial growth factor (VEGF), atrial natriuretic peptide, and tyrosine hydroxylase.

Adrenomedullin (AM), a potent endogenous vasodilating peptide, has recently been isolated from the acid extract of human pheochromocytoma.[3,4] Plasma levels of AM in patients with hypertension, renal failure,[5] or congestive heart failure[6] have been reported to be higher than those of normal volunteers, suggesting that AM participates in blood pressure regulation. In this study, we investigated the effect of hypoxia on AM expression in cultured human umbilical vein endothelial cells (HUVEC).

We found that hypoxic conditions (0–3% oxygen) significantly increased AM mRNA (Fig. 1A) and the secretion of AM protein (Fig. 1B) in HUVEC. This stimulatory effect of low oxygen tension on the AM mRNA levels was reversible upon reexposure to a 21% oxygen environment (Fig. 1C) and was not affected by the presence of five times the normal media glucose concentration (Fig. 1D). Sodium azide, an inhibitor of oxidative phophorylation, had no significant effect on the expression of AM (data not shown). Anisomycin and cycloheximide, potent protein synthesis inhibitors, did not abolish the induction of AM by hypoxia, suggesting that de novo protein synthesis may not be necessary (Fig. 2A). Also, the determination of AM mRNA half-life showed an increase of mRNA stability during hypoxia (Fig. 2B). To better understand the mechanism of hypoxic induction of AM in HUVEC, we have evaluated the effect of cobalt chloride on the induction of AM, which has been shown to induce erythropoietin, or VEGF. Cobalt chloride significantly increased AM mRNA (Fig. 2C) and protein (Fig. 2D) in HUVEC.

These findings suggest a role for AM in the control of regional blood flow in the vasculature in response to changes in oxygen tension. Like erythropoietin and VEGF, the release of which is induced by both hypoxia and cobalt chloride,[7] ad-

From Clark EB, Nakazawa M, Takao A (eds.): Etiology and Morphogenesis of Congenital Heart Disease: Twenty Years of Progress in Genetics and Developmental Biology. Armonk, NY: Futura Publishing Co., Inc.; © 2000.

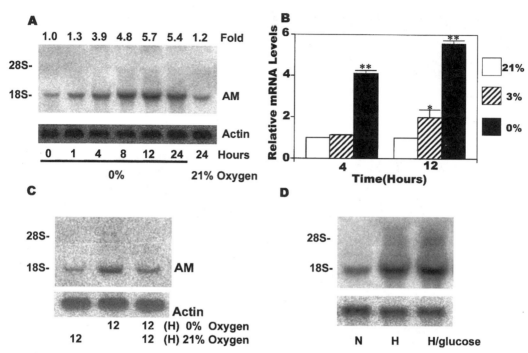

Figure 1. A. Time course of AM mRNA induction by hypoxia in HUVEC. Total RNA was subjected to Northern blot analysis with a ^{32}P-labeled AM probe. The filter was stripped and reprobed with γ-actin. Signal intensities were determined using Bioimage Analyzer BAS2000. The AM mRNA levels at 21% oxygen (time 0) were arbitrarily made equal to 1. **B.** Hypoxia increased the secretion of AM from cultured endothelial cells. Media conditioned by HUVEC under normoxic (21% oxygen; *open bars*) or hypoxic (3% oxygen, *hatched bars* and 0% oxygen, *solid bars*) conditions were collected at the indicated times. **C.** The effect of hypoxia on AM was reversible. Total cellular RNA was harvested from endothelial cells grown in 21% or 0% oxygen environment for 12 hours (*lanes 1* and *2*, respectively) and from cells exposed to 0% oxygen for 12 hours followed by 21% oxygen for 12 hours (*lane 3*). **D.** Effect of glucose on hypoxic induction of AM mRNA in HUVEC. Cells were maintained in the 21% oxygen environment (*lane 1;* N) or exposed to the 0% oxygen environment for 12 hours in the presence of normal media concentrations of glucose (*lane 2;* H) or five times that concentration (*lane 3;* H/glucose).

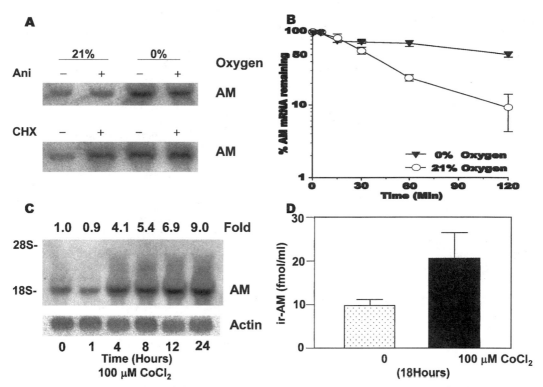

Figure 2. A. Effect of anisomycin or cycloheximide on hypoxic induction of AM mRNA in HUVEC. Cells were maintained in the 21% oxygen environment (*lanes 1* and *2*) or exposed to the 0% oxygen environment (*lanes 3* and *4*) for 12 hours in the presence (+) or absence (−) of 1 μM anisomycin (Ani) and 10 μg/mL cycloheximide (CHX). **B.** Effect of hypoxia on AM mRNA stability. Actinomycin D (5 μg/mL) was added either before exposure to normoxia (*open circles*) or after 12 hours of an initial exposure to hypoxia (*closed triangles*). Using a Bioimage Analyzer, relative intensities of AM and γ-actin mRNA remaining after the indicated time periods of exposure to actinomycin D were determined as a semi-log function of time. **C.** Effect of cobalt chloride (100 μM) on the induction of AM mRNA. **D.** Effect of cobalt chloride on the induction of AM protein in HUVEC.

renomedullin secretion is also induced by both stimuli. Our results suggest that adrenomedullin, erythropoietin, and VEGF may share a common oxygen-sensing mechanism. Hypoxic induction of AM may play a pathophysiological role in vascular systems.

Materials and Methods

Cell Culture and Conditions for Achieving Hypoxia

HUVEC were prepared from umbilical cord veins according to the method described by Jaffe et al.[8] They were plated onto gelatin-coated dishes and grown in MCDB 105 medium supplemented with 10% FBS, 10 ng/mL recombinant human basic fibroblast growth factor, 100 units/mL penicillin, and 100 μg/mL streptomycin at 37°C, under an atmosphere of 5% CO_2/95% air, in a humidified incubator. Cells were used for experiments at passage levels 5–10. Endothelial cells at confluence were exposed to various oxygen tensions in air-tight chambers flushed with preanalyzed gas mixtures and maintained at 37°C. All experiments were performed in MCDB 105 medium containing 5% FBS but no other additives.

Northern Blot Analysis

Total cellular RNA was isolated from HUVEC by the acid-guanidinum phenol-chloroform method. Total RNA was electrophoresed through a 1% agarose gel containing formaldehyde and was transferred to a nylon membrane. Northern blots were hybridized with the human AM cDNA probe labeled with [α-^{32}P]dCTP using random hexanucleotide primers. A 1.4-kb *EcoRI/Xho* I fragment of human AM cDNA was utilized. Human AM cDNA was kindly provided by Dr. Naoto Minamino and Dr. Kenji Kangawa (National Cardiovascular Center Research Institute, Osaka, Japan). The blots were stripped and rehybridized with γ-actin cDNA. The intensity of the bands obtained was quantitated with a Bioimage Analyzer and normalized to the actin transcript levels.

Radioimmunoassay for AM

To quantify the amount of AM protein secreted by the cells, conditioned media were collected in chilled tubes with aprotinin, centrifuged, and stored at −40°C until analysis. A sample was extracted on a Sep-Pak tC18 ODS cartridge and eluted with 70% acetonitrile, containing 0.1% trifluoroacetic acid. Concentrated eluates were then assayed using a specific and sensitive human AM 1-52 RIA kit. The minimal detectable concentration of immunoreactive AM (ir-AM) for the assay was 0.33 fmol per tube, and the standard curve range was from 0.662 to 106 fmol per tube. Recovery was 72 ± 5% and inter- and intraassay variations were 3.0–17.0 and 1.7–10.7%, respectively.

Actinomycin D Chase Experiments

To assess the effect of hypoxia on the half-life of AM mRNA transcripts, confluent HUVEC monolayers were exposed to normoxia (21% oxygen) or hypoxia (0% oxygen). Actinomycin D (5 μg/mL) was added, either before exposure to normoxia or after 12 hours of an initial exposure to hypoxia. Total RNA was extracted at 0, 5, 15, 30, 60, and 120 minutes after the addition of actinomycin D, and Northern blot analysis was performed using human AM and actin cDNA probes. Using the Bioimage Analyzer, relative intensities of signals for AM and actin mRNA remaining after the indicated time periods of exposure to actinomycin D were determined as a semi-log function of time.

Statistics

Values are expressed as mean ± SD. Statistics were performed by using unpaired Student's *t*-test. Significance was determined at the 95% confidence level.

References

1. Heistad DD, Abboud FM. Dickinson W. Richards Lecture: Circulatory adjustments to hypoxia. *Circulation* 1980;61:463–470.
2. Voelkel NF. Mechanisms of hypoxic pulmonary vasoconstriction. *Am Rev Respir Dis* 1986;133:1186–1195.
3. Kitamura K, Sakata J, Kangawa K, et al. Cloning and characterization of cDNA encoding a precursor for human adrenomedullin [published erratum appears in *Biochem Biophys Res Commun* 1994;15;202:643]. *Biochem Biophys Res Commun* 1993;194:720–725.
4. Kitamura K, Kangawa K, Kawamoto M, et al. Adrenomedullin: A novel hypotensive peptide isolated from human pheochromocytoma. *Biochem Biophys Res Commun* 1993;192:553–560.
5. Ishimitsu T, Nishikimi T, Saito Y, et al. Plasma levels of adrenomedullin, a newly identified hypotensive peptide, in patients with hypertension and renal failure. *J Clin Invest* 1994;94:2158–2161.
6. Jougasaki M, Wei CM, McKinley LJ, et al. Elevation of circulating and ventricular adrenomedullin in human congestive heart failure. *Circulation* 1995;92:286–289.
7. Goldberg MA, Schneider TJ. Similarities between the oxygen-sensing mechanisms regulating the expression of vascular endothelial growth factor and erythropoietin. *J Biol Chem* 1994;269:4355–4359.
8. Jaffe EA, Nachman RL, Becker CG, et al. Culture of human endothelial cells derived from umbilical veins. Identification by morphologic and immunologic criteria. *J Clin Invest* 1973;52:2745–2756.

Section VII

55

Overview: Syndromes, Developmental Fields, and Human Cardiovascular Malformations

*John M. Opitz, MD, H. Joseph Yost, PhD,
and Edward B. Clark, MD*

The last decade has brought remarkable advances in our understanding of cardiovascular development. From an era of reductionism, we now begin the process of assembling the information from molecular sources to gain a comprehensive view of the heart and vascular bed. This must be done in light of two histories. A brief developmental history guided by genes and epigenetic forces and an ancient evolutionary history more than 3.8 billion years old. What happens during development, normal or abnormal, is possible because of evolution. The evolutionary (and therefore the developmental) unit is the developmental field, not the cell as often assumed. In this context we will examine some aspects of cardiovascular development and maldevelopment.

Introduction

Cardiac formation in mammals is unusual in several respects.

- It is *precocious* compared to the development of other organs, leading to a functional contractile tubular structure as early as 17 days, a mere 3 or 4 days after the initial appearance of the endocardial tubes in the cardiogenic regions of the embryo.
- It begins individually in two bilaterally symmetrical *distantly located prospective primordia* before fusing in the midline to form a single structure, the *definitive* primordium of the heart. Thus, the final anterior ventral midline position of the early embryonic heart is a *secondary* morphogenetic state. The rare case of a "hemibaby"[1] may well represent an absence of one of the halves with "default" development of the other half.
- Normal cardiac morphogenesis involves a distortion from the initially bilaterally symmetrical midline structure it was at the beginning of the 4th week through a process of *dextral looping* (the first indication of left-right asymmetry of the embryo), which gives the heart its asymmetrical shape at the beginning of the 4th week and ultimate left-of-midline position that it occupies under normal circumstances.
- Cardiac morphogenesis involves not only an *endogenous* self-differentiation mechanism, as is true of all other parts of the body, but also the mor-

From Clark EB, Nakazawa M, Takao A (eds.): Etiology and Morphogenesis of Congenital Heart Disease: Twenty Years of Progress in Genetics and Developmental Biology. Armonk, NY: Futura Publishing Co., Inc.; © 2000.

phogenetic effects of *exogenous* cells, namely the ectomesenchymal cells of the cranial or "cardiac" neural crest that originate from rhombomere 8 and migrate via branchial arches 4 and 6 into the heart to participate in conotruncal septation as one of the final primary morphogenetic events in heart development during the 7th and 8th weeks.

- Cardiac morphogenesis is also unusual in that it involves not only the well-known mechanisms of induction (by signals from adjacent endomesoderm such as *cerberus*),[2] but also *hemodynamic* factors beginning to act at the time of the first heart beat on day 17, before the end of blastogenesis, a mere 3 or 4 days after the initial appearance of the endocardial tubes in the cardiogenic region of the embryo.
- This unusual structure/function interaction in morphogenesis requires unusually early *specification of functional cell lineages,* namely the myocardium (which begins contraction perhaps as early as day 17), and with formation thereafter of the specialized conduction systems.

Thus, the fundamental question arises whether this unusual morphogenetic nature exempts the heart from the developmental field constraints imposed on all other parts of the body? As we shall show below this is not true, the adult heart being the result not only of the above morphogenetic phenomena but also of pattern formation.[3,4]

Development and Morphology

Development is the process whereby *organic* form is produced *epigenetically*, leading to the gradual emergence of the sexually mature adult characteristic of the species and capable of repeating the haplo-diploid life cycle. The formal and causal aspects of development are the focus of the science of *morphology* [Goethe, 1797, Burdach, 1800,[5]], which may be defined as the science of the *form* (anatomy), *formation* (embryology and genetics),

transformation (evolution), and *malformation* ("teratology") of living beings.

When Goethe said: *"Gestaltenlehre ist Verwandlungslehre, "* [The study of the form [of an organism] is simultaneously study of its change. By "change" he meant not only change during its ontogeny (Bildung) but also during its phylogeny (Umbildung)[5]] he alluded to the *two* histories of mature organisms (including that of plants), namely a developmental one and an evolutionary one, as true of the entire organism as it is of all of its parts. With respect to the heart the following summary may be offered.

The evolution of multicellularity and of more complex body plans was accompanied by the simultaneous development of a cardiovascular system to serve cellular nutrition, gas-fluid-ion exchange, and general physiological homeostasis. A heart/pumping mechanism evolved in both groups of animals, namely:

1. Those with a *closed* vascular system and mesoderm-derived tubes lined with a special epi(endo)thelium (annelids with ancestral vascular type, cephalopods and vertebrates); and
2. Those with a hemolymph vascular system which is *open* to body spaces and is *not* lined with a special endothelium (most molluscs and arthropods—derived type).

In vertebrates, a substantial amount of extracellular fluid is returned by frequently contractile lymph vessels. In amphibia, rhythmically contracting lymph hearts are known. In mammals, lymph vessels pass through lymph nodes that filter the lymph fluid through their interstices.

In view of the similarities between both of these (open and closed) vascular systems, it is not surprising that they share ancient, conserved molecular mechanisms of morphogenesis and of cell-lineage specification.

Etienne Geoffroy St-Hilaire (1772–1855) through his profound insight into the nature of homology (not named as such until 1843 by Owen in English biology) noted that the position of the heart ventrally (and of the neural tube dorsally) in vertebrates represented a simple inversion of the dorso-ventral axis from that of an animal ancestral to vertebrates and invertebrates with a ventral nervous system and dorsal heart. This hypothesis was substantiated by the recent analyses of molecular pathways, reviewed by De Robertis and Sasai.[6] Georges Cuvier (1769–1832), who asserted the fixity of species (but allowed their extinction) in only a few *embranchements*, emphasized the primacy of *function* in determining form; however, with respect to the cardiovascular system both of these historic antagonists contributed fundamental insights.[7]

Development and Evolution

To repeat: All living organisms have two histories: A developmental one (brief), and an evolutionary one (some 3.8 billion years long). It is now generally accepted that:

- *All* morphological development occurs in developmental fields;
- The evolutionary change of form from one species to another represents a permanent change of developmental processes;
- Therefore, *the developmental field is the fundamental unit of development and of evolution.* This is in contradistinction to *cells,* which are the fundamental unit of structure and function. Thus, *everything* that develops, whether normal or abnormal, has evolved, or, put another way: Nothing can occur in development whether normal or abnormal, that has not been made possible by evolution.

Mammals, indeed all vertebrates, undergo Type II or direct development[8,9] whereby cleavage, morula, and blastula formation generate the *primary field* consisting of totipotent cells. During gastrulation, the process of *pattern formation* partitions the undifferentiated primary field into several areas of specific morphogenetic fate called *progenitor fields.* Pattern formation, or induction, involves the expression of diffusible *intercellular* morphogens, and the appearance, during mid-or late gastrula-

tion, of transient spatial domains of *upstream* transcription factor expression which specify the major initial parts, or *progenitor* fields of the embryo. Subsequent expression of *downstream* gene batteries refines and partitions the progenitor fields into subregions, the *secondary or epimorphic fields* that give rise to each part of the final structure or organ. Most known histological or molecular markers of differentiated cellular function, indicating *specification of cell lineage,* can be detected in vertebrate embryos only at gastrula stages or thereafter. A common upstream pattern formation mechanism underlies the development of the major parts of *all* bilaterian body plans; it is also important to realize that these upstream molecular systems do not control directly the final differentiation gene batteries although some of the *same* regulators are still operating at later stages. It is a truly remarkable fact, that in spite of evident differences in embryonic processes, at the level of the molecular biology of "morphogenetic gene" regulation, all metazoan embryos use similar or identical systems such as cell signaling factors and their antagonists, zinc finger transcription regulators, various homotypic and heterotypic pairs of helix-loop-helix regulators, and regionally expressed homeodomain regulators, growth factors, and their receptors.

Thus, developmental (or morphogenetic) fields are those parts of the embryo in which final structure is specified. In the words of Spemann[10]: "*Induktion ist nichts anderes als Feldwirkung* " (induction is nothing else than field effect). From a *clinical* perspective, fields are defined on the basis of the criteria of *heterogeneity, homology,* and *phylogeneity.*

Developmental Fields

By now it may be asserted axiomatically that all development occurs in developmental fields and all primary malformations are developmental fields defects. Developmental fields are the morphogenetic units of the embryo in which events are spatially coordinated, temporally synchronized, and epimorphically hierarchical in bringing forth final structure.[11] Developmental field theory arose twice in this century; once in the 1920s out of the school of Entwicklungsmechanik (Alexander G. Gurwitsch, Paul Weiss, and Hans Spemann, the last receiving the Nobel Prize for Physiology or Medicine for his work in 1935), and a second time out of the clinical genetics program at the University of Wisconsin in the 1960s. As emphasized by Stern, genetic concepts were lacking in the work of Weiss and Spemann, and the field concept of Gurwitsch was dismissed, probably correctly, by Spemann in his Silliman lectures[10] as a form of vitalism. Thus, their work concerned itself predominantly with the *formal genesis* of embryonic structure. The Wisconsin school, on the other hand, derived its concept from clinical genetics, hence complementing the earlier formulation through an analysis of *causal genesis* (cause). A unified developmental field concept may be outlined from a genetic perspective as follows:

1. Given that a specific malformation, e.g., cleft palate, extra thumb, marsupial scrotum, atrial isomerism, tetralogy of Fallot, truncus arteriosus, is demonstrably due to two or more different causes (mendelian, aneuploidy, teratogenic) then a *dys*morphogenetic unit of the embryo has been identified, i.e., a unit all of whose component parts react together in an *identical,* highly limited manner to a potentially large number of different causes. It follows logically that the parts of the embryo identified in this manner also constitute morphogenetic units under *normal* conditions. This perspective on fields may be designated the *criterion of heterogeneity.*

2. The inference from the analysis of heterogeneity is strengthened if the given malformation affects "corresponding" parts of the body that are "serially homologous" (Owen) by virtue of similar structure and ontogeny due to shared molecular induction systems in many different species. Such parts include vertebrae, ribs, and corre-sponding digits. A particularly instructive example is the autosomal (or X-linked) dominant Wulfsberg mutation, which caused in a mother and all 3 of her children deficiency of the 5th ray of the hands and feet.[12] This may be designated the *criterion of homology.* Of course, only a special set of anomalies ever fulfills this criterion simply because most anomalies involve nonserially homologous structures.

3. The *criterion of phylogeneity* is confirmatory of the field theory if the same malformation occurs in different species due to the same or different causes. Structural similarity being due to similar ontogeny in different animals *sharing historically homologous* parts by virtue of descent, with modification, from a common ancestor with a prototypic developmental plan. A spectacular early example of phylogeneity, recognized as such during the 19th century, is that of holoprosencephaly in many different animal species including fish, cats, calves, lambs, dogs, guinea pigs, and of course, humans (hence, the legends of the cyclops). (Alobar) holoprosencephaly is extraordinarily heterogeneous in humans; Muenke and his coworkers have identified not only the *Sonic Hedgehog* locus as site of the HPE3 mutation, but almost 3 dozen aneuploid/triploid forms as well.[13,14] Recently, Cooper et al.[15] were able to identify the teratogenic action of jervine, the active compound in *Veratrum californicum,* the ingestion of which by pregnant ewes may cause holoprosencephaly in their lambs, as due to a defect of the ability of cell surface or cytoplasmic receptors to bind the Sonic hedgehog-cholesterol adduct necessary to induce the neural tube.

The relationship between the causal, formal, and evolutionary aspects of development are summarized in Figure 1 and

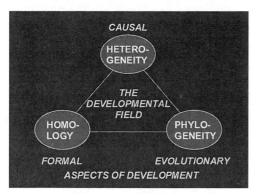

Figure 1. Summarization of the relationship between the causal, formal and evolutionary aspects of development.

appear to constitute a nontautological, noncircular, efficient definition of the development field at all three of its stages. The *primary field* is the entire embryo during early embryogenesis (blastogenesis) preceding the formation of the midline/axes, gastrulation, segmentation, cardiogenesis/lateralization, and neurulation. Morphogenetic events at the midline include formation of the primitive streak/gastrulation, neurulation, lateralization (e.g., of optic field), and fusion of the cardiac tubes.

Cardiac Morphogenesis

The molecular systems involved in cardiac morphogenesis are reviewed by Witte et al.[16] and by Olson and Srivastava,[17] and in this volume. The molecular determinants of laterality formation and cardiac looping and situs are becoming known in several species and provide an elegant explanation for the laterality abnormalities in conjoint twins.[18–25] Recently, Debrus et al.[26] and de Meerus et al.[27] were able to characterize two blastogenesis mutations in humans, one autosomal recessive, one autosomal dominant affecting midline development and cardiac morphogenesis, looping and situs formation. Developmental constraints operate in cardiac development as in all morphogenetic processes of the body, severely limiting the range of normal or abnormal morphogenetic outcomes to a re-

markably limited repertoire of structure. And in view of the fact that the number of our genes ranges in the tens of thousands, of chromosome mutations and contiguous gene syndromes in the hundreds, and of teratogens in the dozens, heterogeneity is not surprising, nor the fact that the heart anomalies seen in such teratogenic disorders as the fetal alcohol syndrome[28] or a metabolic disruption sequence such as maternal phenylketonuria[29] are no different than those seen in Mendelian mutation or aneuploidy syndromes.

Recently, Belmont reviewed the molecular genetics of cardiac morphogenesis and of congenital heart defects,[30] also reviewed elsewhere in volume. Only a few examples will be cited.

The *Hand1 bHLH* transcription factor is essential not only for cardiac morphogenesis but also for placentation.[31] *Hand1* expression is restricted to placental trophoblast and later to embryonic cardiac and neural crest cells. In *Hand1* null mice developmental arrest occurred on day 7.5 with defects of trophoblast giant cell differentiation. In an attempt at rescue through fusion of mutant embryos with wild type tetraploid embryos that contribute wild type cells to the trophoblast, but not to the embryo, survival was ensured until day 10.5 when the chimeric embryos died of heart failure due to abnormal looping and ventricular myocardial differentiation. In humans null *Hand1* mutations would therefore probably be early embryonic lethals.

The work of Srivastava et al.[32] on the related basic helix-loop-helix transcription factors *dHAND* and *eHAND* is particularly effective in demonstrating the genetic control of *dHAND* over the formation of the mesodermal-derived right ventricle and of the neural crest-derived aortic arches. Targeted deletion of *dHand* in mouse embryos resulted in embryonic death at day 10.5 of heart failure with dilatation of the aortic sac, absence of first or second aortic arch arteries, and an abrupt connection between the conotruncus and the left ventricle with no evidence of the intervening right ventricle. Looping occurred normally in these mice.

The gene homologous to the *Drosophila* homeobox gene *tinman* is the human *NKX2–5* gene, mapped to 5q35 and important in early cardiac looping. Mutations of the mouse *Nkx2.5* gene result in heart failure without completion of looping. Genetic studies in four families by Schott et al.[33] with an autosomal dominant nonsyndromal trait producing predominantly secundum atrial septal defects with atrioventricular (AV) block, but also ventricular septal defects, tetralogy of Fallot, subvalvular aortic stenosis, ventricular hypertrophy, pulmonary atresia, and redundant mitral valve leaflets with fenestrations showed 3 different *NKX2–5* mutations. These findings indicate that *NKX2–5* is important for regulation of septation during cardiac morphogenesis, and for maturation and maintenance of AV node function throughout life.

Kosaki et al.[34] recently demonstrated mutations in *ACVR2B*, the gene for human activin receptor type IIB, in rare individuals with left-right axis malformations.

Individuals with deletions of 8p23.1 frequently have congenital heart defects. The gene encoding *GATA4*, another zinc finger transcription factor involved in cardiac morphogenesis, maps to 8p23.1. Pehlivan et al.[35] recently demonstrated by fluorescent in situ hybridization haploinsufficiency of *GATA4* in 4 patients with del (8)(p23.1) and congenital heart defects including secundum atrial septal defect (ASD), valvar pulmonary stenosis (PS), left superior vena cava (LSVC), cardiomyopathy, ventricular septal defect (VSD), AV canal, and tetralogy of Fallot. The *GATA4* gene was not deleted in a 5th patient with del(8)(p23.1) without cardiac anomalies.

One of the most striking pieces of evidence supporting the evolutionary implications of the concept of homology is the fact that the process of pattern formation involves identical conserved gene families over many metazoan phyla from the fruitfly and nematode to all mammals, a phenomenon that may be referred to as *universality*, and seems the most reasonable explanation for the concept of phylogeneity. The best known examples of such universality are the many homeobox genes known to be involved in numerous "homologous" morphogenetic processes in many different phylogenetic forms (e.g. the *tinman* gene mentioned above as involved in *Drosophila* cardiac morphogenesis, and its homolog *NKX2–5* in human cardiac morphogenesis).

The homeobox genes in the various animals participate not only in the specification of the basic axial body plan, but also of other body parts such as fins or limbs. This phenomenon may be referred to as morphogenetic *parsimony* and is the probable explanation of much of *pleiotropy*.[36] Pleiotropy refers to the fact that *one* cause (e.g., mutation) results in multiple manifestations, a virtually universal phenomenon in Mendelian genetics.

Malformations

Malformations are gross defects of blastogenesis or organogenesis, i.e., *qualitative* abnormalities of morphogenesis. Mild malformations (to be distinguished from *minor anomalies*, i.e., defects of phenogenesis) are common in the population, appear to have no selective disadvantage and to be dominantly inherited in many cases. They include cleft of uvula and of xiphisternum, torus palatinus, extra nipples, mild to moderate cutaneous syndactyly of toes 2 and 3, postaxial postminimus polydactyly in certain populations, absence of upper lateral incisors and of third molars, of palmaris longus muscles, of xiphisternum and many others.

From an evolutionary perspective, the largest and most important group of human malformations is the *vestigia*. This term refers to anomalies of *incomplete* formation, i.e., persistence of an embryonic state. These include cleft lip with or without cleft palate, failure of neural tube formation/closure, webbed digits, a tail, extra nipples, omphalocele, hypospadias, imperforate anus, VSD, patent ductus arteriosus (PDA), ASD, and many more. To answer the question whether an anomaly is a vestigium, one must inquire whether it is ever a *normal* state during the morphogenesis of the organism under consideration.

Field formation represents, in part, the consequence of the reduction of metamerism, i.e., the progressive integration of formerly identical, segmentally repeated simpler structures into fewer, non-metameric, more complex parts of the body. Examples are the integration of the three or four most rostral cervical vertebrae of our agnathan ancestors into the neocranium (i.e., occipital bone); the bilaterally symmetrical, metameric branchial arch vascular system into a single aortic arch system; the mammary line with potential for many pairs of mammary glands into a single pair of breasts; or the change from pronephros to serially repeated mesonephros to single metanephric kidney pair.

Atavisms are defined as recurrence of an ancestral morphological (hence morphogenetic) state and were accepted by Darwin as a powerful piece of evidence for the theory of descent with modification. Atavisms may occur naturally (legs on whales, toes on horses) or through artificial selection (Sewall Wright's "atavistic" restoration of the "lost" toes in guinea pigs) or produced through gene manipulation (i.e., atavistic reformation in the mouse of the pterygoquadrate bone of reptiles through targeted disruption of *Hoxa-2*[37]). In humans they were documented convincingly in the many muscle abnormalities seen in aneuploidy, especially 18-trisomy infants dissected with great care.[38,39] Atavisms appear to be rare in humans, vestigia are by far the most common group of malformations. Nevertheless, it is important to keep the phenomenon in mind in case of odd (and some not so odd) anomalies. Is the interstitial (a very uncommon) form of polydactyly, seen in the Pallister-Hall syndrome due to *GLI-3* mutations,[40] an atavism in view of the fact that all of the Devonian ancestral land vertebrates (*Acanthostega, Ichthyostega,* and *Tulerpeton)* were normally polydactylous with 6 to 8 digits per limb? Or is simple cleft palate an atavism in view of the fact that all birds and reptiles (except for crocodiles) have a cleft palate? Or agenesis of the corpus callosum, normal in monotremes, reptiles and marsupials? Or scrotum rostral to penis ("marsupial scrotum"), normal in marsupials and lagomorphs (pikes, rabbits, hares)?

Thus, to answer the question whether a given malformation is an atavism, one must inquire whether it is ever a normal morphological state in another species.

One of the pioneers of the evolutionary perspective of isolated, (i.e. non-syndromal) heart malformations was the late Helen Taussig (1900–1986). In her last paper, Taussig[41] proposed, again, that isolated cardiac anomalies may have an evolutionary origin. With her vast knowledge of mammalian malformations and after a study of over 5000 birds, she concludes that similar/identical malformations in different species "points to either a common external causative factor or a common origin" (the word "origin" here used as in the origin of species). She stated pithily, "Genes that code the malformed heart must be transmitted with that part of the genetic makeup common to all birds and mammals. Malformations caused by teratogens produce widespread organ injury to a potentially normal embryo, whereas the evolutionary malformation is an organ-specific anomaly in an otherwise normal mammal or bird and occurs in widely separated species." A beautiful formulation indeed of the concept of phylogeneity.

Polytopic Anomalies

The phenomenon of parsimony is likely responsible not only for pleiotropy but also for the occurrence of what may be called *polytopic anomalies.* Polytopic anomalies are defined as the nonrandom co-occurrence of two or more defects of blastogenesis in the same individual. The first of these, defined as such, was the acrorenal (polytopic) field defect,[42] i.e., the concurrence of abnormalities of limbs and kidneys, first postulated to share a common developmental basis during the thalidomide epidemic and demonstrated as such by Lash[43] and Geduspan and Solursh.[44,45] A common upstream inductor system of mesonephros and limb buds appears to be fibroblast growth factor 8 (*FGF8*).[46]

Another highly heterogeneous polytopic field defect is the cardiomelic anomaly or complex[47] strikingly seen in the Holt-Oram syndrome due to mutations of the T-box gene *TBX-5*.[48–50] The occurrence of multiple polytopic field defects in one fetus or infant was, and to some extent still is referred to as an *association* (e.g., VATER or "schisis" association). The connotation of association, in this context, being "idiopathic," i.e., cause unknown, with negligibly small (?2%) empiric recurrence risk. If cause (e.g., trisomy 13) is known, then these multiple anomalies represent pleiotropy, and the condition is a syndrome. Gross anomalies of blastogenesis, including polytopic and multiple polytopic anomalies may be seen in the infants of diabetic mothers. Teratogens (e.g., Accutane, thalidomide) may also produce defects of blastogenesis.

Summary

"Ich bin zum Erstaunen da," [very roughly: "I was made to be constantly amazed."] said Goethe, and wonder, Aristotle noted, is the beginning of all knowledge. In our understanding of the phenomenon of organic development we have come far from the fear and superstition of our ancestors who created legends, spoke of monsters (*monstra*) as acts of God and believed in maternal impressions, reincarnations, and matings with animals and the devil to that of the great pioneer investigators, from Aristotle to Spemann, of the phenomenon of normal development, to the present day when, through means of molecular biology, it has become possible to understand better the relationship between development and evolution on the basis of shared, molecular means of induction as the basis of homology of structure and development. In our understanding of this process, clinical geneticist have made substantial contributions in introducing a *causal* understanding of (field) development and of bringing an evolutionary perspective to the phenomenon of normal and dysmorphogenetic developmental phenomena.

The insights that Goethe and Burdach brought 200 years ago to the formulation of the science of morphology still serve well today when defining this newly reunited branch of biology as the science of the form, formation, transformation and malformation of living organisms. The analysis of development from an evolutionary perspective is what unites and gives meaning to all parts of biology.

Acknowledgements: We are grateful to Mrs. Sandie Ramos for expert secretarial collaboration and to the Primary Children's Medical Center Foundation for a generous grant in support of the International Clinical Genetics Research and Consultation Program to the Division of Medical Genetics of the Department of Pediatrics at the University of Utah.

References

1. Carranza A, Gilbert-Barness E, Madrigal F, et al. Complete absence or deficiency of one half of the body. *Am J Med Genet* 1998;76:197–201.
2. Bouwmeester T, Kim S-H, Sasai Y, et al. Cerberus is a head-inducing secreted factor expressed in the anterior endoderm of Spemann's organizer. *Nature* 1996;382:595–601.
3. Opitz JM, Clark EB. Developmental and genetic aspects of syndromal cardiac malformations. In: Herzfehler, Genetik, eds. *Genetics and Cardiopathies.* Stuttgart: Wissenschaftliche Verlagsgesellschaft. 1999; pp. 277–292.
4. Sater AK, Jacobson A. The restriction of the heart morphogenetic field in *Xenopus laevis. Dev Biol* 1990;140:328–336.
5. Schmid G. Über die Herkunft der Ausdrücke Morphologie und Biologie. *Nova Acta Leopoldina (Neue Folge).* Vol. 2, issue 3/4, number 8, 1935:597–620 (also Kuhn D. personal communication to H-R Wiedemann, 10/28/1991, available on request).
6. DeRobertis EM, Sasai Y. A common plan for dorsoventral patterning in Bilateria. *Nature* 1996;380:37–40.
7. Appel TA. *The Cuvier-Geoffroy Debate: French biology in the decades before Darwin.* New York: Oxford University Press; 1987.
8. Davidson EH. Spatial mechanisms of gene regulation in metazoan embryos. *Development* 1991;113:1–26.

9. Davidson EH, Peterson KJ, Cameron RA. Origin of bilaterian body plans: Evolution of developmental regulatory mechanisms. *Science* 1995;270:1319–1325.

10. Spemann H (1936 publication of the Silliman lectures of 1933): Experimentelle Beiträge zu einer Theorie der Entwicklung. Berlin, Julius Springer. (1938 English translation): *Embryonic Development and Induction*. New Haven, Conn: Yale University Press; reprinted 1962, New York: Hafner Publ Co.

11. Opitz JM. Blastogenesis and the "primary field" in human development. *Birth Defects Orig Artic Ser* 1993;29(1):3–37.

12. Wulfsberg EA, Mirkinson LJ, Meister SJ. Autosomal dominant tetramelic postaxial oligodactyly. *Am J Med Genet* 1993;46:579–583.

13. Roessler E, Belloni E, Gaudenz K, et al. Mutations in the human *Sonic hedgehog* gene cause holoprosencephaly. *Nature Genet* 1996;14:357–360.

14. Belloni E, Muenke M, Roessler E, et al. Identification of Sonic Hedgehog as a candidate gene responsible for holoprosencephaly. *Nature Genet* 1996;14:353–356.

15. Cooper MK, Porter JA, Young KG, et al. Teratogen-mediated inhibition of target tissue response to *Shh* signaling. *Science* 1998;280:1603–1607.

16. Witte DP, Aronow BJ, Harmony JAK. Understanding cardiac development through the perspective of gene regulation and gene manipulation. *Pediatr Path Lab Med* 1996;16:173–194.

17. Olson EN, Srivastava D. Molecular pathways controlling heart development. *Science* 1996;272:671–676.

18. Levin M, Roberts DJ, Holmes LB, et al. Laterality defects in conjoined twins. *Nature* 1996;384:321.

19. Levin M, Pagan S, Roberts DJ, et al. Left/right patterning signals and the independent regulation of different aspects of situs in the chick embryo. *Dev Biol* 1997;189:57–67.

20. Danos MC, Yost HJ. Role of notochord in specification of cardiac left-right orientation in Zebrafish and Xenopus. *Dev Biol* 1996;177:96–103.

21. Danos MC, Yost HJ. Linkage of cardiac left-right asymmetry and dorsal-anterior development in *Xenopus*. *Dev Biol* 1995;121:1467–1474.

22. Bower PN, Brueckner M, Yost HJ. Laterality disturbances. *Progr Pediatr Cardiol.* 1996;6:53–62.

23. Hyatt BA, Lohr JL, Yost HJ. Initiation of vertebrate right-left axis formation by maternal *Vg1*. *Nature* 1996;384:62–65.

24. Lohr JL, Danos MC, Yost HJ. Left-right asymmetry of a *nodal*-related gene is regulated by dorsoanterior midline structures during *Xenopus* development. *Development* 1997;124:1465–1472.

25. Ramsdell AF, Yost HJ. Molecular mechanisms of vertebrate left-right development. *Trends Genet* 1998;14:459–465.

26. Debrus S, Sauer U, Gilgenkrantz S, et al. Autosomal recessive lateralization and midline defect: Blastogenesis recessive 1. *Am J Med Genet* 1997;68:401–404.

27. DeMeeus A, Lorda P, Tenconi R, et al. Blastogenesis dominant 1: A sequence with midline anomalies and heterotaxy. *Am J Med Genet* 1997;68:405–408.

28. Clark EB, Ohanian L. Maternal alcohol consumption and developmental defects of the cardiovascular system. In: Zakharis, Wassef M, eds. *Alcohol and the Cardiovascular System*. NIAAA/NIH Res Monogr 1996;31:137–158.

29. Rouse B, Azen C, Koch R, et al. Maternal phenylketonuria collaborative study (APKUCS) offspring: Facial anomalies. Malformations and early neurological sequelae. *Am J Med Genet* 1997;69:89–95.

30. Belmont JW. Recent progress in the molecular genetics of congenital heart defects. *Clin Genet* 1998;54:11–19.

31. Riley P, Anson-Cartwright L, Cross JC. The *Hand1* bHLH transcription factor is essential for placentation and cardiac morphogenesis. *Nat Genet* 1998;18:271–275.

32. Srivastava D, Thomas T, Lin Q, et al. Regulation of cardiac mesodermal and neural crest development by the bHLH transcription factor, dHand. *Nat Genet* 1997;16:154–160 (with News and Views Comments by Overbeck PA: Right and Left go dhand and ehand. ibid, p 119; erratum ibid, p 410).

33. Schott JJ, Benson DW, Basson CT, et al. Congenital heart disease caused by mutations in the transcription factor NKX2.5. *Science* 1998;281:108–111.

34. Kosaki R, Gebbia M, Kosaki K, et al. Left-right axis malformations associated with mutations in *ACVR2B*, the gene for human activin receptor type IIB. *Am J Med Genet* 1999;82:70–76.

35. Pehlivan T, Pober BR, Brueckner M, et al. *GATA4* haploinsufficiency in patients with interstitial deletion of chromosome region 8p23.1 and congenital heart disease. *Am J Med Genet* 1999;83:201–206.

36. Plate L. Vererbungslehre und Deszendenz-theorie. Festschrift für Richard Hertwig. II: 537. *Jena, Fischer.* 1910.

37. Rijli FM, Mark M, Lakkaraju S, et al. A homeotic transformation is generated in the rostral branchial region of the head by disruption *of Hoxa-2*, which acts as a selector gene. *Cell* 1993;75:1333–1349.

38. Barash BA, Freedman L, Opitz JM. Anatomic studies in the 18-trisomy syndrome. *Birth Defects Orig Artic Ser* 1970;6(4):3–15.

39. Opitz JM, Gilbert-Barness EF. Reflections on the pathogenesis of Downs syndrome. *Am J Med Genet* 1990;7(suppl):38–51.

40. Biesecker LG. Strike three for GLI3. *Nat Genet* 1998;17:259–260.

41. Taussig HB. Evolutionary origin of cardiac malformations. *J Am Coll Cardiol* 1988;12:1079–1086.

42. Dieker H, Opitz JM. Associated acral and renal malformations. *Birth Defects Orig Artic Ser* 1969;5(3):68–77.

43. Lash W. Studies on the ability of embryonic mesonephros explants to form cartilage. *Dev Biol* 1963;6:217–232.

44. Geduspan JS, Solursh M. A growth-promoting influence from the mesonephros during limb outgrowth. *Dev Biol* 1992;151:242–250.

45. Geduspan JS, Solursh M. Effects of the mesonephros and insulin-like growth factor I on chondrogenesis of limb explants. *Dev Biol* 1993;156:500–508.

46. Crossley PH, Minowada G, MacArthur CA, et al. Roles for FGF8 in the induction, initiation, and maintenance of chick limb development. *Cell* 1996;84:127–136.

47. Wilson GN. Correlated heart/limb anomalies in Mendelian syndromes provide evidence for a cardiomelic developmental field. *Am J Med Genet* 1998;76:297–305.

48. Basson CT, Bachinsky DR, Lin RC, et al. Mutations in human TBX5 cause limb and cardiac malformation in Holt-Oram syndrome. *Nat Genet* 1997;15:30–35.

49. Li QY, Newbury-Ecob RA, Terrett JA, et al. Holt-Oram syndrome is caused by mutations in TBX5, a member of the *Brachyury* (T) gene family. *Nat Genet* 1997;15:21–29.

50. Papaioannou VE, Silver LM. The T-box gene family. *BioEssays* 1998;20:9–19.

56

Human Cardiac Development

David I. Wilson, BA, MB BS, PhD,
Mark Clement-Jones, MB, BS, Neil Hanley, MB BS,
Karen Piper, BSc, Andy Curtis, BSc,
Susan Lindsay, BSc, PhD, Phil Bullen, MS, BS,
Steven Robson, MS, BS, MD, and Tom Strachan, BSc, PhD

Our understanding about the development of the human heart has come from both studying human embryos and extrapolation from other species, notably the mouse. Most of the human data has come from collections of embryos notably the Carnegie (U.S.), Kyoto (Japan), and Boyd (U.K.) collections. Although these have been valuable for morphological and histological examinations, they have not been suitably fixed for gene expression studies. There has been a consensus that despite humans and mice sharing a common ancestor 60 million years ago, embryogenesis in these two species is sufficiently similar that developmental processes in humans can be extrapolated from murine models or studies in other species (e.g., chick or *Xenopus*).

The mouse has provided a useful genetic model upon which to study human disease. However it is becoming increasingly evident that many important genetic differences exist between the two species.[1] For instance, the expression domains of WNT7A differ in human and mouse embryonic brain[2]; triplet nucleotide repeat expansion does not seem to be a pathogenic mechanism in mice in contrast to humans and there are primate specific genes of developmental importance (e.g., SHOX). Furthermore, the phenotypes of several mouse transgenic knockouts have followed recessive patterns of inheritance whereas the human disease followed a dominant pattern. It is therefore important to include the investigation of human embryonic development including cardiogenesis, rather than rely solely on extrapolated data from other species.

We have undertaken a molecular genetic study of human embryonic development and have collected early human embryos for gene expression studies. Ethical permission for this study has been granted and we follow the Polkinghorne Committee (U.K.) guidelines for the scientific use of human embryonic and fetal tissues.[3] Written consent is requested from women undergoing medical or surgical termination of pregnancy.[4,5] The embryos are examined and staged using the Carnegie staging system[6,7]; trophoblastic tissue is also taken for chromosome analysis. The embryos are suitably fixed for mRNA tissue in situ hybridization,[8] immunocytochemistry, cryosectioning, or mRNA preservation. We have collected over 250 embryos since 1995 using these

From Clark EB, Nakazawa M, Takao A (eds.): Etiology and Morphogenesis of Congenital Heart Disease: Twenty Years of Progress in Genetics and Developmental Biology. Armonk, NY: Futura Publishing Co., Inc.; © 2000.

methods, most of which have been collected intact or with minimal disruption.

The Carnegie staging system uses similar morphological and histological landmarks that are similar to those used in staging embryos from other species (chick and mouse). The temporal reference is ovulation and 23 Carnegie stages (CS) span the 56 day (post-ovulation) embryonic period. We have obtained embryos between CS 8 (18 day) and CS 23 (56 day) together with fetal samples.

We have performed mRNA tissue in situ studies using standard techniques[8–10] (Moorman and Lako), immunocytochemistry and also made stage specific cDNA libraries. The gene expression studies have focused on genes that are of fundamental developmental importance (e.g., WNT gene family), genes that cause human developmental phenotypes or primate specific genes for which there cannot be a murine model. The expression of several genes studied have been important for cardiac development.

Mutations in SOX9 (SRY-related HMG-box) have been identified in patients with camptomelic dysplasia. This phenotype is characterized by a skeletal dysplasia including a severe thoracic dystrophy and 46XY males can have sex reversal; approximately 30% of cases have a cardiac septal defect. A preliminary study has shown SOX9 expression in the truncal cushions of CS17 and CS18 human embryos in addition to the skeletal structures affected and gonads. This would suggest that the cardiac abnormalities seen in camptomelic dysplasia are primary defects rather than secondary to flow disturbance caused by the thoracic dystrophy.

TBX5 is one of the T-box gene family and mutations have been identified in individuals with Holt-Oram syndrome.[11] This is characterized by radial ray limb defects and also cardiac septal defect. We have shown TBX5 expression not only in atrioventricular endocardial cushions, but the atrial wall and coronary sinus. The overall expression pattern is similar to that in mouse although mice have a left

superior vena cava rather than coronary sinus.

SHOX (Short-stature homeobox) is a gene on the human X chromosome that has been implicated in the phenotype of Turner's syndrome (45 XO). Cardiac defects are associated with Turner syndrome and include hypoplastic left heart and coarctation of the aorta. Mutations in SHOX have been found in individuals with short stature and also Leri-Weil syndrome (skeletal dysplasia). A preliminary study has been unable to identify SHOX expression in human embryonic outflow tract, ventricles or aorta which suggests that SHOX is not the gene that causes the heart defects in Turner's syndrome. SHOX is not thought to have a murine orthologue, and therefore this study could not have been performed in mice.

In order to understand more fully the mechanisms that underlie human development, it is important to include human embryo gene expression studies. The embryos that we have collected do not cover the entire period of organogenesis and indeed it may not be possible to obtain embryos from the very early stages; nevertheless we have accessed a developmental window that includes significant cardiogenic events. Furthermore, the challenge that will follow the sequencing of the entire human genome will be the characterization of many novel genes.[12] Where and when these genes are expressed will be an important part of their characterization.

Acknowledgements: We are grateful to David Brook (Nottingham, U.K.) for probes for TBX5, and Hideko Kasahara and Seigo Izumo (Harvard, U.S.) for antibodies to NKX2.5. This work has been supported by Wellcome Trust and MRC (U.K.).

References

1. Strachan T, Lindsay S. Why study human embryos? The imperfect mouse model. In Strachan T, Lindsay S, Wilson DI, eds. *Molecular Genetics of Early Human Development.* Oxford: Bios Scientific Publishers; 1997:13–26.

2. Lindsay S, Bullen P, Lako M, et al. Expression of Wnt genes in postimplantation human embryos. In: Strachan T, Lindsay S, Wilson DI, eds. *Molecular Genetics of Early Human Development*. Oxford: Bios Scientific Publishers; 1997:13–26.

3. Polkinghorne DR. Guidelines on the Research Use of Foetuses and Foetal Material. HMSO Ref. No. CM762; 1989.

4. Soothill P, Rodeck C. First trimester fetal necroscopy after ultrasound-guided aspiration. *Lancet* 1997;343:1096–1097.

5. Cadepond F, Ulmann A, Baulieu E. RU486 (Mifepristone): Mechanisms of action and clinical uses. *Ann Rev Med* 1997;48:129–156.

6. O'Rahilly R, Muller F. *Developmental Stages of Human Embryos*. Washington, D.C.: Carnegie Institution of Washington, Publication No. 637; 1987.

7. Bullen P, Wilson DI. The Carnegie staging of human embryos: A practical guide. In: Strachan T, Lindsay S, Wilson DI, eds. *Molecular Genetics of Early Human Development*. Oxford: Bios, Scientific Publishers; 1997 pp. 371–379.

8. Moorman AFM, De Boer PAJ, Vermeulen JL, et al. Practical aspects of radioisotopic in situ hybridization on RNA. *Histochem J* 1993;25:251–266. Review.

9. Wilson DI. Approaches to study gene expression in early human development. In: Strachan T, Lindsay S, Wilson DI, eds. *Molecular Genetics of Early Human Development*. Oxford: Bios Scientific Publishers; 1997:13–26.

10. Lako M, Lindsay S, Bullen P, et al. A novel mammalian Wnt gene, WNT8b, shows brain-restricted expression in early development, with sharply delimited expression boundaries in the developing forebrain. *Hum Mol Gen* 1998;7:813–822.

11. Li YQ, Newbury-Ecob RA, Terrett JA, et al. Holt-Oram syndrome is caused by mutations in TBX5, a member of the Brachyury (T) gene family. *Nat Genet* 1997;15:21–27.

12. Strachan T, Abitbol M, Davidson D, et al. A new dimension for the Human Genome Project. *Nat Genet* 1997;16:126–132.

57

Role of the bHLH Transcription Factor, dHAND, in Cranial/Cardiac Neural Crest Development

Hiroyuki Yamagishi, MD, and Deepak Srivastava, MD

Cranial and cardiac neural crest (NC) cells arise from the dorsal aspect of the neural tube, migrate to populate branchial arch mesenchyme and vascular mesenchyme of arch arteries, and differentiate to form craniofacial structures and smooth muscle of the great vessels.[1] Defects of this cell lineage are implicated in a number of human congenital syndromes, such as 22q11.2 deletion/DiGeorge syndrome, and congenital conotruncal and aortic arch malformations.[1-3] Elucidating the molecular mechanism which regulates NC development is, therefore, fundamental to understanding the pathogenesis of these disorders.

Transcription factors sharing a basic helix-loop-helix (bHLH) domain serve as regulators of determination and differentiation for diverse cell types including skeletal muscle, hematopoietic cells and some neuronal cells.[4-6] dHAND is a basic helix-loop-helix protein that is expressed in the heart, lateral plate mesoderm, and mesenchyme derived from NC.[7-9] Mice homozygous null for the *dHAND* gene have a hypoplastic right ventricle and die from cardiac failure by embryonic day (E) 11.0.[8] Here we report a role for dHAND in NC development. The data indicate that

From Clark EB, Nakazawa M, Takao A (eds.): Etiology and Morphogenesis of Congenital Heart Disease: Twenty Years of Progress in Genetics and Developmental Biology. Armonk, NY: Futura Publishing Co., Inc.; © 2000.

dHAND is essential for persistence of cranial/cardiac NC-derived mesenchyme which is fated to differentiate into craniofacial/cardiovascular structures.

In NC derivatives, dHAND is first detectable in the first and second branchial arches of E9.0 mouse embryos, specifically in the mesenchyme of the branchial arches and the aortic arch arteries. *dHAND*-null embryos display hypoplasia of the branchial arches.[10] At E9.5, wild-type embryos have good development of the first and second branchial arches and have begun to form the third and fourth arches. However, *dHAND*-null embryos form only a single branchial arch even at E10.0 (Fig. 1). NC markers, including the homeobox genes *Dlx-2, MHox,* and *Msx2* are expressed at normal levels in *dHAND*-null branchial arches, suggesting that NC migration and initial differentiation are unaffected in the absence of dHAND. However, extensive apoptosis, a detected by TUNEL assay and electron microscopy, was evident in the mesenchyme of *dHAND*-null branchial arches. This suggests that dHAND may function in a pathway important for survival of branchial arch mesenchymal cells.

Msx1, another homeobox gene, is normally expressed in the mesenchyme of the branchial arches and limb buds, similar to dHAND. Unlike other homeobox genes, *Msx1* is not expressed in *dHAND*-null branchial arches, but is expressed in the

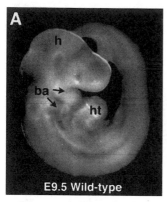
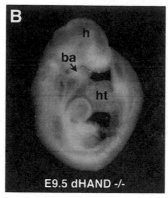
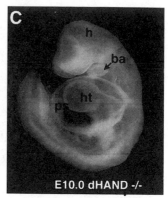

Figure 1. Branchial arch hypoplasia in *dHAND* mutants. Embryonic day 9.5 (E9.5) wild-type (**A**), E9.5 *dHAND*-null (**B**), and E10.0 *dHAND*-null (**C**) mouse embryos are shown in lateral view. Note development of only a single branchial arch (ba) in the mutants, and dilation of the aortic sac (as). h, head; ht, heart; ps, pericardial sac.

limb buds, suggesting that Msx1 may lie downstream of dHAND in a molecular pathway controlling branchial arch growth. The dHAND-independent regulation of *Msx1* in the limb bud is consistent with separable regulatory elements identified in the *Msx1* promoter that controls branchial arch and limb bud expression.[11] *Msx1* and *Msx2* are co-expressed in the subepithelial layer of the distal branchial arch which is the leading edge of the developing arch. Msx2 has been implicated in mediating BMP-4 induced programmed cell death[12] whereas Msx1 may promote cellular proliferation[13]; a balance between the two may be critical to appropriate growth of the branchial arch. *Msx1*-null mice are born alive but have craniofacial malformations, including small mandible and cleft palate.[14] dHAND may play a role in craniofacial development by regulating downstream genes, such as *Msx1*.

NC-derived cells also give rise to the vascular mesenchyme of aortic arch arteries. dHAND is expressed in vascular mesenchymal cells that are fated to differentiate into pericyte and smooth muscle cells. *dHAND*-null embryos display collapse of the aortic arch arteries.[8] To trace development of vascular endothelial cells with an in vivo marker, transgenic mice containing a lacZ marker under control of the endothelial-specific Tie-2 promoter[15] were crossed into the *dHAND*-null background. At E8.5, prior to vascular mesen-

chyme invasion, lac-Z expression revealed that endothelial cells are patterned correctly to form the dorsal aorta and aortic arch arteries in the absence of dHAND. However, the patterning of the aortic arch arteries and rostral dorsal aorta, where dHAND is normally expressed, disintegrated in *dHAND* mutants by E9.5. Tie-2 and the other endothelial markers, Tie-1, Flt-1, and PECAM are expressed at normal levels in *dHAND*-null mice. Thus, dHAND is essential for persistence of arch arteries, but is not required for initial development and formation of the endothelial cells.

In *dHAND* mutants, vascular mesenchymal cells had migrated around endothelial cells, but were fewer in number compared with wild-type, as demonstrated by electron microscopy. Wild-type mesenchymal cells develop cytoplasmic process to contact endothelial cells, however, *dHAND*-null mesenchymal cells remained rounded without making appropriate contact with endothelial cells. The vascular mesenchymal marker, angiopoietin-1,[16] is expressed in *dHAND*-null mesenchymal cells, however, no expression of the vascular smooth muscle cell marker, SM22,[17] is detectable in *dHAND*-null aortic arch arteries, suggesting that *dHAND*-null vascular mesenchymal cells fail to differentiate into smooth muscle cells. Similar to that observed in the branchial arches and *dHAND*-null right

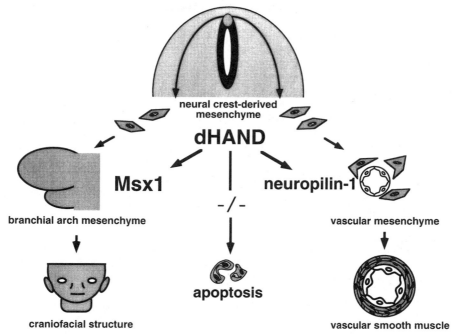

Figure 2. Role of dHAND in neural crest development. dHAND is required for survival of post-migratory neural crest-derived mesenchyme, and regulates Msx1 in branchial arches and neuropilin-1 in aortic arch arteries during development.

ventricle, vascular mesenchyme cells displayed cytoplasmic blebbing and underwent apoptosis.

In an effort to understand the molecular mechanisms through which dHAND functions, we sought to identify dHAND-dependent genes by suppressive subtractive hybridization, where *dHAND*-null heart cDNA was subtracted from wild-type heart cDNA. One dHAND-dependent gene encoded neuropilin-1, a vascular endothelial growth factor (VEGF) receptor involved in vascular development,[18] that also functions as a semaphorin III receptor in neuron development.[19,20] Our analyses indicate that neuropilin-1 is normally expressed in the heart, branchial arches, aortic-arch arteries and dorsal aorta at E9.5, coincident with dHAND expression. In *dHAND* mutants, neuropilin-1 is down-regulated in heart, branchial arches, arch arteries and rostral portion of the dorsal aorta, but not in the caudal portion. Down-regulation of neuropilin-1 specifically in the rostral but not caudal aorta correlates with dHAND expression and function. The disruption

of a VEGF-mediated pathway may be playing a role in the pathogenesis of the vascular defects in *dHAND*-null mice.

In conclusion, we propose a model for a molecular mechanism where dHAND regulates development of cranial/cardiac NC-derived mesenchyme (Fig. 2). In this model, dHAND functions in post-migratory NC development, and is required for cell survival of NC-derived mesenchyme. dHAND regulates Msx1 in branchial arch mesenchyme, and the VEGF receptor, neuropilin-1, in the vascular mesenchyme of aortic arch arteries. It will be important to determine if these pathways are disrupted in any of the well-described NC syndromes in humans.

References

1. Kirby ML, Waldo KL. Role of neural crest in congenital heart disease. *Circulation* 1990;82:332–340.
2. Kirby ML. Cellular and molecular contributions of the cardiac neural crest to car-

diovascular development. *Trends Cardiovasc Med* 1993;3:18–23.

3. Emanuel BS, Budarf PJ, Scambler PJ. The genetic basis of conotruncal cardiac defects: The chromosome 22q11.2 deletion. In: Harvey RP, Rosenthal N, eds. *Heart Development*. New York: Academic Press; 1998:463–478.

4. Olson EN, Klein WH. bHLH factors in muscle development: Dead lines and commitments, what to leave in and what to leave out. *Genes Dev* 1994;8:1–8.

5. Shivdasani RA, Mayar EL, Orkin SH. Absence of blood formation in mice lacking the T-cell leukaemia oncoprotein tal-1/SCL. *Nature* 1995;373:432–434.

6. Jan YN, Jan LY. HLH proteins, fly neurogenesis, and vertebrate myogenesis. *Cell* 1993;75:827–830.

7. Srivastava D, Cserjesi P, Olson EN. A subclass of bHLH proteins required for cardiogenesis. *Science* 1995;70:1995–1999.

8. Srivastava D, Thomas T, Lin Q, et al. Regulation of cardiac mesodermal and neural crest by the bHLH protein, dHAND. *Nat Genet* 1997;16:154–160.

9. Srivastava D. Segmental regulation of cardiac development by the basic helix-loop-helix transcription factors dHAND and eHAND. In: Rosenthal N, Harvey R, eds. *Heart Development*. 1998:143–155.

10. Thomas T, Kurihara H, Yamagishi H, et al. A signaling cascade involving endothelin-1, dHAND and Msx 1 regulates development of neural crest-derived branchial arch mesenchyme. *Development* 1998;125:3005–3014.

11. MacKenzie A, Purdie L, Davidson D, et al. Two enhancer domains control early aspects of the complex expression pattern of Msx1. *Mech Dev* 1997;62:29–40.

12. Marazzi G, Wang Y, Sassoon D. Msx2 is a transcriptional regulator in the BMP4-mediated programmed cell death pathway. *Dev Biol* 1997;186:127–138.

13. Song K, Wang Y, Sassoon D. Expression of Msx1 on myoblasts inhibits terminal differentiation and induces cell transformation. *Nature* 1992;360:477–481.

14. Satokata I, Maas R. Msx1 deficient mice exhibit cleft palate and abnormalities of craniofacial and tooth development. *Nat Genet* 1994;6:348–356.

15. Schlaeger TM, Qin Y, Fujiwara Y, et al. Vascular endothelial cell lineage-specific promoter in transgenic mice. *Development* 1995;121:1089–1098.

16. Suri C, Jones PF, Patan S, et al. Requisite role of angiopoietin-1, a ligand for the Tie2 receptor, during embryonic angiogenesis. *Cell* 1996;87:1171–1180.

17. Li L, Miano JM, Mercer B, et al. Expression of the SM22alpha promoter in transgenic mice provides evidence for distinct transcriptional regulatory programs in vascular and visceral smooth muscle cells. *J Cell Biol* 1996;132:1–11.

18. Soker S, Takashima S, Miao HQ, et al. Neuropilin-1 is expressed by endothelial and tumor cells as an isoform-specific receptor for vascular endothelial growth factor. *Cell* 1998;92:735–745.

19. He Z, Tessier-Lavigne M. Neuropilin is a receptor for the axonal chemorepellent semaphorin III. *Cell* 1997;90:739–751.

20. Kitsukawa T, Shimizu M, Sanbo M, et al. Neuropilin-semaphorin III/D-mediated chemorepulsive signals play a crucial role in peripheral nerve projection in mice. *Neuron* 1997;19:995–1005.

58

Human Genetic Analysis of Cardiac Proliferation and Differentiation

Mairead Casey, BSc, Jordan Winter, BA,
Cathy J. Hatcher, PhD Carl J. Vaughan, MD,
Caroline S. Mah, BA, Alfred E. Denio, MD,
Alan D. Irvine, MD, Anne Hughes, PhD,
Diana M. Eccles, MD, Richard S. Houlston, MD, PhD,
J. Aidan Carney, MD, PhD,
Constantine A. Stratakis, MD, PhD,
and Craig T. Basson, MD, PhD

Cardiac myxomas are heart tumors that arise from pluripotent primitive mesenchymal cells that reside in the adult subendocardial myocardium and which have the capacity to differentiate along multiple lineages.[1-4] Such tumors express protein markers and exhibit morphologic features consistent with human cardiac muscle, skeletal muscle, epithelial tissues, and even osseous structures.[1-4] These tumors arise in approximately 0.07% of individuals.[5] Molecular genetic analysis of cardiac myxomas may provide an opportunity to modulate cardiomyocyte precursors and to identify genetic approaches to therapy for human ischemic heart disease and heart failure. To date, it remains unknown what genetic events activate proliferation and drive differentiation of these subendocardial mesenchymal cells. However, if such genetic pathways could be manipulated in

man to stimulate proliferation of such cells and to direct their differentiation into cardiomyocytes, regeneration of cardiac muscle might be feasible.

In the autosomal dominant syndrome Carney complex, intracardiac myxomas develop in the setting of lentiginosis and endocrinopathy. In the autosomal dominant syndrome Carney complex,[5-9] affected individuals exhibit cutaneous disease (lentigines, ephelides, and blue nevi) in the setting of intracardiac myxomas. Intracardiac myxomas are usually atrial, but ventricular neoplasia also occurs. Such atrial myxomas have been estimated[5] to account for 7% of all atrial myxomas, and they represent a tumor type that is particularly refractory to therapy. Although sporadic atrial myxomas occur most commonly as isolated left atrial lesions in middle aged women, familial atrial myxomas occur in young individuals without gender preference and are often bilateral and/or multicentric. In addition, while sporadic atrial myxomas are usually highly amenable to curative surgical resection, familial lesions frequently

From Clark EB, Nakazawa M, Takao A (eds.): Etiology and Morphogenesis of Congenital Heart Disease: Twenty Years of Progress in Genetics and Developmental Biology. Armonk, NY: Futura Publishing Co., Inc.; © 2000.

recur, often at locations distant to the initial operative site.[8,9]

Although most myxomas are intracardiac, extracardiac myxomas and nonmyxomatous tumors may also occasionally occur.[7-9] Carney complex may also present with nonneoplastic endocrine abnormalities, most commonly Cushing syndrome secondary to primary pigmented nodular adrenocortical hyperplasia.[7] A variety of hematologic, immunologic, and rheumatologic disorders (e.g., anemia, polycythemia, fever, rheumatoid arthritis, vasculitis, systemic lupus erythematosus, and Raynaud's phenomenon) have all been associated with atrial myxomas.[5]

Such systemic abnormalities are thought to be secondary to secretion of the cytokine interleukin 6 by the cardiac tumor itself, and frequently resolve with resection of the tumor.[10-13] The relationship of such cytokine release to reversible heart failure seen in such patients is unknown. Histopathological studies of Carney complex lentigines and myxomas have failed to demonstrate features unique to this syndrome.[8]

The gene defect that produces cutaneous and cardiovascular disease in Carney complex remains unknown. No cytogenetic abnormalities have been consistently associated with the Carney com-

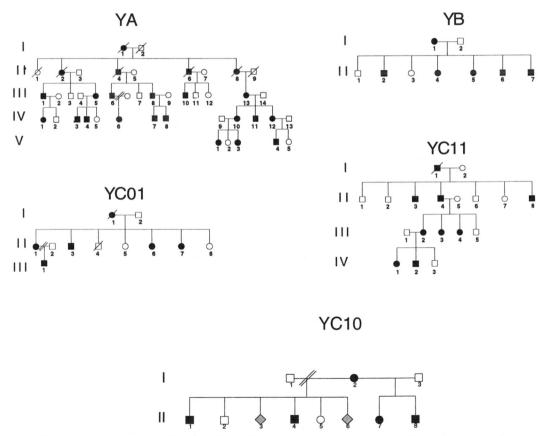

Figure 1. Pedigrees of five families affected by Carney complex. The subject number and disease status of each family member analyzed are indicated. Squares denote male family members, and circles females. Affected and unaffected individuals are represented by closed and open symbols, respectively, and indeterminate or unknown diagnoses by stippled symbol. Slashes denote deceased family members. Pedigrees and clinical characteristics of these families have been previously described.[18-20]

plex to assist in identifying a chromosomal locus that might contribute to such a defective regulatory process.[14-16] Efforts[17] to identify mutations in the protooncogene Gsα have been unsuccessful. Telomeric rearrangements in sporadic atrial myxomas have been occasionally noted[14-16] to involve chromosomes 2, 12, and 17. Thus, Stratakis et al.[18] employed linkage analysis with genetic markers on the short arm of chromosome 2 to evaluate kindreds affected by the Carney complex and have proposed a chromosomal locus in a 6.4 cM interval on chromosome 2p. However, their haplotype analysis[18] questioned the universal applicability of this locus. Our initial studies demonstrated that Carney complex was at least genetically heterogeneous.[19]

We have, therefore, used linkage analysis and positional cloning to identify the chromosomal location of the gene defect that causes cardiac myxomas and Carney complex in five unrelated kindreds (Fig. 1).[20] We initially confirmed genetic heterogeneity of Carney complex; none of the 5 families was linked to the previously proposed chromosome 2p locus.[18] After then performing a random genome search, we[20] observed linkage to human chromosome 17q2 (Fig. 2). Analysis with microsatellite polymorphisms on the long arm of chromosome 17 reveals maximal pairwise LOD scores of 5.8, 1.5, 1.8, 1.5, and 2.9 for families YA, YB, YC01, YC10, and YC11, respectively. Haplotype analysis excludes a founder effect at this locus. These data identify a major 17 cM locus (CAR) at chromosome 17q2 (Fig. 2)[20] that, with odds of 2 trillion:1 contains the Carney complex disease gene. Moreover, genotyping with

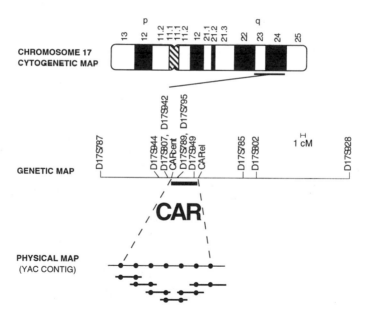

Figure 2. Map location of the CAR locus for familial cardiac myxomas and the Carney complex. The cytogenetic map depicts an ideogram of chromosome 17 with Giemsa banding pattern. Positive bands are black and the pericentromeric region is hatched. Numbers indicate cytogenetic designations for bands. The genetic map locations of polymorphic loci analyzed from 17q2 are given. One centimorgan (cM) is indicated. Initial linkage studies[20] demonstrated that the gene responsible for Carney complex (CAR) resides in a 17-cM interval. More recent haplotype analysis suggests that CAR is located in the refined approximately 5-cM interval between CARcent and CARtel. This interval, as shown on the physical map schematic, has been cloned into a contiguous array of 6 YAC clones.

chromosome 17q2 CAR locus polymorphisms has now enabled us to perform preclinical diagnosis of individuals at risk for development of cardiac myxomas and has prompted altered approach to surveillance echocardiography in members of families affected by Carney complex.

Our current refined mapping studies with these and other newly identified families affected by cardiac myxomas have further reduced the minimal genetic interval containing the disease gene to approximately 5 cM. To identify specific gene mutations that cause Carney complex, we have established a contig of 6 YAC clones (Fig. 2) encompassing the complete CAR locus. A variety of known genes map to this locus, and novel transcripts are also now being isolated from the CAR locus. CAR locus candidate genes are being subjected to mutational analysis by cycle sequencing of exon segments amplified from genomic DNA.

Identification of the Carney complex disease gene will foster new concepts in regulation of cardiac cell growth and differentiation. Controlled activation of the Carney complex disease gene within cardiac tissue may suggest novel therapies for myocardial regeneration in ischemic and idiopathic cardiomyopathies.

Acknowledgements: We are grateful to family members and their physicians for their participation in this study. This work was supported by an American Heart Association Student Scholarship in Cardiovascular Disease and Stroke (J.W.), by the Wendy Will Case Cancer Fund (C.T.B.), and by a Grant-in-Aid from the American Heart Association, New York City Affiliate, Inc. (C.T.B.).

References

1. Lie JT. The identity and histogenesis of cardiac myxomas: A controversy put to rest. *Arch Pathol Lab Med* 1989;113:724–726.
2. Ferrans VJ, Roberts WC. Structural features of cardiac myxomas: Histology, histochemistry, and electron microscopy. *Hum Pathol* 1973;4:111–146.
3. Johansson L. Histogenesis of cardiac myxomas. *Arch Pathol Lab Med* 1989;113:735–741.
4. Burke AP, Virmani R. Cardiac myxomas: A clinicopathologic study. *Am J Clin Pathol* 1993;100:671–680.
5. Reynen K. Cardiac myxomas. *N Engl J Med* 1995;333:1610–1617.
6. Online Mendelian Inheritance in Man, OMIM™. Center for Medical Genetics, Johns Hopkins University (Baltimore, Md), and National Center for Biotechnology Information, National Library of Medicine (Bethesda, Md). World Wide Web URL: http://www.ncbi.nlm.nih.gov/omim/, 1996.
7. Carney JA, Gordon H, Carpenter PC, et al. The complex of myxomas, spotty pigmentation, and endocrine overactivity. *Medicine* 1985;64:270–283.
8. Carney JA. Differences between nonfamilial and familial cardiac myxoma. *Am J Surg Pathol* 1985;9:53–55.
9. McCarthy PM, Piehler JM, Schaff HV. The significance of multiple, recurrent, and "complex" *cardiac myxomas*. *J Thorac Cardiovasc Surg* 1986;91:389–396.
10. Soeparawata R, Poeml P, Schmid C, et al. Interleukin-6 plasma levels and tumor size in cardiac myxoma. *J Thorac Cardiovasc Surg* 1996;112:1675–1677.
11. Kanda T, Umeyama S, Sasaki A, et al. Interleukin-6 and cardiac myxoma. *Am J Cardiol* 1994;74:965–967.
12. Parissis JT, Mentzikof D, Georgopoulou M, et al. Correlation of interleukin-6 gene expression to immunologic features in patients with cardiac myxomas. *J Interferon Cytokine Res* 1996;15:589–593.
13. Vaughan CJ, Gallagher MM, Murphy MB. Left ventricular myxoma presenting with constitutional symptoms and raised serum interleukin-6 both suppressed by naproxen. *Eur Heart J* 1997;18:703.
14. Richkind KE, Wason D, Vidaillet HJ. Cardiac myxoma characterized by clonal telomeric association. *Genes Chrom Cancer* 1994;9:68–71.
15. Dewald GW, Dahl RJ, Spurbeck JL, et al. Chromosomally abnormal clones and nonrandom telomeric translocations in cardiac myxomas. *Mayo Clin Proc* 1987;62:558–567.
16. Dijkuizen T, van den Berg E, Molenaar WM, et al. Cytogenetics of a case of cardiac myxoma. *Cancer Genet Cytogenet* 1992;63:73–75.

17. DeMarco L, Stratakis CA, Boson WL, et al. Sporadic cardiac myxomas and tumors from patients with Carney complex are not associated with activating mutations of the Gsα gene. *Hum Genet* 1996;98:185–188.

18. Stratakis CA, Carney JA, Lin JP, et al. Carney complex, a familial multiple neoplasia and lentiginosis syndrome: Analysis of 11 kindreds and linkage to the short arm of chromosome 2. *J Clin Invest* 1996;97:699–705.

19. Basson CT, MacRae CA, Korf B, et al. Genetic heterogeneity of familial atrial myxoma syndromes (Carney complex). *Am J Cardiol* 1997;79:994–995.

20. Casey M, Mah C, Merliss AD, et al. Identification of a novel genetic locus for familial cardiac myxomas and Carney complex. *Circulation* 1998;98:2560–2566.

59

Blocks of Duplicated Sequence Define the Endpoints of DGS/VCFS 22q11.2-Deletions

Beverly S. Emanuel, PhD, Elizabeth Goldmuntz, MD,
Marcia L. Budarf, MD, Tamim Shaikh, PhD,
James McGrath, MD, PhD, Donna McDonald-McGinn, MS,
Elaine H. Zackai, MD, Deborah A. Driscoll, MD,
and Laura Mitchell, PhD

Clinical and molecular studies have demonstrated that deletions of chromosome 22 occur with an extremely high frequency, making the 22q11.2 deletion syndrome a significant clinical problem in the general population. The disorders associated with deletions of chromosomal region 22q11.2, DGS/VCFS/CTAFS, have been collectively referred to as the 22q11.2 deletion syndrome.[1,2] The development of fluorescence in situ hybridization (FISH) assays for diagnostic purposes has greatly improved detection of the deletion such that recent estimates indicate that the incidence of the 22q11 deletion is approximately 1:4,000 live births.[3]

Patient Cohort

At the Children's Hospital of Philadelphia we are currently following a sample of more than 250 deletion-positive individuals who are enrolled in a prospective study of this disorder. Fifty-nine per-

cent of patients were ascertained through Genetics, 25% from Cardiology, and 10% from the Cleft Palate Team. All patients had microdeletions diagnosed by FISH with N25. The characteristics of deleted patients with a congenital heart defect (CHD) were compared to those without CHD. This analysis indicates that the two groups do not differ from each other with respect to either maternal or paternal age, gestational age, or birth weight. In this deletion positive sample, there is a non-significant excess of males with a heart defect, 53.3% with versus 47.1% without a heart defect. This slight male excess is consistent with findings for CHD in general.

A total of 130 deleted individuals in our prospective sample have had detailed molecular analysis to determine the size of their deletion. Further, we have analysed the cardiac data on 103 of the individuals with "sized deletions." The cardiac evaluation included either a physical exam, chest x-ray, electrocardiogram, or an echocardiogram, or some combination of these modalities. Of the patients with "sized" deletions, 81 of 103 (78.6%) had cardiac anomalies. The most common cardiac anomaly was tetralogy of Fallot (TOF) (34.6% of patients with a CHD),

From Clark EB, Nakazawa M, Takao A (eds.): Etiology and Morphogenesis of Congenital Heart Disease: Twenty Years of Progress in Genetics and Developmental Biology. Armonk, NY: Futura Publishing Co., Inc.; © 2000.

followed by interrupted aortic arch type B (17.3%), conoventricular septal defect (14.8%), truncus arteriosus (13.6%), and aortic arch anomalies (12.3%). The frequency of CHD in patients with "sized" deletions is similar to that in the total deletion positive sample, suggesting that this is a representative subset of patients. Further, we have no evidence that cardiac status is influenced by size or location of the deletion.

From the opposite perspective, we recently examined the frequency of 22q11.2 deletion in 251 patients ascertained with one of seven conotruncal defects.[4] Of these 251 patients, 45 (17.9%) had a deletion. However, the proportion of CHD patients with versus without a deletion varied by the primary cardiac diagnosis. Deletions were most common in patients with interrupted aortic arch type B (12/24 = 50%), truncus arteriosus (10/29 = 34.5%) and TOF (20/126 = 15.9%) as well as in patients with posterior malalignment type ventricular septal defect (2/6 = 33.3%). Only one of twenty patients with a double-outlet right ventricle (DORV) had a 22q11 deletion. Based on these findings, we believe that it is clinically important to test for the 22q11 deletion in infants within these "high-risk" groups because they are at risk for multiple extracardiac anomalies that warrant early detection and intervention.

It is also important to identify the infant with a 22q11 deletion for family counseling purposes as a significant proportion of cases are familial in origin. Several investigators have demonstrated that a proportion of deletions are inherited, with the majority of familial deletions being inherited from the mother.[5–7] Despite the potential for heritability of a deletion, the vast majority of deletions appear to occur as de novo lesions indicating an extremely high "mutation" rate within the 22q11.2 genomic region ($\sim2.5 \times 10^{-4}$). Although the 22q11.2 deletion occurs with a high frequency, the molecular mechanism by which it takes place is largely unknown.

Mechanism of Deletion

We and others have previously noted the presence of gene-related duplicated sequences within 22q11.[8,9] We have positioned these duplicated sequences within 22q11 by mapping using our somatic cell hybrid panel.[10,11] Initially, we worked with mapping the 3′ end of the BCR gene and noted that GGT-like sequences mapped similarly in the hybrids. It now appears as though the number and complexity of these duplicated sequence blocks were underestimated. Although the duplicated regions were initially identified as being comprised of BCR-like and GGT-like elements, as we constructed contigs of the region, we found that we encountered numerous other duplicated elements including numerous ESTs such as HMPLP.[12] From our mapping efforts it has become evident that that there are at least four of these large duplicated blocks within the region denoted as the 22q11.2 deleted region. In addition, there are several blocks which map distal and at least one which is located proximal to the common large deletion.

Our goal was to utilize the aforementioned map resources for gene discovery. Further, we wished to characterize our patient cohort in an attempt to determine the smallest region of deletion overlap (SRO) to aid in identification of critical genes. To date 25 genes within the large commonly deleted region have been identified (Fig. 1).[2] Although most of these genes have been suggested as potential candidates for the disorder, it has not been possible to unequivocally identify any of the genes as being responsible for the observed phenotype or for any of the individual features in isolation. At this point a question which remains unanswered is whether haploinsufficiency of a single gene is sufficient to produce the complete DGS/VCFs phenotype or whether reduced dosage for several genes is necessary. The identification of numerous genes has merely served to emphasize the challenge inherent in determining which gene(s) is etiologically related to the features seen in affected individuals.

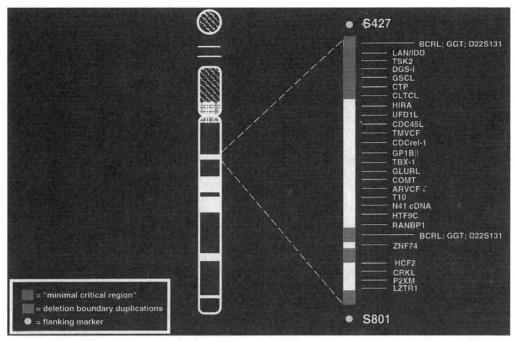

Figure 1. Genes identified in the region most consistently deleted in VCFS. Genes opposite the pink block are in the minimal critical region. Yellow circles identify the flanking markers. Green areas represent the regions containing duplicated sequenced.

In order to determine whether there is an SRO that might indicate a relevant gene, we have analyzed the size of the deletion in numerous patients. We have utilized unique cosmids for anchor loci, and FISH to examine the size and endpoints of the deletions in N25 deleted patients (Fig. 2). We have used a sequential FISH assay using paired FISH probes in two colors to determine the deletion endpoint boundaries. Thus a probe which maps within the deletion at the proximal end, D22S36, and one which flanks the deletion at the distal end, D22S801, are paired in one experiment with a distal 22q cosmid as a control. The companion experiment employs a proximal flanking marker S427 and a distal deleted marker,

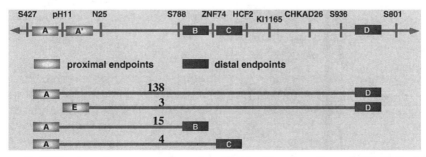

Figure 2. DiGeorge chromosomal region illustrating location of 22q11.2 deletion boundaries. Regions that contain the deletion endpoints are indicated as rectangles. Above the top line are the genes and markers used to identify the cosmids used for FISH experiments. The four lines on the bottom indicate recurrent deletion sizes. The numbers above these lines represent the number of patients identified with those deletion boundaries.

HCF2. In each case one of the two probes from the test region is deleted. This result defines the common large deletion. If one of the internal test probes is not deleted in the first set of FISH experiments, additional markers are applied which are selected from the centromeric or telomeric end of the deletion region as appropriate until a deleted marker is identified.

Using FISH, we have examined the position of the deletion endpoints (DEPs) in 160 patients. One hundred-thirty are part of the sample followed clinically at the Children's Hospital of Philadelphia and 30 were referred from outside institutions. The vast majority of patients (138 or 86.1%) have the common large (~3 Mb) deletion diagnosed by FISH. The deletion is flanked proximally by D22S427 and distally by D22S801 (Fig. 2). Three individuals (2.0%) have deletions which are slightly skewed on the proximal end (A'–D) as they are not deleted for D22S36 but have the same distal endpoint. Fifteen or 9.4% of patients have A–B deletions whose distal deletion endpoints are more centromeric. Four patients (2.5%) have A–C deletions. All of these deletion endpoints appear to cluster in the vicinity of the aforementioned large blocks of duplicated DNA sequence within 22q11.2. Although the numbers are small, we detect no phenotypic differences between the patient groups. From these studies one would be inclined to conclude that the minimal region of deletion overlap should extend from D22S36 to D22S788, the region common to the recurrent breakpoints.

However, we have recently identified a patient (CJ) with a novel deletion which does not overlap with the recurrent deletions. He has features consistent with the 22q11.2 deletion including truncus arteriosus, a broad nasal bridge and tip, hypoplastic alae nasae, a bifid uvula, mild micrognathia, feeding problems, short stature, hypospadias, speech delay, and articulation delay. We performed FISH analysis on the CJ deletion and were surprised to find that the patient was not deleted for any of the markers within the commonly deleted region including D22S75 (N25), D22S788, ZNF74, HCF2, and cHKAD26. However, he is deleted for D22S801. His deletion has as its proximal boundary the distal endpoint of the commonly deleted region whereas his distal deletion endpoint is in the vicinity of another more distal duplicated sequence block which contains the BCRL4 and GGTL repeats. The location of duplicated sequence blocks in the vicinity of his and the other 22q11.2 DEPs strongly implicates the duplicated sequence blocks in the events leading to deletion.

Thus, a composite 22q11 breakpoint map is beginning to emerge, which begins to confound the concept of a SRO for the 22q11 deletion. There are numerous typical deletions and several recurrent variants. However, there are several unique patients whose deletions do not overlap the SRO, including the patients reported by Kurahashi et al.,[13] O'Donnell et al.,[14] McQuade et al.,[15] and patient "g" reported by Levy et al.[16] In addition, new and intriguing deletions are those of CJ and that of a family reported by Rauch et al. at the David Smith meeting (1998) whose deletions appear not to overlap with the others which have been seen. These two novel deletions would appear to involve the more distal duplicated sequence blocks. The significance of these deletions with regard to genes etiologic to the phenotype remains to be determined. Thus, several nonoverlapping regions can now be implicated in the etiology of the phenotype. These deletions are seen in patients with conotruncal cardiac defects. Thus, this suggests that it is unlikely that a single gene within the common deletion region is responsible either for the entire phenotype or for the cardiac defects and indicates that perhaps a more complex mechanism may need to be sought.

Acknowledgements: These studies were supported in part by DC02027 and HL51533 from the National Institutes of Health, Grant H9605 from the W.W. Smith Charitable Trust (L.M.) and funds from the Letitia Scott endowed chair of the Children's Hospital of Philadelphia (B.S.E.).

References

1. Driscoll DA, Emanuel BS. DiGeorge and velocardiofacial syndromes: The 22q11 deletion syndrome. *Ment Retard Dev Dis Res Rev* 1996;2:130–138.
2. Budarf ML, Emanuel BS. Progress in the autosomal segmental aneusomy syndromes (SASs): Single or multi-locus disorders? *Hum Mol Genet* 1997;6:1657–1665.
3. Burn J, Goodship J. Congenital heart disease. In *Emery and Rimoin's Principles and Practice of Medical Genetics*. New York: Churchill Livingstone; 1996:767–803.
4. Goldmuntz E, Clark BJ, Mitchell LE, et al. Frequency of 22q11 deletions in patients with conotruncal defects. *J Am Coll Cardiol* 1998;32:492–498.
5. Leana-Cox J, Pangkanon S, Eanet KR, et al. Familial DiGeorge/velocardiofacial syndrome with deletions of chromosome area 22q11: Report of five families with a review of the literature. *Am J Med Genet* 1996;65:309–316.
6. Ryan AK, Goodship JA, Wilson DI, et al. Spectrum of clinical features associated with interstitial chromosome 22q11 deletions: A European collaborative study. *J Med Genet* 1997;34:798–804.
7. McDonald-McGinn DM, LaRossa D, Goldmuntz E, et al. The 22q11.2 deletion: Screening, diagnostic workup, and outcome of results; report on 181 patients. *Genetic Testing* 1997;1:99–108.
8. Budarf M, Canaani E, Emanuel BS. Linear order of the four BCR-related loci in 22q11. *Genomics* 1988;3:168–171.
9. Collins JE, Mungall AJ, Badcock KL, et al. The organization of the γ-glutamyl transferase genes and other low copy repeats in human chromosome 22q11. *Genome Res* 1997;7:522–531.
10. Emanuel BS, Budarf ML, Scambler PJ. The genetic basis of conotruncal cardiac defects: The chromosome 22q11.2 Deletion. Chapter in R Harves, N Rosenthal (eds) *Heart Development*. Academic Press, New York.
11. Budarf ML, Eckman B, Michaud D, et al. Regional localization of over 300 loci on human chromosome 22 using a somatic cell hybrid mapping panel. *Genomics* 1996;35:275–288.
12. Gong W, Emanuel BS, Collins J, et al. A transcription map of the DiGeorge and velo-cardio-facial syndrome minimal critical region on 22q11. *Hum Mol Genet* 1996; 5:789–800.
13. Kurahashi H, Nakayama T, Osugi Y, et al. Deletion mapping of 22q11 in CATCH22 syndrome: Identification of a second critical region. *Am J Hum Genet* 1996;58: 1377–1881.
14. O'Donnell H, McKeown C, Gould C, et al. Detection of a deletion within 22q11 which has no overlap with the DiGeorge syndrome critical region. *Am J Hum Genet* 1997;60:1544–1548.
15. McQuade LR, Christodoulou J, Sachdev R, et al. Two further cases of 22q11 deletions with no overlap to the DiGeorge syndrome critical region. *Am J Hum Genet* 1998;63: A335.
16. Levy A, Demczuk S, Aurias A, et al. Interstitial 22q11 deletion excluding the ADU breakpoint in a patient with DGS. *Hum Mol Genet* 1995;4:2417–2418.

60

Genotype-Phenotype Correlations in del 22q11.2 Syndrome and Long QT Syndrome

Rumiko Matsuoka, MD, Michiko Furutani, BSc,
Misa Kimura, MS, Kaoru Akimoto, MD, PhD,
Gail A. Robertson, PhD Shin-ichiro Imamura, DVM, PhD,
Toshimitsu Shibata, MD, Shinsei Minoshima, PhD,
Nobuyoshi Shimizu, PhD, Peter J. Scambler, PhD,
Hiroyuki Yamagishi, MD, Kunitaka Joh-o, MD,
Atsuyoshi Takao, MD, and Kazuo Momma, MD

To investigate molecular and clinical aspects of conotruncal anomaly face (CAF), we studied the correlation between deletion size and phenotype and the mode of inheritance in 183 CAF syndrome (CAFS) patients. For the phenotypic study, we added dysmorphism of the nose, which appears to be divided into two parts (upper part and lower part) at the joint of the wing and sides of the nose, to the typical facial features of CAF (Fig. 1a).[1] This makes physical diagnosis of del22q11.2 syndrome more certain, and indicates that CAFS is the same pathological entity as velocardiofacial syndrome (VCFS).[2] In our study, the clinical condition of DiGeorge syndrome (DGS) patients, such as the frequency of cardiovascular anomalies and increased susceptibility to some infectious diseases, was more variable and severe than that of CAFS patients. In CAFS patients, the most frequently observed anomaly was tetralogy of Fallot (TOF) (74%). Conversely, in DGS probands with deletion of 22q11.2, the most frequent cardiovascular anomalies found were interruption of the aortic arch type B (41%), and TOF (29%).[2]

Hemizygosity for a region of 22q11.2 was found in 180 (98%) of the patients with CAFS by fluorescent in situ hybridization (FISH), using 20 DiGeorge critical region probes. Figure 1b shows 180 of the patients with CAFS (162) or DGS (18). Ninety-one percent had a distal breakpoint (type A), 4% had an intermediate breakpoint (type B), and 6% more proximal breakpoints (types C, D, and E). All DGS and CAFS patients with schizophrenia fell into the type-A group. Nineteen of 143 families (13%) had familial CAFS and 16 affected parents (84%) were mothers. However, no familial cases were found among CAFS patients with absent thymus/DGS, which indicates that extragenic factors may play a role in the genesis of phenotypic variability, especially in patients with cardiovascular anomalies. Also, no difference in deletion size was

From Clark EB, Nakazawa M, Takao A (eds.): Etiology and Morphogenesis of Congenital Heart Disease: Twenty Years of Progress in Genetics and Developmental Biology. Armonk, NY: Futura Publishing Co., Inc.; © 2000.

a

CAFS

DGS

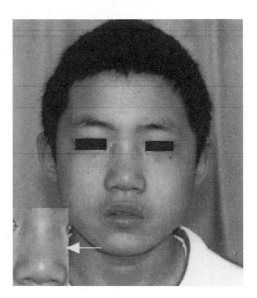

b

	Type		Deletion size(MB)	Probes	Patient number	Frequency
CAFS	A-I	1	3		141	87% (141/162)
		2	2.8		2	1% (2/162)
		3	1.3		1	1% (1/162)
	A-II	1	2.8		3	2% (3/162)
	B	1	2.5		5	3% (5/162)
		2	2		1	1% (1/162)
	C	1	2		6	4% (6/162)
	D	1	1.5		1	1% (1/162)
	E	1	1.3		2	1% (2/162)
DGS	A-I	1	3		17	100% (18/18)
		2	2.5		1	

Probes: a b c d e f g h i j k l m n o p q r s t u

Figure 1. Typical conotruncal anomaly face of conotruncal anomaly face syndrome (CAFS) and DiGeorge syndrome (DGS) patients. Arrows show the new description of nose that appears to be divided into two parts (upper part and lower part) at the joint

found among the same family members in the familial CAFS cases, although they had different phenotypes (type A, 53%; type B, 32%; type C, 16%). The findings of this study indicated that CAF was almost always associated with the deletion of 22q11.2. As well as the major features of the syndrome, other notable extracardiac anomalies were found to be susceptibility to infection, schizophrenia, atrophy or dysmorphism of the brain, thrombocytopenia, short stature, facial palsy, anal atresia, and mild limb abnormalities. An overlap of similar but varied phenotypes, including both the facial characteristics and structural anomalies, was seen in CAFS, DGS, VCFS, and Opitz GBBB syndrome. We named the four syndromes with a deletion of the 22q11.2 region (i.e., CAFS, VCFS, DGS, and Opitz GBBB) del22q11.2 syndrome.

Congenital long QT syndrome (LQTS) includes LQT1, LQT2, and LQT3, in which the syndrome is linked to chromosome 15, 7, and 3, respectively.[7] Four disease genes of LQTS were reported.[7] Interestingly, each different mutation of the disease genes shows different clinical features. For example, some mutations of the SCN5A gene will represent LQTS and another mutation of this gene represents idiopathic ventricular fibrillation, so-called Brugada syndrome.[8] In order to make criteria for the types of LQTS, before we start to analyze a gene, we have the patient take an exercise test with a Holter-electrocardiogram and then we calculate the QaT/RR interval correlation.[9] The slope of LQT1 seems to be gentle. Patients with this gentle QaT/RR slope (less than 0.2) were prone to have a cardiac accident during exercise. On the other hand, patients with LQT2 who underwent the exercise test showed a similar slope to normal controls. These criteria are very useful for identifying which of the four disease genes are involved in LQTS. Before we start to analyze a gene, we check the QaT slope during exercise, evaluate LQT1 or LQT2 and then perform gene analysis. Figure 2a shows electrocardiograms of a patient. The tracings of the II, aVF, and V5 leads show a low T-wave, which is characteristic for LQT2. This patient had episodes of syncope and the QaT slope during exercise was within normal limits, indicating that this patient may have a human *ether-a-go-go*-related gene *(HERG)* mutation.

Mutations in the *HERG*, which is responsible for the rapid component of the delayed rectifier current (I_{Kr}), cause the disease in the LQT2 families.[7] We recently reported a novel missense mutation of *HERG* (G601S) in an LQTS family.[10] In order to find genotype-phenotype correlations, we performed an electrocardiographic analysis on members of this family using Holter recording during exercise. Also, to elucidate their electrophysiological properties, we expressed the G601S mutant channels in mammalian cells and *Xenopus* oocytes. The properties of the G601S mutant current in human embryonic kidney 293 (HEK293) cells showed a characteristic inward rectifying outward current similar to the wild-type HERG, but the current density was only 15.5% of that of the wild-type HERG. Our results with *Xenopus* oocytes are consistent with those in cultured cells. Doubling the amount of RNA injected from 1.25 to 2.5 ng resulted in a 78% increase for wild-type currents and a 75% increase for G601S currents. The currents from coinjected oocytes as expected exhibited an

of the wing and side of nose (**a**). The deletion size of 22q11.2 in 162 CAFS patients and 18 DGS patients (**b**). Five types (A, B, C, D, and E) of deletion on the telomere side of the chromosome were observed. All DGS patients had the same A type of deletion (gray) on the telomere side. Chromosome 22q11.2 region probes for fluorescent in situ hybridization: a, N72H9 (D22S181)[2]; b, KeioBAC298H8; c, scl1.1a (D22S139)[2]; d, 46A9(ADU)[3]; e, 87H3[3]; f, 18C3[3]; g, 111F11[3]; h, N25 (D22S75)[2]; i, 79H12[3]; j, 15A10[3]; k, 59C10[3]; l, C443 (D22S941)[2]; m, H160b[4]; n, D0832[5]; o, sc4.1 (D22S134)[2]; p, R32[3]; q, scl1.1b (D22S139)[2]; r, N19B3 (D22S264)[2]; s, N122B5 (D22S934)[2]; t, CHKAD26[6]; and u, N77F7 (D22S939)[2]. KeioBAC298H8 clone (**b**) was screened from the Keio BAC library.

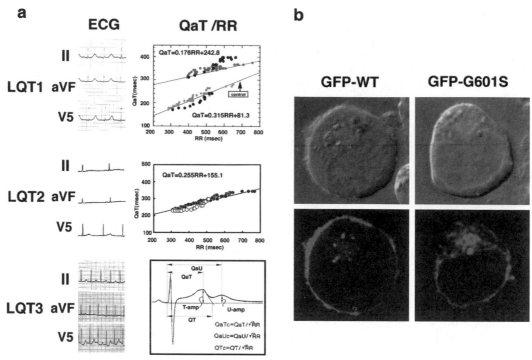

Figure 2. Electrocardiogram and QaT/RR slope of long QT syndrome patients (**a**). Confocal imaged GFP-tagging of G601S and wild-type HERG channels (**b**). The upper panels exhibit merged images of Nomarski with GFP fluorescence; and the lower panels, GFP fluorescence images. A wild-type HERG protein (GFP-WT) signal was present intracellularly in the endoplasmic reticulum and perinuclear space, and in the plasma membrane. The unstained region within the cell is the nucleus. For the G601S mutation (GFP-G601S), the signal was present, intracellularly, but with a reduced plasma membrane signal. See color appendix.

additive effect of the two RNA species alone, thus indicating that the G601S mutant subunit does not interact in a dominant-negative manner with HERG. This mutant produces less current than wild-type channels, with no change in kinetic properties and without the dominant-negative suppression of the wild-type subunits. Also, to examine the cellular trafficking of mutant HERG channel subunits, enhanced green fluorescent protein tagging analysis was performed. A decreased percentage of the G601S mutant HERG channel on the cell surface was observed compared to that of the wild-type HERG channel (Fig. 2b).

Our results from both the *Xenopus* oocyte and HEK293 cell expression systems support the idea that HERG G601S is a hypomorphic mutation resulting in a reduced current amplitude, suggesting an additional, novel mechanism underlying LQT2.

Materials and Methods

Patients

CAFS: 148 probands including 127 de novo patients (86%) and 21 familial CAFS patients (14%) (75 males and 73 females; ages ranged from one month to 35 years) and 147 of their family members (55 fathers, 84 mothers, 5 brothers, 2 sisters, and 1 child). CAFS with completely absent thymus/DGA: 18 probands (10 males and 8 females; ages ranged from 10 days to 18 years) and 26 of their family members (12 fathers and 14 mothers).

FISH

FISH was performed as described previously[2] using 20 DiGeorge critical region probes.[2-6]

QaT Measurement

The measurements of QaT on electrocardiograms of LQTS patients were performed as described previously.[9]

Transfection and Voltage Clamp

For expression in mammalian cells, we used HEK293 cells. The cells were transfected using the lipofectamine method (Gibco-BRL, Sparks, MD) with 2.5 mg of the following: wild-type HERG/pcDNA3, G601S HERG/pcDNA3, the GFP tagged wild-type HERG channel (GFP-WT), G601S mutant HERG (GFP-G601S), and pEGFP-C2. Electrical recording was performed 48 hours after initiation of the transfection. The whole-cell voltage-clamp method used was the same as that described previously.[11-13] Oocytes cells injected with 1.25 ng of RNA were injected with 18.4 nL of the same batch of RNA. Oocytes were stored at 18°C in ND-96 solution[14] supplemented with 1mM gentamycin and 1mg/mL BSA. Two-electrode voltage clamp recordings were performed at room temperature, 1 to 4 days postinjection, as previously described.[15]

Laser Confocal Microscopy

Cells were cultured for 36 to 48 hours after transfection and photographed at 1,000 magnification under a microscope LSM510 (Zeiss, North York, Ontario). Confocal analysis was performed using an argon-krypton laser. The cells were observed after being treated with 0.1% trypsin (which causes the cells to become round) and resuspended in phosphate buffered saline.

References

1. Kinouchi A, Mori K, Ando M, et al. Facial appearance of patients with conotruncal anomalies. *Pediatr Jpn* (in Japanese) 1976;17:84.
2. Matsuoka R, Kimura M, Scambler PJ, et al. Molecular and clinical study of 183 patients with conotruncal anomaly face syndrome. *Hum Genet* 1998;103:70–80.
3. Gong W, Emanuel BS, Collins J, et al. A transcription map of the DiGeorge and velo-cardio-facial syndrome minimal critical region on 22q11. *Hum Mol Genet* 1996; 5:789–800.
4. Goldmuntz E, Driscoll D, Budarf ML, et al. Microdeletions of chromosomal region 22q11 in patients with congenital conotruncal cardiac defects. *J Med Genet* 1993;30:807–812.
5. Halford S, Wadey R, Roberts C, et al. Isolation of a putative transcriptional regulator from the region of 22q11 deleted in DiGeorge syndrome, Shprintzen syndrome and familial congenital heart disease. *Hum Mol Genet* 1993;2:2099–2107.
6. Kurahashi H, Akagi K, Karakawa K, et al. Isolation and mapping of cosmid markers on human chromosome 22, including one within the submicroscopically deleted region of DiGeorge syndrome. *Hum Genet* 1994;93:248–254.
7. Roden DM, Lazzara R, Rosen M, et al. Multiple mechanisms in the long-QT syndrome: Current knowledge, gaps, and future directions. *Circulation* 1996;94:1996–2012.
8. Schott J-J, Benson DW, Basson CT, et al. Congenital heart disease caused by mutations in the transcription factor NKX2–5. *Science* 1998;281:108–111.
9. Shibata T, Yamaoka K, Iwamoto M, et al. QaT interval-heart rate relation during exercise in long QT syndrome. Proceedings of the Second World Congress of Pediatric Cardiology and Cardiac Surgery. Armonk, New York: Futura Publishing; 1998:877.
10. Akimoto K, Moro T, Nakazawa R. Novel missense mutation (G601S) of HERG in a Japanese long QT syndrome family. *Hum Mut* Mutation in Brief #75 On-line; 1997. (http://journals.wiley.com/1059–7794/humuann.htm).

11. Hamill OP, Marty A, Neher E, et al. Improved patch-clamp techniques for high-resolution current recording from cells and cell-free membrane patches. *Pflugers Arch* 1981;391:85–100.

12. Hagiwara N, Irisawa H, Kasanuki H, et al. Background current in the sino-atrial node cells of the rabbit heart. *J Physiol* 1992;448:53–72.

13. Matsuda N, Hagiwara N, Shoda M, et al. Enhancement of the L-type Ca2+ current by mechanical stimulation in single rabbit cardiac myocytes. *Circ Res* 1996;78:650–659.

14. Rudy B, Iverson LE. Ion channels. *Methods Enzymol* 1992;207:225–338.

15. London B, Trudeau MC, Newton KP, et al. Two isoforms of the mouse ether-a-go-go-related gene coassemble to form channels with properties similar to the rapidly activating component of the cardiac delayed rectifier K$^+$ current. *Circ Res* 1997;81:870–878.

61

Combined Missense Mutations of the Mitochondrial DNA Gene, β-Cardiac Myosin Heavy-Chain Gene and Cardiac Troponin T Gene in Familial Hypertrophic Cardiomyopathy

Shoichi Arai, BSc, Kunitaka Joh-o, MD,
Michiko Furutani, BSc, Shin-ichiro Imamura, DVM, PhD,
Atsuyoshi Takao, MD, Kazuo Momma, MD,
and Rumiko Matsuoka, MD

Familial hypertrophic cardiomyopathy (HCM) often shows familial aggregation with autosomal dominant inheritance, and is one of the major causes of sudden death in young adults. The severity and distribution of cardiac hypertrophy found in affected individuals varies widely and correlates poorly with the clinical symptoms of dyspnea, angina, or sudden death. Mutations in the human β-cardiac myosin heavy chain (MHC) gene, human cardiac/skeletal essential light chain gene, regulatory light chain gene, α tropomyosin gene and myosin binding protein C gene, cardiac troponin T gene, or cardiac troponin I gene are responsible for familial HCM.[1-9]

We screened for mutations in the β-cardiac MHC gene and cardiac troponin T genes in two HCM families. In one family (family D), all affected members (n = 4) with HCM had a missense mutation of the β-cardiac MHC gene at exon 20 (Gly741 → Trp),[1] and one affected son and his unaffected father had a missense mutation of the cardiac troponin T gene at exon 14 (Lys253 → Arg). The Gly741 → Trp mutation of the β-cardiac MHC gene was not present in 100 unrelated normal subjects. However, the Lys253 → Arg mutation of the cardiac troponin T gene was present in 2 of 100 unrelated normal subjects, and therefore is assumed to be an uncommon neutral polymorphism.[2] In another family (family G), all affected members (n = 4) with HCM and chest pain (n = 1) had the same missense mutation of the β-cardiac MHC gene at exon 20 (Gly741 → Trp).

In these families, various phenotypes were seen in the affected members with HCM. This suggests that the possibility of HCM developing may be determined by some other gene(s) contributing to HCM. Some studies reported that mtDNA mutation is responsible for mitochondrial cardiomyopathy. Therefore, in this study, we performed the screening for mtDNA mutations and histological analyses in affected members of families D and G.

From Clark EB, Nakazawa M, Takao A (eds.): Etiology and Morphogenesis of Congenital Heart Disease: Twenty Years of Progress in Genetics and Developmental Biology. Armonk, NY: Futura Publishing Co., Inc.; © 2000.

a

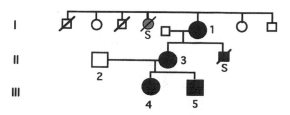

Patient Number	Age(years)/Sex	Clinical Diagnosis	2D-echocardiography				Crisis Age	Missense Mutation		
			PWT (mm)	IVST (mm)	SAM	ASH		β-MHC Gly741Trp	Tn-T Lys253Arg	mtDNA Tyr3394His
1.	63/F	HCM	9	14	+	+	51	+	–	–
2.	45/M	Normal	–	–	–	–	–	–	+	–
3.	44/F	HCM	7	14	+	+	36	+	–	–
4.	19/F	HOCM	7	29	+	+	11	+	–	–
5.	17/M	HOCM ASD	7	22	+	+	9	+	+	–

b

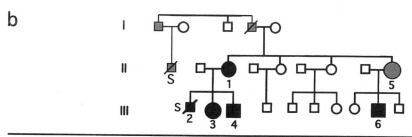

Patient Number	Age(years)/Sex	Clinical Diagnosis	2D-echocardiography				Crisis Age	Missense Mutation	
			PWT (mm)	IVST (mm)	SAM	ASH		β-MHC Gly741Trp	mtDNA Tyr3394His
1.	58/F	HCM	9	14	–	+	47	+	+
2.	13/M	HCM, sudden death					12		
3.	26/F	HCM	9	13	+	+	11	+	+
4.	22/M	HOCM	11	26	+	+	7	+	+
5.	49/F	Chest pain	7	12	–	–	–	+	+
6.	33/M	HOCM	14	30	+	+	13	+	+

Figure 1. a. Results of the pedigree, clinical analysis, and genetic analyses of family D. Two-dimensional echocardiographic findings. PWT, posterior wall thickness; IVST, interventricular septum thickness; SAM, systolic anterior motion of the mitral valve; ASH, asymmetric septal hypertrophy. **b.** The results of the pedigree, clinical analysis, and genetic analyses of family G. Symbols denote sex and disease status: boxes, males; circles, females; solid, affected; clear, unaffected; slashed, deceased; S, sudden death; number, patient number; solid, familial hypertrophic cardiomyopathy; open, normal; gray, suspected hypertrophic cardiomyopathy; HCM, hypertrophic cardiomyopathy; HOCM, hypertrophic obstructive cardiomyopathy; ASD, atrial septal defect.

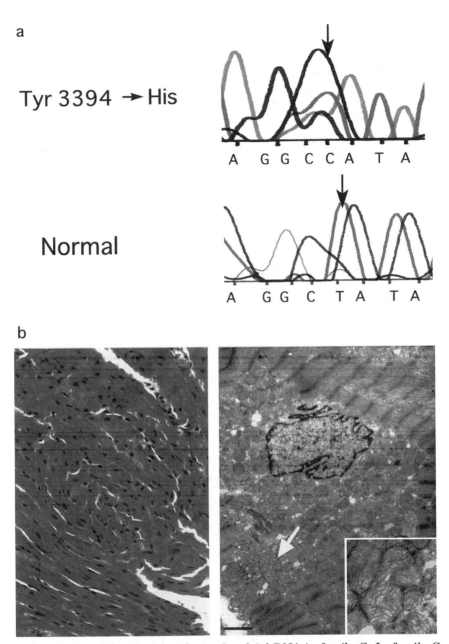

Figure 2. a. Missense mutations of mitochondrial DNA in family G. In family G, one mutation at the evolutionary conservative region at nt 3394 of mtDNA (T-to-C converted) can be detected by the appearance of restriction sites. **b.** The electron micrograph of family G, patient 2. The left panel shows hematoxylin staining. The right panel shows an electron micrograph.

Materials and Methods

Clinical Analysis

Clinical evaluation of family members from these HCM families was performed by history-taking, physical examination, 12-lead electrocardiography, and 2-dimensional echocardiography with a Doppler study. Echocardiographic measurements of wall thickness and cavity dimensions and the presence or absence of systolic anterior motion (SAM) of the mitral valve were determined according to established protocols.[1]

mt-DNA Analysis

We analyzed the direct full sequencing of mtDNA (16569bp) of unaffected members in these two HCM families. DNA was prepared from peripheral blood. The mtDNA amplification was performed as described previously.[10] To identify the mutations, the products were sequenced using an ALF DNA sequencer II (Pharmacia LKB, Gaithersburg, MD). The sequences were compared to the standard Cambridge sequence.[11]

Histological Analysis

Myocardial muscle biopsy samples were stained by hematoxylin and eosin (HE). Electron microscopy of myocardial muscle biopsy samples were also performed.

In the two HCM families, the clinical findings and mitochondrial mutations of family members with HCM, who had the same mutation of the β-cardiac MHC gene were compared (Fig. 1a, b).

In family D, electron micrography was within the normal limits and showed 50 mtDNA mutations, including 8 missense mutations. One mutation was at the evolutionary conservative region (at nt 10398). This missense mutation at nt 10398 of mtDNA (A-to-G) converted the evolutionary conservative amino acid Thr to Ala in the ND3 gene product, and has been previously reported in HCM patients. However, we concluded that this mutation is polymorphic, since more than 30% of normal controls have this mutation. Pathological examinations showed myocyte hypertrophy, and disarray in HE staining, but did not show abnormal mitochondria in an electron micrograph (data not shown).

On the other hand, in family G, one mutation at the evolutionary conservative region at nt 3394 of mtDNA (T-to-C) converted the evolutionary conservative amino acid Tyr to His in the ND1 gene product (Fig. 2a). Pathological examinations showed myocyte hypertrophy and disarray in HE staining and an increased number of pleomorphic giant mitochondria in an electron micrograph (Fig. 2b).

These findings indicate that somatic mtDNA mutations coexist with gene mutations of sarcomeric contractile proteins, such as that of the β-cardiac MHC gene in HCM patients, and may interact, or modify the phenotypes of hypertrophic cardiomyopathy.

References

1. Arai S, Matsuoka R, Takao A, et al. Missense mutation of the β-cardiac myosin heavy-chain gene in hypertrophic cardiomyopathy. *Am J Med Genet* 1995;58:267–276.
2. Watkins H, McKenna WJ, Thierfelder L, et al. Mutations in the genes for cardiac troponin T and α-tropomyosin in hypertrophic cardiomyopathy. *N Engl J Med* 1995; 332:1058–1064.
3. Arbustini E, Fasani R, Morbini P, et al. Coexistence of mitochondrial DNA and β myosin heavy chain mutations in hypertrophic cardiomyopathy with late congestive heart failure. *Heart* 1998;80:548–558.
4. Fananapazir L, Dalakas MC, Cyran F, et al. Missense mutations in the β-myosin heavy-chain gene cause central core disease in hypertrophic cardiomyopathy. *Proc Natl Acad Sci U S A* 1993;90:3993–3997.
5. Marian AJ, Yu Q, Mare A Jr, et al. Detection of a new mutation in the β myosin heavy chain gene in an individual with hypertrophic cardiomyopathy. *J Clin Invest* 1992;90:2156–2165.

6. Watkins H, Thierfelder L, Anan R, et al. Independent origin of identical β cardiomyopathy. *Am J Hum Genet* 1993;53:1180–1185.

7. Thierfelder I, Watkins H, MacRae C, et al. α-tropomyosin, and cardiac troponin T mutations cause familial hypertrophic cardiomyopathy: A disease of the sarcomere. *Cell* 1994;77:701–712.

8. Bonne G, Carrier L, Bercovici J, et al, Cardiac myosin binding protein C gene splice acceptor site mutation is associated with familial hypertrophic cardiomyopathy. *Nat Genet* 1995;11:438–440.

9. Warkins H, Rosenzweig A, Hwang D, et al. Characteristics and prognostic implications of myosin missense mutations in familial hypertrophic cardiomyopathy. *N Engl J Med* 1992;326:1108–1114.

10. Tanaka M, Ozawa T. In: Longstaff R, Revest S, eds. *Protocols in Molecular Neurology*. The Human Press, Totawa, New Jersey; 1992:25–53.

11. Anderson S, Bankier AT, Barrel BG, et al. Sequence and organization of the human mitochondrial genome. *Nature* 1981;290:457–465.

62

Efficient Finding of Disease Genes by Genomic Sequencing of Targeted Chromosomal Regions

Nobuyoshi Shimizu, PhD

Since its official start in 1991, the international human genome project (HGP) has made rapid progress and has accomplished its initial goal, mapping of the human genome. However, there are still enormous tasks to reach the final goal, sequencing of the entire human genome consisting of 3,000 Mb as well as complete understanding of the estimated 100,000 human genes.[1] To facilitate this challenging task, we are taking a systematic gene hunting approach through the Keio strategy which combines several advanced molecular techniques such as exon trapping, cDNA capture and genomic sequencing (Fig. 1). We have cloned and characterized over 150 new human genes (Table 1). Here, we briefly describe the strategies of gene isolation and characteristics of the newly discovered genes.

Strategies of Gene Isolation

We constructed a high quality BAC library and chromosome-specific cosmid libraries[2] and developed efficient PCR screening and high fidelity digital hybridization methods to construct BAC/cosmid DNA contigs.[3] We utilize the shotgun se-

quencing method to completely determine the genomic sequence of each cloned DNA with no gaps and high accuracy (>99.999%) (Kawasaki et al., unpublished). The genomic sequence is routinely subjected to homology search and analysis of protein coding potential using computer programs GRAIL and GENSCAN. Predicted exon sequences are used as probes to screen corresponding cDNA clones or as primers to amplify cDNA fragments from appropriate cDNA libraries by PCR. Eventually, the entire gene structure is determined and the function of its product is predicted by domain analysis.

To complement this approach, we are also performing a cDNA isolation by differential hybridization using a tissue (retina)-enriched cDNA library.[4]

SIM1, SIM2, and MNB for Down Syndrome

SIM2 (single-minded 2) and MNB (minibrain) were the first two genes discovered from the Down syndrome critical region of chromosome 21 and considered to be involved in the mental retardation of the patients.[5,6] SIM2 encodes a PAS family transcription factor and MNB encodes a dual specific protein kinase. Mouse homolog of human SIM2 (mSIM2) was isolated from mouse chromosome 16 and its expression was found to be preferential in

From Clark EB, Nakazawa M, Takao A (eds.): Etiology and Morphogenesis of Congenital Heart Disease: Twenty Years of Progress in Genetics and Developmental Biology. Armonk, NY: Futura Publishing Co., Inc.; © 2000.

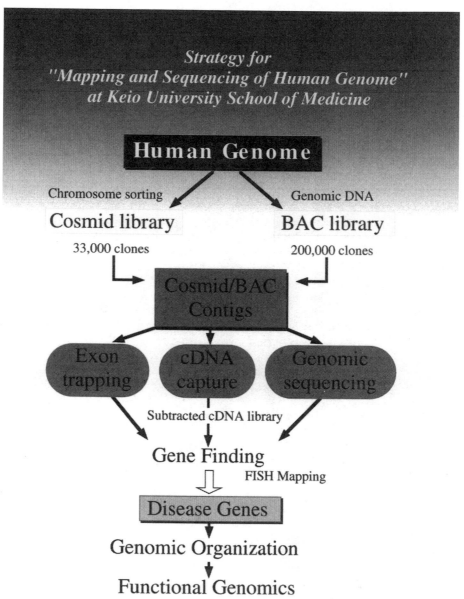

Figure 1. Keio strategy of efficient gene finding.

Table 1
The Newly Discovered Genes and the Genomically Characterized Known Genes
Through Keio Genome Strategy

Genes	Location	Characteristics
SIM2 (single-minded 2/DS)	21q22.2	Transcription factor, 55kb/11 exons
MNB (minibrain/DS)	21q22.2	Dual protein kinase, 150kb/13 exons
HCS (holocarboxylase synthetase)	21q22.2	Biotin-utilizing metabolic pathways
ETS2 (v-ets oncogene homolog)	21q22.2	Oncogene, 17.6 kb/10 exons
TMEM1 (transmembrane protein 1)	21q22.3	Ion channel, 94kb/23 exons
PWP2 (periodic tryptophan protein 2)	21q22.3	Signal Transduction, 24kb/21 exons
KNP-1 (keio novel protein 1)	21q22.3	E. coli SCRP-27A homolog, 12kb/7 exons
KRPC7	21q22.3	Ion channel, 95 kb/32 exons
AIRE (APECED)	21q22.3	Transcription factor, 13kb/15 exons
PFKL (phosphofructokinase, liver)	21q22.3	Glycolysis, 28 kb/22 exons
CSTB (cystatin B/EPM1)	21q22.3	Protease inhibitor, EPM1, 2.5 kb/3 exons
IGLC 1-7 (Igλ constant region 1-7)	22q11	Immunoglobulin light chain λ
IGLV1-69 (Igλ variable region 1-6)	22q11	Immunoglobulin light chain λ
Gene 1	22q11	Protein phosphatase
Gene 2	22q11	DNA topoisomerase
TGFB1P1	22q11	TGF-β1 pseudogene
Gene 3	22q11	Unknown
VPREB1	22q11	V1 related gene
5OY11.1	22q11	Sheep/bovine 5'-OY11.1 homolog
3OY11.1	22q11	Sheep/bovine 3'-OY11.1 homolog
BCRL4	22q11	BCR pseudogene
POM121	22q11	Rat POM121 homolog pseudogene
GGTP1	22q11	GGT pseudogene
GGTP2	22q11	GGT pseudogene
Gλ1	22q11	J-C1 related gene
Parkin (PARK2)	6q25.2-q27	Juvenile Parkinsonism/12 exons
MYOC (myocilin/GLC1A)	1q23-q24	Myosin like protein, 3 exons, Glaucoma
RAO (retina amine oxidase)	17q21	Amine oxidase, 6 kb/4 exons
ISLR (immunoglobulin superfamily containing leucine rich repeat)	15q23-q24	Membrane protein, 2 exons
pMEL17 (melanoma antigen)	12q13-q14	Tyrosinase, Melanin synthesis
SIM1 (single-minded 1)	6q16.3-q21	Transcription factor
GLUL (glutamine synthetase)	1q25	Glutamine synthesis
GLULP (GLUL pseudogene)	9p13	GLUL pseudogene
GLULL1 (GLUL related gene 1)	5q33	GLUL related gene
GLULL2 (GLUL related gene 2)	11p15	GLUL related gene
GLULL3 (GLUL related gene 3)	11q24	GLUL related gene

DS, down syndrome; APECED, autoimmune polyendocrinopathy-candidiasis-ectodermal dystrophy; EPM1, progressive myoclonus epilepsy of Unverricht-Lundborg type; GLC1A, Primary Open Angle Glaucoma (POAG).

diencepharon of the mouse brain whereas MNB is expressed rather ubiquitously in various tissues.[7,8] SIM1 and its mouse homolog was isolated from human chromosome 6q16.3-q21 and mouse chromosome 10, respectively.[9]

AIRE for Autoimmune Disease

AIRE (autoimmune regulator) was isolated from human chromosome 21q22.3 and proven to be a pathogenic gene for an autoimmune disease called APECED (autoimmune polyendocrinopathy-candidiasis-ectodermal dystrophy) and it was the first transcription factor found to be involved in the mechanism of immune tolerance.[10–13] AIRE encodes a transcription factor with SAND and PHD finger motifs and its expression is restricted to thymus, lymphnode and fetal liver which are responsible for the auto immune response (Heino et al., in press). Various mutations were found in the APECED patients of different ethnic origins.[14,15]

PARKIN for Parkinson's Disease

PARKIN (PARK2) was isolated from human chromosome 6q25.2-q27 as a gene responsible for an inherited Parkinson's disease (PD) called AR-JP (autosomal-recessive juvenile parkinsonism).[16] PARKIN is likely to be involved in the sporadic PD, which is now the second most common form of neurodegenerative disease after Alzheimer's, affecting at least 120,000 people in Japan. PARKIN encodes a protein of a relative molecular mass (Mr) 51,652, which has moderate similarity to ubiquitin at the N-terminus, is rich in Cys, and has a motif similar to a RING-finger at the C-terminus. The PARKIN gene consists of 12 exons flanked with unusually large introns, implicating at least 1 Mb in size, a second largest gene ever known after dystrophin. Interestingly, most AR-JP patients have large deletion mutations.[17,18] The Parkin gene

expression is rather ubiquitous among tissues but the AR-JP is pathologically characterized by the loss of nigral and locus coeruleus neurons.[19]

MYOC for Glaucoma

MYOC (myocilin) located on human chromosome 1q23-q24 produces a novel cytoskeletal protein and is now identified to be identical to TIGR, which is the pathogenic gene for a primary open angle glaucoma.[4,20] Mouse homolog of human MYOC was isolated and its expression in ocular tissues was studied.[21]

RAO, ISLR TRPC7 as Candidate Genes

RAO (amine oxidase, retina) located on human chromosome 17q21 is expressed preferentially in ganglion cell layer of retina and proposed to be a strong candidate gene for a hereditary ocular disease.[22,23] ISLR (immunoglobulin superfamily containing leucine-rich domain) located on human chromosome 15q23-q24 appears to be expressed in various tissues and is considered as a candidate gene for Bardet-Biedl syndrome type 4 (Nagasawa et al., unpublished).[24] TRPC7 (transient receptor potential-related channels 7) isolated from human chromosome 21q22.3 encodes a putative Ca^{++} channel transmembrane protein.[25] TRPC7 is considered to be a good candidate gene for bipolar affective disorder.

Other New Genes KNP-I, PDE9A, and BID

KNP-I (Keio novel protein I) isolated from human chromosome 21q22.3 is homologous to the *E. coli* SCRP-27A protein of which function is unclear.[26] PDE9A is also isolated from the 21q22.3 and it encodes a novel cyclic nucleotide phosphodiesterase.[27] BID is a death agonist maps on the duplicated region of 22q11.2 that is associated with the cat eye syndrome.[28]

Genomic Structures of ETS2, HCS, TMEM1, PWP2, CSTB, and PFKL

The contiguous genomic sequences of over 1-Mb regions occassionally locates the previously known cDNA sequences and immediately determines its genomic exon/intron structure. Several genes were in fact analyzed in this way, including the genes such as ETS2 (v-ets oncogene), HCS (holocarboxylase synthetase), TMEM1 (transmembrane protein 1), PWP2 (periodic tryptophan protein 2), CSTB (cystatin B) and PFKL (phosphofructokinase, liver) (see ALIS, http://www-alis.jst.go.jp/). The genomic structure with precise sequence information is being utilized for precise DNA diagnosis of corresponding diseases, particularly HCS deficiency and an epilepsy (CSTB).

Immunoglobulin Light Chain λ (IGL) Gene Cluster

We established the precise genomic organization of immunoglobulin light chain λ (IGL) gene cluster located in human chromosome 22q11 by determining the contiguous genomic sequence of over 1 Mb.[29,30] We found 69 variable segments (IGLV) genes and 7 constant segments (IGLC) genes together with the VpreB gene in this cluster. Unexpectedly, a dozen of non-Ig genes and pseudogenes were found within or outside of the IGL gene cluster, including two novel genes, one for a protein phosphatase and the other for a DNA topoisomerase. These substantial amounts of sequence information are now being analyzed in terms of the generation of gene diversity and distribution of various repeat sequences during molecular evolution.

Prospects

The prospected goal of finishing genomic DNA sequencing has been shifted to the year 2003 and massive efforts are in progress. Meanwhile, we will gain a much better understanding of the human genome which contains a blueprint of our life. The nucleotide sequence information will undoubtedly serve as an essential foundation of the human biology, including the molecular mechanisms of cardiogenesis and heart diseases.

Acknowledgements: The author thanks all the individuals listed as authors of the references for their contributions to the Keio strategy. This study was supported in part by the Ministry of Education, Science, Sports and Culture, Japan Society of Promotion of Science, and Science and Technology Agency.

References

1. Shimizu N. Human genome project: Current status, keio strategy and prospects, In: Uyemura K, Kawamura K, Yazaki T, eds *Frontiers of Neural Development.* Tokyo: Springer/Verlag, 1998:535–540.
2. Asakawa S, Abe I, Kudoh Y, et al. Human BAC library: Construction and rapid screening. *Gene* 1997;191:69–79.
3. Asakawa S, Shimizu N. High-fidelity digital hybridization screening. *Genomics* 1998;49:209–217.
4. Kubota R, Noda S, Wang Y, et al. A nobel myosin-like protein (myocilin) expressed in connecting cilium of photoreceptor: Molecular cloning, tissue expression and chromosomal mapping. *Genomics* 1997;41:360–369.
5. Kudoh J, Chrast R, Rossier C, et al. Single-minded and Down syndrome? *Nat Genet* 1995;10:9–10.
6. Shindoh N, Kudoh J, Maeda H, et al. Cloning of a human homolog of the *Drosophila* minibrain/rat Dyrk gene from "the Down syndrome critical region" of chromosome 21. *Biochem Biophys Res Commun* 1996;225:92–99.
7. Yamaki A, Noda S, Kudoh J, et al. The Mammalian single-minded (SIM) gene: Mouse cDNA structure and diencephalic expression indicate a candidate gene for Down syndrome. *Genomics* 1996;35:136–143.

8. Wang J, Kudoh J, Shintani A, et al. Identification of two novel 5′ noncoding exons in human MNB/DYRK gene and alternatively spliced transcripts. *Biochem Biophys Res Commun* 1998;250:704–710.

9. Chrast R, Scott HS, Chen H, et al. Cloning of two human homologs of the *Drosophila* single-minded gene SIM1 on chromosome 6q and SIM2 on 21q within the Down syndrome chromosomal region. *Genome Res* 1997;7:615–624.

10. Nagamine K, Peterson P, Scott HS, et al. Positional cloning of a novel zinc finger protein, AIR, mutated in autoimmune polyglandular disease type I (APECED). *Nat Genet* 1997;17:393–398.

11. Kudoh J, Nagamine K, Asakawa S, et al. Localization of 16 exons to a 450-kb region involved in the autoimmune polyglandular disease type I (APECED) on human chromosome 21q22.3. *DNA Res* 1997;4:45–52.

12. Peterson P, Nagamine K, Scott H, et al. APECED: A monogenic autoimmune disease providing new clues to self tolerance. *Immunol Today* 1998;19:384–386.

13. Nagamine K, Kudoh J, Kawasaki K, Minoshima S, Asakawa S, Ito F, and Shimizu N. Genomic Organization and Complete Nucleotide Sequence of the TMEM1 Gene on Human Chromosome 21q22.3, Biochem. Biophys. Res. Commun., 235(1):185–190 (1997).

14. Scott HS, Heino M, Peterson P, et al. Common mutations in autoimmune polyendocrinopathy-candidiasis-ectodermal dystrophy (APECED) patients of different origins. *Mol Endocrinol* 1998;12:1112–1119.

15. Rosatelli MC, Meloni A, Devoto M, et al. A common mutation in sardinian autoimmune polyendocrinopathy-candidiasis-ectodermal dystrophy (APECED) patients. *Hum Genet* 1998;103:428–434.

16. Kitada T, Asakawa S, Hattori N, et al. Deletion mutation in PARKIN gene causes autosomal recessive juvenile parkinsonism (AR-JP). *Nature* 1998;392:605–608.

17. Hattori N, Matsumine H, Asakawa S, et al. Point mutations (Thr240Arg and Ala311Stop) in the Parkin gene. *Biochem Biophys Res Commun* 1998;249:754–758.

18. Hattori N, Kitada T, Matsumine H, et al. Molecular genetic analysis of a novel Parkin gene in Japanese families with AR-JP: Evidence for variable homozygous deletions in the Parkin gene in affected individuals. *Ann Neurol,* in press.

19. Shimura H, Hattori N, Kubo S, et al. Immunohistochemical and subcellular localization of Parkin: Absence of protein in AR-JP patients. *Ann Neurol,* 1999; 45:668–672.

20. Kubota R, Kudoh J, Mashima Y, et al. Genomic organization of the human myocilin gene (MYOC) responsible for primary open angle glaucoma. *Biochem Biophys Res Commun* 1998;242:396–400.

21. Takahashi H, Noda S, Imamura Y, et al. Mouse myocilin (Myoc) gene expression in ocular tissues. *Biochem Biophys Res Commun* 1998;248:104–109.

22. Imamura Y, Kubota R, Wang Y, et al. Human retina-specific amine oxidase (RAO): cDNA cloning, tissue expression and chromosomal mapping. *Genomics* 1997;40:277–283.

23. Imamura Y, Noda S, Mashima Y, et al. Human retina-specific amine oxidase: Genomic structure of the gene (AOC2), alternatively spliced variant, and mRNA expression in retina. *Genomics* 1998;51:293–298.

24. Nagasawa A, Kubota R, Imamura Y, et al. Cloning of the cDNA for a new member of the immunoglobulin superfamily (ISLR) containing leucine-rich repeat (LRR). *Genomics* 1997;44:273–279.

25. Nagamine K, Kudoh J, Minoshima S, et al. Molecular cloning of a novel putative Ca2+ channel protein (TRPC7) highly expressed in brain. *Genomics* 1998;540:124–131.

26. Nagamine K, Kudoh J, Minoshima S, et al. Isolation of cDNA for a novel human protein KNP-I that is homologous to the *E. coli* SCRP-27A protein from the autoimmune polyglandular disease type I (APECED) region of chromosome 21q22.3. *Biochem Biophys Res Commun* 1996;225:608–616.

27. Guipponi M, Scott HS, Kudoh J, et al. Identification and characterization of a novel cyclic nucleotide phosphodiesterase gene (PDE9A) that maps to 21q22.3; alternative splicing of mRNA transcripts, genomic structure and sequence. *Hum Genet* 1998;103:386–392.

28. Footz TK, Birren B, Minoshima S, et al. The gene for death agonist BID maps to the region of human 22q11.2 duplicated in cat eye syndrome chromosomes and to mouse chromosome 6. *Genomics* 1998;51:472–475.

29. Kawasaki K, Minoshima S, Schooler K, et al. The organization of the human immunoglobulin λ gene locus. *Genome Res* 1995;5:125–135.

30. Kawasaki K, Minoshima S, Mine E, et al. One megabase sequence analysis of the human immunoglobulin λ gene locus. *Genome Res* 1997;7:250–261.

63

Genetics of Ventricular Arrhythmias

Jeffrey A. Towbin, MD

Ventricular arrhythmias are common pathways leading to sudden death, with 300,000 to 400,000 sudden deaths attributed to ventricular arrhythmias every year in the United States alone.[1] Until recently, the underlying causes of these devastating clinical disorders were unknown. The goal of this presentation is to outline the current understanding of the genetic aspects of ventricular arrhythmias.

The best understood disorder responsible for primary ventricular arrhythmias is the long QT syndromes (LQTS),[2] which typically present clinically with syncope (commonly associated with emotional or physical stress or acoustic triggers), seizures, and ventricular tachyarrhythmias including polymorphous ventricular tachycardia or torsade de pointes. In these patients, the electrocardiogram (ECG) usually is characterized by prolongation of the QT interval corrected for heart rate (QTc) to >460 msec, abnormal T waves, and bradycardia.[2] Most commonly, patients with LQTS are sporadic or demonstrate an autosomal dominant inheritance pattern[2] as initially described by Romano et al.[3] in 1963 and O.C. Ward[4] in 1964. Less commonly, autosomal recessive inheritance associated with sensorineural deafness, as initially described in 1957 by Jervell and Lange-Nielsen,[5] may be observed. Furthermore in sporadic

cases, LQTS may be an acquired phenomenon, particularly when associated with various medications such as antiarrhythmic agents (quinidine, procainamide, etc.), antibiotics such as erythromycin, cisapride, and terfenadine (antihistamine), amongst others.[2]

During the past decade, the molecular mechanisms underlying LQTS have started to become unraveled. After the initial mapping of the first LQTS locus to chromosome 11 by Keating et al.[6] and the subsequent identification of genetic heterogeneity by Towbin et al.,[7] five genetic loci and four genes responsible for LQTS were identified. These genes, all of which have been shown to encode ion channels (Table 1), result in abnormal repolarization when mutated. The first gene, KVLQT1, also known as LQT1, was initially mapped to chromosome 11p15.5 by Keating et al.[6] and later cloned by Wang et al.[8] Sequence analysis identified a potassium channel-encoding gene and, since its identification, KVLQT1 has been shown to be the most common cause of LQTS, with more than 50 separate mutations identified thus far. Electrophysiological and biophysical analysis has shown that the KVLQT1 channel has the electrophysiological characteristics of the slowly activated delayed rectifier potassium channel I_{Ks} but requires the association of a β subunit in order to function properly. This β subunit was shown by Barhanin et al.[9] and Sanguinetti et al.[10] to be encoded by the KCNE1 gene on chromosome 21q22, which encodes the minK potassium channel, now known as LQT5. Not only is

From Clark EB, Nakazawa M, Takao A (eds.): Etiology and Morphogenesis of Congenital Heart Disease: Twenty Years of Progress in Genetics and Developmental Biology. Armonk, NY: Futura Publishing Co., Inc.; © 2000.

Table 1
Characteristics of the Genes Responsible for the Long QT Syndromes

Locus Name	Location	Gene Name	Gene Product
LQT1	11p15.5	KVLQT1	K$^+$ Channel (I$_{Ks}$)
LQT2	7q35	HERG	K$^+$ Channel (I$_{Kr}$)
LQT3	3p21.3	SCN5A	Na$^+$ Channel (I$_{Na}$)
LQT4	4q25-q27	?	?
LQT5	21q22	minK (KCNE1)	K$^+$ Channel (I$_{Ks}$)
JLN1	11p15.5	KVLQT1	K$^+$ Channel (I$_{Ks}$)
JLN2	21q22	minK (KCNE1)	K$^+$ Channel (I$_{Ks}$)

minK required for proper functioning of KVLQT1 and hence I$_{Ks}$, but mutations in minK itself can also result in the LQTS phenotype,[11] albeit an uncommon cause of LQTS. In both KVLQT1 and KCNE1 (minK), the most common type of mutation is missense and is heterozygous, resulting in the Romano-Ward syndrome with autosomal dominant inheritance. However, when either of these genes have homozygous mutations, the Jervell and Lange-Nielsen syndrome[12–14] with its associated sensorineural deafness occurs. Most commonly, the deafness appears to have autosomal recessive inheritance (in other words, it requires both alleles to be mutated in order for deafness to occur), while LQTS is autosomal dominant with a more severe phenotype occurring with the homozygous mutations. We recently identified an Amish family, however, in which both deafness and LQTS appeared to behave as autosomal recessive traits.[15]

Another gene responsible for LQTS, the LQT2 gene, was initially mapped to chromosome 7q35-q36 before being identified as the *human ether-a-go-go-related gene* (HERG), a potassium channel-encoding gene, via positional candidate gene cloning by Curran et al.[16] Biophysical analysis identified this gene to encode the rapidly activated delayed rectifier potassium channel I$_{Kr}$,[17] the channel that is blocked by the majority of drugs that cause the acquired form of LQT2. This gene appears to be the second most commonly mutated gene causing LQTS and, in most cases, results from a dominant negative mechanism. Potassium channels require formation of a tetrameric unit, which occurs by the coalescence of four separate α subunits. When an abnormal α subunit is utilized along with the wild-type α subunits, the abnormal α subunit can act as a "poison pill," causing abnormal functioning of the entire tetramer. This mechanism, which may also occur in KVLQT1, appears to depend somewhat on the position of the mutation. Also notable, minK appears to interact with HERG in a regulatory fashion, although the details of this interaction are not yet certain.

The final gene thus far identified and characterized in LQTS is the so-called LQT3 gene, which was initially mapped to chromosome 3p21 before positional candidate gene cloning determined it to be the cardiac sodium channel gene SCN5A.[18] This gene, which appears to be responsible for a small number of LQTS cases, most commonly results in the LQTS phenotype via a gain-of-function mechanism. Here, the mutation causes a defect in the inactivation gate, which results in persistent flow of sodium ions across the channel, resulting in prolongation of the QT interval and a risk of torsade de pointes. SCN5A is a large gene that encodes the entire tetrameric sodium channel protein I$_{Na}$. Recently it has been shown by my laboratory that mutations in certain positions of this gene may result in a completely different phenotype than LQTS (Fig. 1) but still result in ventricular tachyarrhythmias.[18] We showed that certain mutations result in ECG findings of ST segment elevation in leads V1–V3, a right bundle branch pattern in some cases, and ventricular fibrillation.[19] This series of findings were previously described by Brugada and Brugada,[20] and is

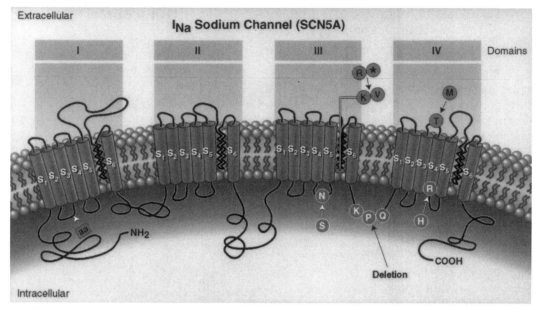

Figure 1. The cardiac sodium channel gene (INa), a tetrameric protein encoded by SCN5A, is mutated in different portions of the gene in LQT3 (S→N, ΔKPQ deletion, H→R amino acid changes) and Brugada syndrome (aa insertion, R*→KV, and M→T), resulting in different clinical phenotypes. (Reprinted with permission from Reference 19.)

now known as the Brugada syndrome. A similar disorder common to Southeast Asia, known as sudden unexpected nocturnal death syndrome (SUNDS), is believed likely to be due to mutations in this gene as well. Interestingly, mutations in SCN5A causing Brugada syndrome appear to result in different biophysical abnormalities when compared to LQT3. In fact, one of the mutants has been shown to cause a more rapid channel inactivation, a nearly opposite effect to that reported for some LQT3 mutations.[19]

To date, the LQT4 gene, mapped by Schott et al.[21] to chromosome 4, has remained elusive. In addition, a sixth gene (and probably others) remains to be identified, as several families are not linked to LQT1-LQT5 loci.

Genotype-phenotype correlations in these ion channelopathies have been reported during the past several years. Moss et al.[22] evaluated the ECGs of patients with known genotypes and demonstrated different ECG patterns based on genotype. Although not completely correl-

ative, the ability to predict the abnormal gene by ECG is reasonably high. However, the best predictor appears to be the T wave. Vincent et al.[23] showed that the QTc interval is problematic for the diagnosis in that a significant percentage of gene carriers have QTc intervals within the normal range of 410–460 msec. The underlying reason for this normal QTc despite abnormal genes is not yet known. In some families with known genetic mutations, in fact, some gene carriers have distinctly prolonged QTc intervals while others are within this normal range. It is not clear whether there are differences in outcome.

Schwartz et al.[24] first showed the clinical utility of genotype analysis when they correlated mutant gene status and potentially specific therapeutic options. Comparing patients with LQT3 (SCN5A) and LQT2 (HERG), they showed that addition of mexiletine (a sodium channel blocker) to the therapeutic regimen resulted in a dramatic shortening of the QTc in LQT3 and, in some cases, T wave normalization. In addition, they also showed that exercise shortened the QTc in the LQT3 patients. LQT2 patients were unaffected by both mexiletine and exercise. This has been confirmed by others using other sodium channel blockers (lidocaine, tocainide). Later, increasing the serum potassium level to >4.5–4.8 using exogenous potassium and/or potassium-sparing agents, was found to shorten the QTc in LQT2 patients and potassium channel openers have also been shown to shorten the QTc in these patients. In none of these studies, however, has improvement in symptoms or reduction in sudden death been shown thus far.

Finally, Zareba et al.[25] recently showed that genotype correlates with clinical presentation and outcome. Studying 541 members of 38 families, 112 LQT1 mutations, 72 LQT2 mutations, and 62 LQT3 mutations were identified and phenotype correlations were performed. The frequency of cardiac events was highest among LQT1 mutation carriers (63%) and LQT2 mutation carriers (46%) versus those with mutations in LQT3 (18%). The genotype and QTc were significant independent predictors of a first cardiac event as well. The cumulative mortality through age 40 years was similar for all three gene carriers but the likelihood of dying during an event was significantly higher among those with mutations of LQT3 (20%) than among those with LQT1 (4%) or LQT2 (4%) mutations. These data also suggest that the severe nature of the clinical findings of Brugada syndrome are due, in significant part, to the mutations in this same gene.

In summary, excellent progress in the understanding of the molecular basis of ventricular arrhythmias has been seen during the decade of the 1990s. The results of this progress include the understanding that the final common pathway to ventricular arrhythmias is related to ion channel abnormalities and this knowledge is likely to lead to improved premorbid diagnosis and new therapeutic options.

References

1. Willich SN, Levy D, Rocco MB, et al. Circadian variation in the incidence of sudden cardiac death in the Framingham heart study population. *Am J Cardiol* 1987;60: 801–806.
2. Schwartz PJ, Locati EN, Napolitano C, et al. The long QT syndrome. In: Zipes DP, Jalife J, eds. *Cardiac Electrophysiology from Cell to Bedside*. New York: WB Saunders; 1995:788–811.
3. Romano C. Congenital cardiac arrhythmia. *Lancet* 1965;I:658–659.
4. Ward OC. A new familial cardiac syndrome in children. *J Ir Med Assoc* 1964;54: 103–106.
5. Jervell A, Lange-Nielsen F. Congenital deaf mutism, functional heart disease with prolongation of the QT interval, and sudden death. *Am Heart J* 1957;54:59–78.
6. Keating MT, Atkinson D, Dunn C, et al. Linkage of a cardiac arrhythmia, the long QT syndrome, and the Harvey *ras-1* gene. *Science* 1991;252:704–706.
7. Towbin JA, Li H, Moss AJ, et al. Evidence of genetic heterogeneity in Romano-Ward Long QT Syndrome: Analysis of 23 families. *Circulation* 1994;90:2635–2644.
8. Wang Q, Curran ME, Splawski I, et al. Positional cloning of a novel potassium channel gene: *KVLQT1* mutations cause cardiac arrhythmias. *Nat Genet* 1996;12: 17–23.
9. Barhanin J, Lesage F, Guillemare E, et al. *KVLQT1* and *IsK* (*minK*) proteins associate to form the I_{Ks} cardiac potassium current. *Nature* 1996;384:78–80.
10. Sanguinetti MC, Curran ME, Zou A, et al. Coassembly of *KVLQT1* and *minK* (*IsK*) proteins to form cardiac I_{Ks} potassium channel. *Nature* 1996;384:80–83.
11. Splawski I, Tristani-Firouzi M, Lehmann MH, et al. Mutations in the *hminK* gene cause long QT syndrome and supress I_{Ks} function. *Nat Genet* 1997;17:338–340.
12. Neyroud N, Tesson F, Denjoy I, et al. A novel mutation on the potassium channel gene *KVLQT1* causes the Jervell and Lange-Nielsen cardioauditory syndrome. *Nat Genet* 1997;15:186–189.
13. Schulze-Bahr E, Wang Q, Wedekind H, et al. KCNE1 mutations cause Jervell and Lange-Nielsen syndrome. *Nat Genet* 1997; 17:267–268.
14. Tyson J, Tranebjaerg L, Bellman S, et al. IsK and KvLQT1: Mutation in either of the two subunits of the slow component of

the delayed rectifier potassium channel can cause Jervell and Lange-Nielsen syndrome. *Hum Mol Genet* 1997;12:2179–2185.

15. Chen Q, Zhang D, Gingell RL, et al. Homozygous deletion in KVLQT1 associated with Jervell and Lange-Nielsen Syndrome. *Circulation* 1999;99(10):1344–1347.

16. Curran ME, Splawski I, Timothy KW, et al. A molecular basis for cardiac arrhythmia: *HERG* mutations cause long QT syndrome. *Cell* 1995;80:795–803.

17. Sanguinetti MC, Jiang C, Curran ME, et al. A mechanistic link between an inherited and an acquired cardiac arrhythmia: *HERG* encodes the I_{Kr} potassium channel. *Cell* 1995;81:299–307.

18. Wang Q, Shen J, Splawski I, et al. *SCN5A* mutations associated with an inherited cardiac arrhythmia, long QT syndrome. *Cell* 1995;80:805–811.

19. Chen Q, Kirsch GE, Zhang D, et al. Genetic basis and molecular mechanisms for idiopathic ventricular fibrillation. *Nature* 1998;392:293–296.

20. Brugada P, Brugada J. Right bundle branch block, persistent ST segment elevation and sudden cardiac death: A distinct clinical and electrocardiographic syndrome. *J Am Coll Cardiol* 1992;20:1391–1396.

21. Schott J, Charpentier F, Peltier S, et al. Mapping of a gene for long QT syndrome to chromosome 4q25–27. *Am J Hum Genet* 1995;57:1114–1122.

22. Moss AJ, Zareba W, Benhorin J, et al. T-wave patterns in genetically distinct forms of the hereditary long-QT syndrome. *Circulation* 1995;92:2929–2934.

23. Vincent GM, Timothy KW, Leppert MF, et al. The spectrum of symptoms and QT intervals in carriers of the gene for the long QT syndrome. *N Engl J Med* 1992;327:846–852.

24. Schwartz PJ, Priori SG, Locati E, et al. Long QT syndrome patients with mutations of the *SCN5A* and *HERG* genes have differential responses to Na^+ channel blockade and to increases in heart rate. Implications for gene-specific therapy. *Circulation* 1995;92:3381–3386.

25. Zareba W, Moss AJ, Schwartz PJ, et al. Long QT syndrome: Clinical course by genotype. *N Engl J Med* 1998;339:960–965.

64

Down Syndrome Congenital Heart Disease: Narrowed Region and DSCAM as a Candidate Gene

J. R. Korenberg, PhD, MD, G. M. Barlow, PhD,
X.-N. Chen, MD, Gary Lyons, PhD, C. Mjaatvedt, PhD,
M. Pettenati, PhD, A. J. VanRiper, MS,
and M. Vekemens, MD

Summary

Down syndrome (DS) is a major cause of congenital heart disease (CHD) affecting the welfare of millions worldwide. Because endocardial cushion defects constitute 60% of DS-CHD, it may provide important clues for understanding normal cardiogenesis and for defining modes of intervention. Studies of rare individuals with DS and partial duplications of chromosome 21 have defined the genetic basis of DS-CHD critical region as a single gene or cluster in band q22.13, flanked by the markers D21S267 and the telomere. We have generated a physical map of this region in bacterial and P1 artificial chromosomes (BACs and PACs), and have used this both to aid large-scale sequencing efforts and for the construction of a transcriptional map. The map now spans about 4 Mb and contains more than 30 expressed genes. We now report clinical and molecular data that narrow the candidate region and support Down syndrome cell adhesion molecule (DSCAM) as a strong candidate for DS-CHD.

To do this, 27 subjects in our panel of individuals with partial trisomy 21 were evaluated using quantitative Southern blot dosage analysis and fluorescence in situ hybridization (FISH) with subsets of 32 BACs spanning the region 21q11.2-ter and 20 molecular markers including D21S3, ETS2, MX1/2, and collagens VI a1/a2 and XVIII. The results indicated that twenty individuals are duplicated for a narrowed DS-CHD region, of whom 10 (50%) have the characteristic spectrum of DS-CHD. These include atrioventricular septal defect (AVSD), ventricular septal defect (VSD), atrial septal defect (ASD), and tetralogy of Fallot (ToF). DUP21BA and DUP21NA, both of whom are duplicated from D21S267-ter, have an AVSD and a primary ASD respectively, DUP21SM (dup. D21S55-ter) has pulmonic stenosis, and DUP21SW (dup. D21S29-collagen VI) has ToF. One case, DUP21PM, is duplicated for 21q22.3 and a small part of chromosome 13, and has a posterior VSD. Seven further individuals are duplicated for the region from the cen-

From Clark EB, Nakazawa M, Takao A (eds.): Etiology and Morphogenesis of Congenital Heart Disease: Twenty Years of Progress in Genetics and Developmental Biology. Armonk, NY: Futura Publishing Co., Inc.; © 2000.

tromere through 21q22.1 above D21S267. None of these subjects have CHD.

These data suggest a narrowed DS-CHD candidate region including the markers D21S3 through collagen VI a1/a2, and excluding the telomere and the region of D21S55. Taken together with the data from the trisomy 16 mouse, these data support a candidate region of D21S3-MX1/2, an interval of approximately 2.5 Mb.

The endocardial cushion defects (ECDs) associated with DS-CHD are thought to be due to altered cell adhesion during cushion morphogenesis. We have generated a transcriptional map of 30 cDNAs in this region, only one of which, DSCAM, encodes a cell adhesion molecule. DSCAM covers more than 750 Mb (40%) of the narrowed region and is expressed in the fetal heart in the mouse and in humans. Given these properties, we propose that DSCAM may play a significant role in cushion development and, when overexpressed, may contribute significantly to the DS-CHD phenotype. The construction of murine models will allow the investigation of DSCAM for a role in cushion morphogenesis and as a cause of DS-CHD. Finally, such models will also provide opportunities studying intervention and possible prevention of CHD.

Introduction

Malformations of the cardiovascular system account for the majority of premature deaths caused by congenital anomalies.[1] The recent revolution in human molecular genetics has provided the tools with which to begin to identify the genes involved and to understand the disturbances in developmental pathways that lead to these defects. Down syndrome (DS), which is normally caused by trisomy 21, is a major cause of congenital heart disease (CHD)[2] and therefore provides an important model with which to link indi-

vidual genes to the pathways controlling heart development.

More than 60% of DS individuals have congenital heart defects, of which the majority involve defects of the atrioventricular septae (AVSDs),[3] and account for more than 70% of all AVSDs.[4] These data strongly suggest that the overexpression of a single gene or gene cluster on chromosome 21 contributes to DS-CHD and may also play a key role in valvuloseptal morphogenesis. It has been suggested that DS-CHD results from a disturbance of cell adhesion,[5] leading to the search for chromosome 21 genes involved in these interactions.

In order to define the genes for DS-CHD, a series of rare individuals with CHD and partial duplications of chromosome 21 was analyzed and the results suggested that the candidate region was located in chromosome band 21q22, defined by the marker D21S55 to the telomere.[6–8] We then generated a contig composed of BACs (bacterial artificial chromosomes) and PACs (P1 artificial chromosomes) covering 3.5 Mb of the 4–5 Mb interval from D21S55 to MX1/2.[9] This contig was then used to construct a transcriptional map of the DS-CHD candidate region.[10] We have identified and evaluated more than 40 cDNAs to date, of which we now propose DSCAM as a strong candidate for DS-CHD.

In order to further narrow the DS-CHD candidate region, and to evaluate DSCAM as a candidate, we have determined the molecular breakpoints present in three individuals with partial trisomy 21 and DS-CHD.[11] Southern blot dosage analysis and fluorescence in situ hybridization (FISH) with 32 BAC clones and molecular markers spanning the region 21q11.2-ter were employed as described for five cases previously reported.[12,13] Figure 1 shows an example of a FISH experiment, and the results of the molecular analyses are summarized graphically in Figure 2.

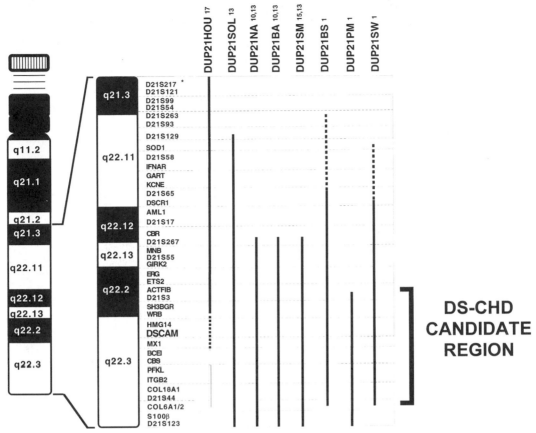

Figure 1. FISH on chromosomes from patient DUP21SW. Two copies of the gene encoding PFKL are seen on the abnormal chromosome 21, and one copy is seen on the normal chromosome 21.

Figure 2. Definition of the candidate region and genes for CHD in DS. A graphic summary of molecular analyses from eight individuals with partial trisomy 21 and CHD defines the region. Solid lines indicate regions of known duplication; dotted lines indicate regions of duplication inferred from cytogenetic findings; white open box indicates one deleted region. *Symbols for genes mapping in the region are listed and descriptions are available through http://www.expasy.ch/cgi-bin/lists?humchr21.txt. Superscripts indicate published studies. See color appendix.

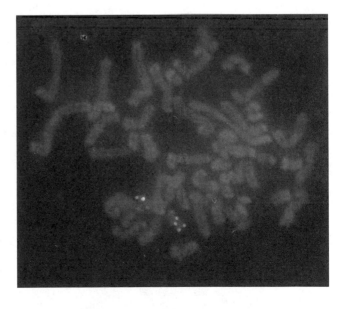

Subjects With Heart Defects and Partial Trisomy 21

DUP21SW has tetralogy of Fallot (ToF), including an ASD, a large VSD, an overriding aorta with outflow tract stenosis, and a stenotic pulmonary valve. He carries a chromosome 21 duplication derived from a maternal rearrangement and defined by the gene markers AML-1 through collagen VI A1/A2.[11] DUP21BS has a large ostium primum defect and an inlet VSD occluded by a tricuspid valve leaflet tissue. She carries a de novo partial duplication of chromosome 21, and carries three copies of the region of 21q22 from KCNE through D21S44.[11] DUP21PM has a moderately sized posterior inlet VSD of the AV canal type, with two distinct AV valves. The VSD was located immediately beneath the tricuspid valve, with valve tissue overlying much of the defect. This was accompanied by moderate pulmonary hypertension, patent ductus arteriosus and mitral valve insufficiency. He carries an unbalanced translocation t(13;21)(q14; q22) resulting in chromosome 21 duplication from D21S3 through the telomere. Although full trisomy 13 is also associated with CHD,[14] it is not the inlet canal type of AVSD seen both in DS and in this case.[4] These data suggest that the heart defects of DUP21PM result from his chromosome 21 rather than his small chromosome 13 duplication.[11]

Down Syndrome Congenital Heart Disease Candidate Region

In view of the evidence supporting a single gene or cluster in 21q22,[7] the minimal DS-CHD candidate region defined by the eight human subjects may be narrowed to D21S3 through collagen VI a1/a2 (see Fig. 2). Most importantly, these results exclude the region of D21S55, which was previously thought to be responsible for many of the features of DS, including the heart defects.[8] Moreover, collagen VI and collagen XVIII remain candidates, although genes located in the subtelomeric regions are excluded. The validity of a single candidate region is supported by the analysis of the full panel of 27 subjects with partial trisomy 21, in which the incidence and spectrum of CHD found in those with duplications including the candidate region (50%) is similar to that associated with full trisomy 21 (60%)[11] and duplications that exclude the candidate region (0/7) do not result in CHD.

The trisomy 16 mouse model of DS[15] has been used to further subdivide the human DS-CHD region[12] but more recent MMU16 partial trisomies[16,17] that lack the mouse region homologous to DiGeorge and Velo Cardio Facial Syndrome (VCFS) regions, have not shown any of the 100% AVSDs seen in full Ts16. Although this may be due to strain differences, it weakens the rationale for excluding all genes telomeric to MX.[12]

Candidate Genes for DS-CHD

Although many genes occupy the DS-CHD candidate region, many of which are ubiquitously expressed, only two will be considered here, collagen VI and DSCAM. Collagen VI has been proposed as a candidate for DS-CHD, as it is both expressed in the endocardial (atrioventricular) cushions and may be involved in adhesion. However, its deletion in humans leads to no apparent cardiac defects, and individuals without collagen VI duplications still get cardiac defects,[18,19] suggesting a lack of sensitivity to the dosage effects suspected for DS-CHD.

DSCAM was isolated and defined as the most significant gene occupying the DS-CHD candidate region.[20] A novel member of the immunoglobulin (Ig) superfamily of cell adhesion molecules, the human form is 99% homologous to the mouse (unpublished data) and spans approximately 1 Mb of the region between

D21S3 and MX. Although studies of AV segmentation have yet to define the pathways of development, changes in cell adhesion appear to underlie DS-CHD. It is clear that these involve effects on migration, proliferation and differentiation of interacting populations of cells derived from myocardium, endothelium, mesenchyme and neural crest, with possible roles recently indicated for epicardium-derived cells.[21] RT-PCR analyses have shown that DSCAM is expressed in mouse fetal heart tissues at E10.5 p.c. and in pooled human fetal heart tissues representing 7.5 to 10 weeks (Korenberg, unpublished data). Further, the strongest expression of DSCAM is seen in neurons of the CNS and in the neural crest and its derivatives, including the cardiac ganglion and the nerves of the heart.[20] It is expected that, similar to its pattern in the CNS, DSCAM may only be expressed briefly during inductive processes, making it difficult to detect in the AV cushions. Nonetheless, DSCAM expression and structure support a role in DS-CHD.

Future studies will examine the role of DSCAM in the endocardial cushions directly using the collagen gel explant system.[22] For the current work, the central questions include whether DSCAM overexpression results in DS phenotypes, which embryonic heart tissues are involved (neural crest, endocardium/mesenchyme and myocardium), the nature of the interactions mediating these effects, such as homophilic and heterophilic adhesion and signaling interactions, and the roles of molecules known to be involved in valvuloseptal morphogenesis, such as NCAM and FGFRs.[23–25] The results of our current investigations should elucidate the role played by chromosome 21 genes such as DSCAM in generating DS phenotypes, particularly DS-CHD.

References

1. Clark EB. Mechanisms in the pathogenesis of congenital heart defects. In: Pierpoint MEM, Moller JH, eds. *The Genetics of Cardiovascular Disease*. Boston, Mass: Martinus-Nijoff; 1987: 3–11.
2. Epstein CJ. *The Consequences of Chromosomal Imbalance*. Cambridge: Cambridge University Press; 1986.
3. Rehder H. Pathology of trisomy 21—with particular reference to persistent common atrioventricular canal of the heart. *Hum Genet* 1981;2(suppl):57–73.
4. Ferencz C, Loffredo CA, Correa-Villasenor A, et al. Genetic and environmental risk factors of major cardiovascular malformations: The Baltimore-Washington Infant Study: 1981–1989. In *Perspectives in Pediatric Cardiology*. Vol. 5. Armonk, NY: Futura Publishing Co.; 1997.
5. Wright TC, Orkin RW, Destrempes M, et al. Increased adhesiveness of Down syndrome fetal fibroblasts in vitro. *Proc Natl Acad Sci U S A* 1984;81:2426–2430.
6. Korenberg JR, Kawashima H, Pulst SM, et al. Molecular definition of a region of chromosome 21 that causes features of the Down syndrome phenotype. *Am J Hum Genet* 1990;47:236–246.
7. Epstein CJ, Korenberg JR, Anneren G, et al. Protocols to establish genotype-phenotype correlations in Down syndrome. *Am J Hum Genet* 1991;49:207–235.
8. Korenberg JR, Chen XN, Schipper R, et al. Down syndrome phenotypes: The consequences of chromosomal imbalance. *Proc Natl Acad Sci U S A* 1994;91:4997–5001.
9. Hubert RS, Mitchell S, Chen XN, et al. BAC and PAC contigs covering 3.5 Mb of the Down syndrome congenital heart disease region between D21S55 and MX1 on chromosome 21. *Genomics* 1997;41:218–226.
10. Korenberg JR. Unpublished data.
11. Barlow G, et al. unpublished data.
12. Korenberg JR, Bradley C, Disteche C. Down Syndroem: Molecular mapping of the congenital heart disease and duodenal stenosis. *Am J Hum Genet* 1992;50:294–302.
13. Korenberg JR, Chen XN, Doege K, et al. Assignment of the human aggrecan gene (ACG1) to 15q26 using fluorescence in situ hybridization analysis. *Genomics* 1993;16:546–548.
14. Hyett J, Mosoco G, Nicolaides K. Abnormalities of the heart and great arteries in first trimester chromosomally abnormal fetuses. *Am J Med Genet* 1997;69:207–216.

15. Reeves RH, Gearhart JD, Littlefield JW. Genetic basis for a mouse model of Down syndrome. *Brain Res Bull* 1986;16:803–814.

16. Reeves RH, Irving NG, Moran TH, et al. A mouse model for Down syndrome exhibits learning and behaviour deficits. *Nat Genet* 1995;11:177–184.

17. Sago H, Carlson EJ, Smith DJ, et al. Ts1Cje, a partial trisomy 16 mouse model for Down syndrome, exhibits learning and behavioral abnormalities. *Proc Natl Acad Sci U S A* 1998;95:6256–6261.

18. Palmer CG, Blouin JL, Bull MJ, et al. Cytogenetic and molecular analysis of a ring (21) in a patient with partial trisomy 21 and megakaryocytic leukemia. *Am J Med Genet* 1995;57:527–536.

19. Delabar JM, Theophile D, Rahmani Z, et al. Molecular mapping of 24 features of Down Syndrome on chromosome 21. *Eur J Hum Genet* 1993;1:114–124.

20. Yamakawa K, Huot YK, Haendelt MA, et al. DSCAM: A novel member of the immunoglobulin superfamily maps in a Down syndrome region and is involved in the development of the nervous system. *Hum Mol Genet* 1998;7:227–237.

21. Poelmann RE, Gittenberger-de Groot AC. A subpopulation of apoptosis-prone cardiac neural crest cells targets to the venous pole: Multiple functions in heart development? *Dev Biol* 1999;207:271–286.

22. Mjaatvedt CH, Markwald RR. Induction of an epithelial-mesenchymal transition by an in vivo adheron-like complex. *Dev Biol* 1989;136:118–128.

23. Oosthoek PW, Wenink AC, Vrolijk BC, et al. Development of the atrioventricular valve tension apparatus in the human heart. *Anat Embryol* 1998;198:317–329.

24. Gittenberger-de Groot AC, Vrancken Peeters MP, Mentink MM, et al. Epicardium-derived cells contribute a novel population to the myocardial wall and the atrioventricular cushions. *Circ Res* 1998;82:1043–1052.

25. Miyazaki K, Yamanaka T, Ogasawara N. A boy with Down's syndrome having recombinant chromosome 21 but no SOD-1 excess. *Clin Genet* 1987;32:383–387.

65

Studies on the Function of the Exocytosis-Relating Protein, HPC-1/Syntaxin 1A and Its Relation to Williams Syndrome

Kimio Akagawa, MD

Introduction

HPC-1/syntaxin1A was originally found as a neuronal membrane protein.[1,2] This molecule belongs to syntaxin protein family mediating intracellular membrane transport in many types of cells and can bind many other so-called "exocytosis-relating proteins," such as synaptobrevin, SNAP25 (23 kD synaptosomal-associated protein) and synaptotagmin.[3] In order to explain molecular mechanism of exocytosis, SNARE hypothesis has been proposed.[4] According to SNARE hypothesis, the complex of NSF (N-ethylmaleimide sensitive fusion protein) and SNAP (soluble NSF attachment protein) in the cytoplasm mediates exocytotic process by binding to SNAP receptors (SNARE) on exocytotic vesicle and the plasma membrane, and HPC-1 functions as one of SNAREs. However, precise physiological function of HPC-1 is not so clear since this protein is distributed widely on the axonal membrane where no exocytosis occurs. In this context, we have carried out cell biological studies on the function of HPC-1 to elucidate this question. This paper reviews our recent works on HPC-1 and indicates a

possible relevancy to a human congenital disease, Williams syndrome (WS).

Suppressive Role of HPC-1 in Exocytosis

In order to investigate the physiological meaning of HPC-1/syntaxin 1A in exocytosis, several distinct types of experiments were attempted. First of all, application of the anti-HPC-1 IgG into the permeabilized pheochromocytoma cells (PC12) was tried to find increase of catecholamine secretion.[5] Also, intracellularly applied antibody enhanced the amplitude of excitatory postsynaptic current by increasing transmitter release from the presynaptic terminals in vitro.[6] In βTc cells, a cell line of the β cell of Langerhans islet, overexpression of HPC-1 decreased insulin release in response to extracellular glucose stimulation.[7] However, syntaxin1B, an isoform of HPC-1/syntaxin 1A in the nervous system, did not show any suppressive effect on insulin release. By injecting the cRNA into fertilized oocytes, HPC-1 protein was ectopically expressed on the plasma membrane of the early embryos of the newt (Fig. 1).[8] It was observed by an electron microscopical study that in the cytoplasm of the ectodermal cells secretory vesicles con-

From Clark EB, Nakazawa M, Takao A (eds.): Etiology and Morphogenesis of Congenital Heart Disease: Twenty Years of Progress in Genetics and Developmental Biology. Armonk, NY: Futura Publishing Co., Inc.; © 2000.

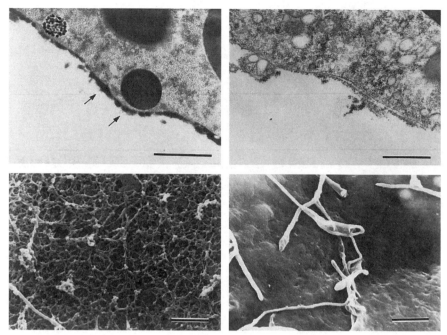

Figure 1. Reduction of ECM secretion by ectopic HPC-1 expression in early amphibian embryos. HPC-1cRNA was injected into 2-cell stage embryos of Japanese newt to express ectopic HPC-1 protein. The surface of ectodermal cells were studied with an electron microscope 48 hours after injection.[8] Upper figures; Electron micrographs of control (left) and HPC-1 expressing embryo (right). The ectodermal cells of the control embryo do not express HPC-1 at this developmental stage. Deposit of electron-dense ECM (arrows) is visible in the control. In case of HPC-1, no ECM deposit is present and secretory vesicles containing ECM accumulate in the vicinity of the plasma membrane. Lower figures: Scanning electron microscopic observations of the cell surfaces of the same regions as the upper figures. ECM is observed as mesh-like materials in the control (left). The cell surface of HPC-1-expressing embryo (right) is devoid of ECM. Scale bars: 0.5 um.

taining extracellular matrix (ECM) accumulated in the vicinity of plasma membrane, resulting in reduction of ECM deposit on the cell surface. Furthermore, in the transformed PC12 cells in which HPC-1 expression was partially suppressed by transfecting the antisense RNA-expressing vector, catecholamine secretion stimulated by secretagogues increased.[9] These results indicated that HPC-1 would play an inhibitory role in exocytosis, possibly by suppressing membrane fusion process between intracellular exocytotic vesicles and plasma membrane. This suppressive function appeared to localize on the N-terminal region of HPC-1 because the mutant molecules lacking N-terminal region revealed no suppressive effect on exocytosis.

Enhancement of Neurite-Sprouting by Suppression of HPC-1 in Neurons

It has been postulated, on the other hand, that HPC-1 might have other functions than exocytosis since distribution of HPC-1 protein was not restricted to the synaptic region of neurons, but also on the axonal plasma membrane where no exocytosis occurred.[10] Interestingly, it was demonstrated that suppression of HPC-1 expression by applying the antisense oligonucleotides against HPC-1 mRNA elicited enhancement of axonal sprouting in cultured dorsal root ganglion neurons (Fig. 2).[11] Neuronal sprouting was also elicited in a similar experiment using cer-

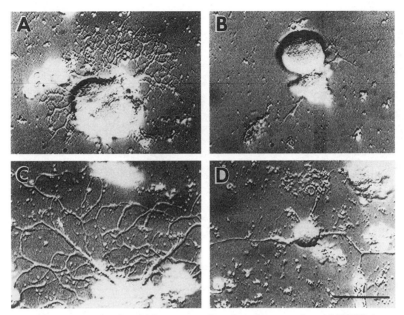

Figure 2. Enhancement of neurite sprouting by suppression of HPC-1 expression. Dorsal root ganglion cells were cultured with 30 uM HPC-1/syntaxin 1A antisense oligonucleotide against HPC-1mRNA (**A, C**) or the sense oligonucleotide (**B, D**), and viewed with contrast enhanced video system[11] one day (**A, B**) and 2 days (**C, D**) after treatment. Scale bar: 50 um. Suppression of HPC-1 expression by the antisense oligonucleotide enhanced formation of fine branchings (neurite sprouting), but the number of main processes was not affected compared to the control.

ebellar granule cells in vitro. In the transformed PC12 cells in which expression of HPC-1 protein was almost completely abolished, abundant microprocess formation and degranulation of catecholamine-containing vesicles were observed.[12] These results indicated that HPC-1 would also be closely related to the mechanism of neuronal sprouting in neurons. Involvement of the other exocytosis-relating proteins in neuronal process formation have also been reported,[13,14] and it was postulated that these could be due to expansion of plasma membrane by accelerating intracellular membrane transport and fusion. In case of HPC-1, neuronal sprouting by HPC-1 suppression was supposed to be due to enhancement of intracellular membrane fusion as well, and possibly to rearrangement of the cytoskeletal structures since HPC-1 could interact with the cytoskeletal protein.[15] Because it was generally accepted that neuronal sprouting could be one of the fundamental properties in long term memory and learning

process in CNS, these results suggested a possible involvement of HPC-1 in the memory-acquiring process of CNS.

Hemizygous Deletion of HPC-1 Gene in WS Patients

In order to examine a possible relationship between HPC-1 gene and human genetic disorders, fluorescent in situ hybridization (FISH) analysis with a genomic probe was performed. The result of FISH revealed that the locus of human HPC-1 gene (STX1A) was mapped to the chromosome 7band q11.2.[16] Because this locus was located within the common chromosome region deleted in patients with WS,[17] which showed cardiovascular disease and peculiar neuropsychological symptoms, the lymphocytes of WS were studied as well. FISH study clearly demonstrated that all 46 patients with WS, so far studied, had hemizygous deletion of HPC-1 gene (Fig. 3).[18] These findings sug-

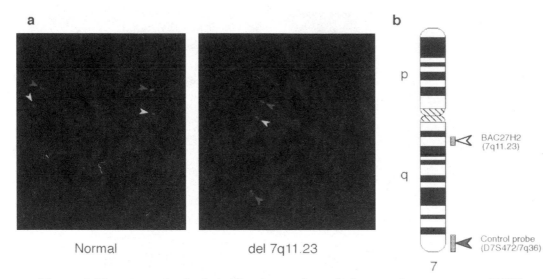

Figure 3. Fluorescent in situ hybridization study on the human chromosomes. **a.** FISH analysis on human lymphocytes was carried out.[18] The hybridization signals were viewed with a confocal laser microscope. The chromosomes are shown in blue. Red points indicate the signals of the chromosome 7 marker (D7S472, green arrow heads) or the HPC-1 probe (BAC27H2, white), respectively. All the No.7 chromosome have HPC-1 signal in the normal control (left), but a No.7 chromosome without HPC-1 signal is present in WS (right, del7q11.23), indicating hemizygous deletion of HPC-1 (STAX1A) gene in WS. **b.** Schematic representation of localization of genome probes on No.7 chromosome. See color appendix.

gested that HPC-1 might be one of the genes responsible for the neuropsychological symptoms of WS because reduction of HPC-1 could regulate transmitter release and neuronal sprouting in vitro. It was also likely that decrease of HPC-1 protein might be a possible cause of abnormalities of endocrine function in WS. However, further studies are clearly necessary to know the pathological mechanism underlying the unique symptoms in WS.

Summary

Function of HPC-1/syntaxin 1A in exocytosis was studied using various types of cells that had exocytotic process. Suppression of HPC-1 expression in neurons or PC12 cells increased transmitter release, whereas overexpression of this protein in the β cells resulted in decrease of insulin secretion. These results indicated that HPC-1 played a suppressive role in regulated exocytosis. In addition, suppression of HPC-1 in neurons enhanced neuronal sprouting, implying the involvement of HPC-1 in the memory-acquiring process of CNS. Fluorescent in situ hybridization studies revealed that HPC-1 gene was hemizygously deleted in WS patients, suggesting that HPC-1 might be a candidate gene responsible for the neuropsychological symptoms in WS.

References

1. Barnstable CJ, Hofstein R, Akagawa K. A marker of early amacrine cell development in rat retina. *Dev Brain Res* 1985;20:286–290.
2. Inoue A, Obata K, Akagawa K. Cloning, and sequence analysis of cDNA for a neuronal cell membrane antigen, HPC-1. *J Biol Chem* 1992;267:10613–10619.
3. Bennett MK, Garcia-Arraras JE, Elferink LA, et al. The syntaxin family of vesicular transport receptors. *Cell* 1993;74:863–873.

4. Sollner T, Rothman JE. Neurotransmission: Harnessing fusionmachinery at the synapse. *Trends Neurosci* 1994;17: 344–348.

5. Kushima Y, Fujiwara T, Morimoto T, et al. Involvement of HPC-1/syntaxin 1A in transmitter release from PC12h cells. *Biochem Biophys Res Comm* 1995;212:97–103.

6. Yamaguchi K, Takada M, Fujimori K, et al. Enhancement of synaptic transmission by HPC-1 antibody in cultured hippocampal neuron. *NeuroReport* 1997;8:3641–3644.

7. Nagamatsu S, Fujiwara T, Nakamichi Y, et al. Expression and functional role of syntaxin 1/HPC-1 in pancreatic β cells: Syntaxin 1A but not 1B play a negative role in regulatory insulin release pathway. *J Biol Chem* 1996;271:1160–1165.

8. Komazaki S, Fujiwara T, Takada M, et al. Rat HPC-1/syntaxin 1A and syntaxin 1B interrupt intracellular membrane transport and inhibit secretion of the extracellular matrix in embryonic cells of an amphibian. *Exp Cell Res* 1995;221:11–18.

9. Akagawa K, Watanabe T, Fujiwara T, et al. Activation of dopamine release from HPC-1/syntaxin 1A reduced PC12h cells. *Neurosci Res* 1977;21(suppl): S88.

10. Koh S, Yamamoto A, Inoue A, et al. Immunoelectron microscopic localization of the HPC-1 antigen in the rat cerebellum. *J Neurocytol* 1993;22:995–1005.

11. Yamaguchi K, Nakayama T, Fujiwara T, et al. Enhancement of neuronal sprouting by suppression of HPC-1/syntaxin 1A activity in the cultured vertebrate nerve cells. *Brain Res* 1996;740:185–192.

12. Akagawa K. Functional analysis of HPC-1/syntaxin 1A and its relation to Williams syndrome. In: Uyemura K, Kaneko A, eds. *Neural Development.* Tokyo: Springer-Verlag; 1999, pp. 371–378.

13. Osen-Sand A, Catsicas M, Staple JK, et al. Inhibition of axonal growth by SNAP-25 antisense oligonucleotides in vitro and in vivo. *Nature* 1993;364:445–447.

14. Ferreira A, Kosik P, Greengard P, et al. Aberrant neurites and synaptic vesicle deficiency in synapsin II-deleted neurons. *Science* 1994;264:977–979.

15. Fujiwara T, Yamaguchi K, Yamamori T, et al. Interaction of HPC-1/syntaxin 1A with the cytoskeletal protein, tubulin. *Biochem Biophys Res Comm* 1997;231:352–355.

16. Nakayama T, Fujiwara T, Miyazawa A, et al. Mapping of the human HPC-1/syntaxin 1A gene (STX1A) to chromosome 7 band q11.2. *Genomics* 1997;42:173–176.

17. Osborn LR, Martindale D, Scherer SW, et al. Identification of genes from a 500-kb region at 7q11.23 that is commonly deleted in Williams syndrome patients. *Genomics* 1996;36:328–336.

18. Nakayama T, Matsuoka R, Kimura M, et al. Hemizygous deletion of the HPC-1/syntaxin 1A gene(STX1A) in patients with Williams syndrome (WS). *Cytogenet Cell Genet* 1998;82:49–51.

66

Mutations in the *JAG1*, a Ligand for a Notch Receptor, Are Responsible for AGS

Takaya Oda, MD, PhD and
Settara C. Chandrasekharappa, PhD

Alagille syndrome (AGS, MIM 118450) is an autosomal dominant developmental disorder affecting liver, heart, eye, face, and vertebrae.[1] Although rare, an estimated 1 in 70,000 live births, AGS is one of the most common genetic causes of chronic liver disorders in infants. Histological findings of bile duct paucity on liver biopsy, associated with three of five major clinical findings are considered as diagnostic of AGS. The five clinical features include cholestasis, heart defects (most commonly, peripheral pulmonary arterial stenosis), posterior embryotoxon (a defect of the anterior chamber of the eye), vertebral abnormalities ("butterfly-shaped" vertebrae) and characteristic face (a high, broad forehead; widely spaced, deep-set eyes; and a prominent, pointed chin). The cardiac anomalies may range from mild to as complex defect as tetralogy of Fallot. The identification of rare AGS patients with cytogenetic and submicroscopic deletions, and translocations had allowed mapping of the AGS locus to a 1.3-Mb region at 20p12.[2,3] Our efforts, described below, narrowed the AGS critical region to 250 kb,[4] identified the *Jagged1* gene (*JAG1*) from this interval,[5] and demonstrated that mutations in *JAG1* are responsible for AGS.[4,6]

From Clark EB, Nakazawa M, Takao A (eds.): Etiology and Morphogenesis of Congenital Heart Disease: Twenty Years of Progress in Genetics and Developmental Biology. Armonk, NY: Futura Publishing Co., Inc.; © 2000.

Figure 1a shows the location of the original 1.3-Mb AGS critical region at 20p12. Three overlapping YAC (yeast artificial chromosome) clones identified from a previously reported YAC contig spanning this region[7] are also shown. We generated a BAC (bacterial artificial clone) contig for the telomeric half (600 kb) of the AGS critical region as shown in Figure 1b. The BAC clones from this contig were used as probes to search for submicroscopic deletions in metaphase spreads from cytogenetically normal AGS patients by fluorescent *in situ* hybridization (FISH). Complete deletion of the region represented by BAC clones b255F12, b19H8, and b204H22 but partial retention of the b334G22 region was observed in an AGS patient. This defined a new centromeric boundary for AGS critical region. Further analysis showed that the deletion in this patient extended to 600 kb. This result, along with a new telomeric boundary observed in another patient, reduced the size of the critical region to a 250-kb interval (Fig. 1b).

Cloning a CpG island located in this critical region led us to the identification and isolation of *JAG1*.[5] The *JAG1* cDNA is 5,942 bp long and possesses three alternative polyadenylation sites, all of which were utilized in multiple tissues. Northern blot analysis of RNA from adult tissues indicated that *JAG1* was widely expressed as a 5.9-kb message in multiple tissues. The *JAG1* encoded a ligand for

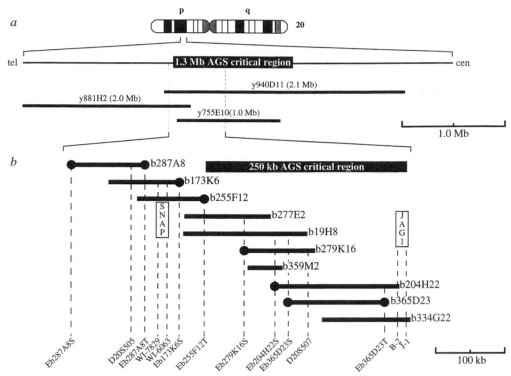

Figure 1. YAC and BAC clone contig for the AGS critical region. **a.** The location of the original 1.3 Mb AGS critical region at 20p12 is shown. Three overlapping YAC clones (y881H2, y755E10, and y940D11) spanning this region, and their size in parenthesis are shown. **b.** A contig for the telomeric half of the 1.3-Mb AGS critical region consisting of ten BAC clones (names with prefix b) and 14 STSs (shown at the bottom). The dashed line connecting the STS to the clone shows the presence of an STS in a BAC clone. Locations of the two genes, *SNAP* and *JAG1* are indicated. The new 250-kb AGS critical region, based on the submicroscopic deletions in two AGS patients, is shown.

a Notch receptor. The importance of Jagged/Notch interactions in cell fate determination during early development made *JAG1* an attractive candidate gene for a developmental disorder such as Alagille syndrome.

The genomic structure of the *JAG1* gene was determined by assembling sequences from the BAC clone b334G22. The sequence analysis indicated that *JAG1* stretches across 36 kb and has 26 exons ranging in size from 28 bp to 2,284 bp. Intron sizes vary from 89 bp to nearly 9 kb.[4] A total of 31 PCR were performed to amplify the complete coding region (3,657 bp) of *JAG1* for mutation detection by SSCP analysis. Variant SSCP fragments were identified and analyzed by direct sequencing.[4] Figure 2 shows the *JAG1* mu-

tations observed by SSCP/sequencing analysis of six kindreds (B to G). Kindred A was found to have lost most of the *JAG1* gene due to a submicroscopic deletion of 600 kb (described above). Three frameshift (kindreds B–D) and three splice donor mutations (kindreds E–G) were identified. Only proband was available from kindred B who showed a 4-bp deletion (1950del4) in exon 12. In kindred C, a frame-shift due to a 2-bp (GT) deletion in exon 22 (3098delGT) was observed in the proband. Both her mother and sister carried the same mutation although they were not known to be diagnosed with AGS. In kindred D, both the proband and his unaffected father showed an extremely subtle variation in the SSCP band pattern and were found to have a

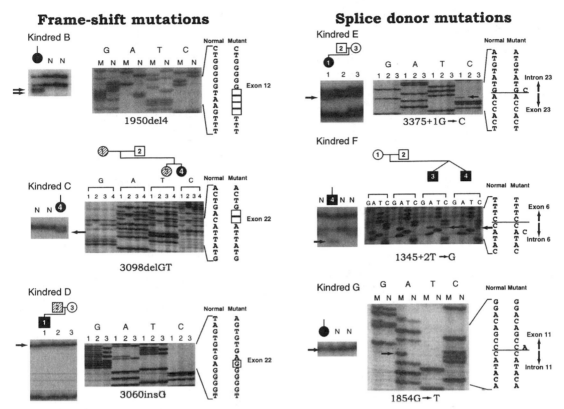

Figure 2. Mutation detection in six AGS kindreds by SSCP and sequence analysis. Arrows indicate the locations of the variant SSCP bands. N and M refer to normal and mutant samples. Frame-shift mutations observed in kindreds B–D are shown on the left, and the splice donor mutations observed in kindreds E-G are shown on the right. Only proband DNA was available for kindreds B and G. Unaffected individuals harboring the same mutation as proband (in kindreds C and D) are shaded.

single nucleotide insertion (3060insG) in exon 22. In kindred E, a new mutation, unique to the affected offspring, changing the normal splice donor signal GT to CT (3375+1G→C) at the junction of exon 23 and intron 23 was observed. A splice donor change from GT to GG (1345+2T→G) in intron 6 was found in affected identical twins in kindred F; neither parent carried this mutation demonstrating another sporadic mutation. In kindred G, a G→T change in the last nucleotide of exon 11 (1845G→T) initially appeared to be a silent mutation, since the substitution did not alter the encoded amino acid, arginine. However, this sequence alteration occurs immediately upstream of the junction of exon 11 and intron 11, changing this from GTCGG/gtatgt to GTCGT/

gtatgt, which could result in abnormal splicing. RNA analysis demonstrated loss of expression of the 1845G→T mutant allele in this patient. None of the 100 chromosomes from normal individuals showed this sequence variation.

The phenotype of patients with point mutations, whether frame-shift and splice alterations (as in kindreds B–F) or lack of expression of the mutant allele (as in kindred G), did not seem different from patients with submicroscopic or large cytogenetic deletions eliminating the entire *JAG1* gene. This suggests that AGS probably arises, as a consequence of haploinsufficiency of the Jagged1 protein. A total of nearly 50 independent mutations, spread throughout the *JAG1* gene in AGS patients have been reported so far.[4,6,8,9]

However, there appears to be no phenotype-genotype correlation.

The Notch signaling pathway has been extensively studied in *Drosophila* and *C. elegans* and is shown to be of importance in cell-fate determination in early embryonic development.[10] AGS is the first developmental disorder to be associated with a member of this pathway. However, involvement of *NOTCH1* in a T-cell leukemia,[11] and *NOTCH3* in CADASIL, a rare cause of stroke and dementia[12] has been described. Detailed study of this pathway promises to yield a better understanding of the human development and associated disorders.

Acknowledgements: We would like to thank our collaborators, Abdel Elkahloun, Kazuki Okajima, Brian Pike, Nancy Spinner, and Francis Collins.

References

1. Alagille D, Estrada A, Hadchouel M, et al. Syndromic paucity of interlobular bile ducts (Alagille syndrome or arteriohepatic dysplasia): review of 80 cases. *J Pediatr* 1987;110:195–200.
2. Spinner NB, Rand EB, Fortina P, et al. Cytologically balanced t(2;20) in a two-generation family with alagille syndrome: cytogenetic and molecular studies. *Am J Hum Genet* 1994;55:238–243.
3. Krantz D, Rand EB, Genin A, et al. Deletions of 20p12 in Alagille syndrome: Frequency and molecular characterization. *Am J Med Genet* 1997;70:80–86.
4. Oda T, Elkahloun AG, Pike BL, et al. Mutations in the human Jagged1 gene are responsible for Alagille syndrome. *Nat Genet* 1997;16:235–242.
5. Oda T, Elkahloun AG, Meltzer PS, et al. Identification and cloning of the human homolog (JAG1) of the rat Jagged1 gene from the Alagille syndrome critical region at 20p12. *Genomics* 1997;43:376–379.
6. Li L, Krantz ID, Deng Y, et al. Alagille syndrome is caused by mutations in human Jagged1, which encodes a ligand for Notch1. *Nat Genet* 1997;16:243–251.
7. Pollet N, Dhorne-Pollet S, Deleuze JF, et al. Construction of a 3.7-Mb physical map within human chromosome 20p12 ordering 18 markers in the Alagille syndrome locus. *Genomics* 1995;27:467–474.
8. Krantz ID, Colliton RP, Genin A, et al. Spectrum and frequency of jagged-1 (JAG1) Mutations in Alagille Syndrome patients and their families. *Am J Hum Genet* 1998;62:1361–1369.
9. Yuan ZR, Kohsaka T, Ikegaya T, et al. Mutational analysis of the Jagged 1 gene in Alagille syndrome families. *Hum Mol Genet* 1998;7:1363–1369.
10. Artavanis-Tsakonas S, Matsuno S, Fortini ME. Notch signaling. *Science* 1995;268:225–232.
11. Ellisen LW, Bird J, West DC, et al. TAN-1, the human homolog of the Drosophila notch gene, is broken by chromosomal translocations in T lymphoblastic neoplasms. *Cell* 1991;66:649–661.
12. Joutel A, Corpechot C, Ducros A, et al. Notch3 mutations in CADASIL, a hereditary adult-onset condition causing stroke and dementia. *Nature* 1996;383:707–710.

67

Chromosomal Deletion and Phenotype Correlation in Patients With Williams Syndrome

Misa Kimura, MS, Hamao Hirota, MD, PhD
Toshio Nishikawa, MD, Shigeru Ishiyama, MD,
Shin-ichiro Imamura, DVM, PhD,
Julie R. Korenberg, PhD, MD Kensaku Mizuno, PhD,
Toshio Nakayama, MD, Kimio Akagawa, MD,
Nobuyoshi Shimizu, PhD, Kunitaka Joh-o, MD,
Carlos Diaz, MD, Mariko Tatsuguchi, MD,
Keiko Komatsu, BSc, Masahiko Ando, MD,
Atsuyoshi Takao, MD, Kazuo Momma, MD,
and Rumiko Matsuoka, MD

Williams syndrome (WS) is a developmental disorder (incidence:1 of 20,000–50,000 live births) with characteristic facial features (Elfin face), congenital heart defects (mostly supravalvular aortic stenosis and peripheral stenosis), mental retardation, a typical cognitive profile, outgoing personality, low birth weight, short stature and infantile hypercalcemia. Previously, hemizygous microdeletion at the elastin locus localized to chromosome 7q11.23 was found in WS.[1, 2] The genes *HPC-1/Syntaxin 1A (STX1A)* and *LIM-kinase 1 (LIMK1)*, which are expressed in brain, have been identified in the same chromosomal region, 7q11.23.[3–5] In addition, three transcripts (*WSCR2, 3, and 5*)[6] and genes, including one gene containing an RNA-binding motif (*WSCR1*)[6] and another gene with similarity to restin (*WSCR4*),[6] the replication factor C subunit 2 (*RFC2*),[7] the human frizzled homologue (*FZD3*),[8] and *FKBP6*, which shows homology to the FK-506 binding protein (FKBP) gene family,[9] have been mapped within the common WS deletion region. Thus, these genes could be involved in the pathogenesis of the unexplained neurological features of WS. The purpose of our present study was to identify a regional deletion size involving the *ELN, HPC-1/ STX1A, LIMK1, WSCR1–5, RFC2, FZD3* and *FKBP6* loci, to provide the basis for determining a possible correlation between deletion size (gene content) and the spectrum of phenotypes, including neuroanatomy and histology as well as blood vessel architecture in patients with WS.

From Clark EB, Nakazawa M, Takao A (eds.): Etiology and Morphogenesis of Congenital Heart Disease: Twenty Years of Progress in Genetics and Developmental Biology. Armonk, NY: Futura Publishing Co., Inc.; © 2000.

We examined 60 WS patients (28 males and 32 females) whose ages ranged from 5 months to 35 years. All patients were sporadic. Of the 60 patients, 26 had been seen at Tokyo Women's Medical University, and 34 were from other institutions. The clinical findings of the 60 patients with WS are as follows: a congenital heart defect (59/60, 98%), typical facial features (56/60, 93%), mental retardation (58/60, 97%), outgoing personality (56/60, 93%), small for date at birth (28/60, 47%), and inguinal hernia (12/60, 20%). Of the cardiovascular findings, supravalvular aortic stenosis was most frequently seen (51/60, 85%). Twenty of the 51 patients with supravalvular aortic stenosis had peripheral pulmonary stenosis (20/51, 40%). Pulmonary stenosis was seen in 10, mitral valve prolapse in 6, ventricular septal defect in 5 and persistent left superior vena cava was seen in 3 patients. Ebstein's anomaly, interruption of the aortic arch, Wolff-Parkinson-White syndrome, double-outlet right ventricle, coarctation of the aorta, right ventricular outflow tract obstruction and hypertrophic cardiomyopathy were each seen in one patient.

The fluorescent in situ hybridization (FISH) was performed with 6 probes (Fig. 1a): BAC 1008H17 (*FKBP6* and *FZD3*), BAC 27H2 (*HPC-1/STX1A*), WSCR (*ELN*), PAC 117G9 (*LIMK1*), BAC 363B4 (*RFC2, WSCR5, 3, and 4*) and BAC 1184P14 (*GTF2I*), in all patients. FISH analysis revealed that 56 of the 60 patients showed hemizygosity with all 6 probes except BAC 1008H17 (Fig. 1b). One of the 60 patients was found to be hemizygous with 5 probes except BAC 1184P14 and 2 of the 60 patients were found to be hemizygous with 5 probes except BAC363B4 and BAC 1184P14. Three patients, who had a smaller deletion, did not have typical facial features, an outgoing personality and their birth weight was within the normal range. However, deletion for all the re-

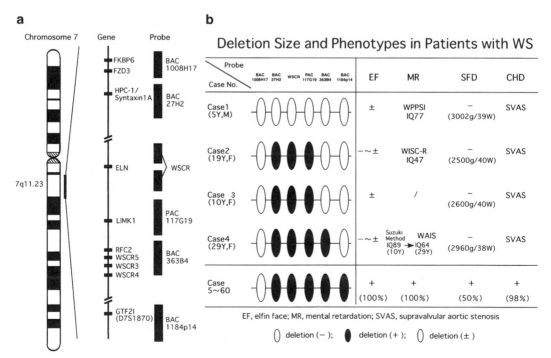

Figure 1. a. Chromosome 7q11.23 region probes and genes. BAC 1008H17 (*FKBP6* and *FZD3*), BAC 27H2 (*HPC-1/STX1A*), WSCR (*ELN*), PAC 117G9 (*LIMK1*), BAC 363B4 (*RFC2, WSCR5, 3, and 4*), and BAC 1184P14 (*GTF2I*) are probes for FISH. **b.** The FISH results and phenotypes in patients with WS.

gions, defined by *ELN*, *HPC-1/STX 1A* and *LIMK1* was found in 59 out of 60 patients with WS. One patient, who did not have cardiac defects, had the same deletion region as the other 55 patients. One patient showed nondeletion at all 6 probes.

Histochemical and immunohistochemical techniques were used to examine elastin and smooth muscle of the aorta and of the mesenteric, subclavian, coronary, pulmonary and brain arteries, vena cava, and lung and kidney blood vessels in autopsy specimens of WS patients. The results of a histological study showed hypertrophied smooth muscle and disorganized structure of the elastic lamellae not only in the aortic wall but also in all the arteries, veins and blood vessels of the organs from the WS patients' autopsy specimens (Fig. 2a, b). In patients with WS, a lower concentration of LIMK1 antibodies was observed in the cerebellar cortex and in the hippocampus compared with the normal control.

Recent reports have shown that point mutations of *ELN* cause autosomal dominant supravalvular aortic stenosis.[10,11] So our FISH results suggest that *HPC-1/STX1A*, *LIMK1* and other genes may affect the cognitive profile and other phenotypes, such as mental retardation and hypercalcemia, in patients with WS. Deletion for all the regions, defined by BAC 27H2 (*HPC-1/STX1A*), WSCR (*ELN*), PAC 117G9 (*LIMK1*) showed tipical WS phenotypes. Interestingly, 3 out of 60 patients who had a smaller deletion, did not have an outgoing personality. This may suggest that some genes, related with an outgoing personality, may be located in the region between *RFC2* to *GTF2I*. The histological study showed that patients with WS had elastin deficiency and hypertrophy of the smooth muscle of all their blood vessels.

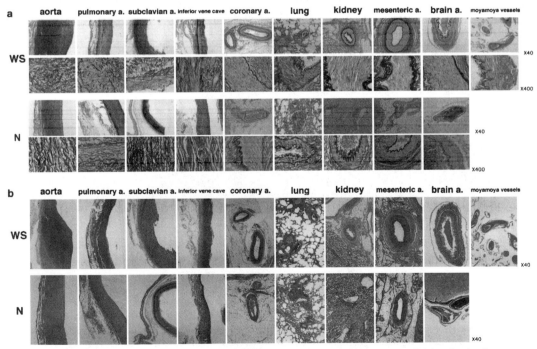

Figure 2. a. Photomicrographs of Victoria blue-van Gieson stained histological sections. In WS the thickening of the media was observed with intimal proliferation and the media shows a marked disarray of elastic fibers. **b.** Photomicrographs of Masson's trichrome-stained histological sections. In WS shows hypertrophied smooth muscle. WS, histological sections from a patient with WS; N, histological sections from normal control. See color appendix.

In conclusion, WS not only includes cardiac defects or mental retardation but also generalized deficiency, such as a typical cognitive profile, outgoing personality, low birth weight, short stature infantile hypercalcemia and inguinal hernia caused by hemizygosity with 7q11.23.

Materials and Methods

FISH

Human metaphase chromosome slides prepared from Epstein-Barr virus-transformed lymphoblastoid cell lines and/or peripheral blood by standard methods. The FISH was performed with 6 probes: BAC 1008H17 (*FKBP6* and *FZD3*), BAC 27H2 (*HPC-1/STX1A*), WSCR (*ELN*), PAC 117G9 (*LIMK1*), BAC 363B4 (*RFC2, WSCR5, 3, and 4*), and BAC 1184P14 (*GTF2I*), in all patients, as described previously.[12]

Histochemical Study

Histochemical and immunohistochemical techniques were used to examine elastin and smooth muscle of the aorta and of mesenteric, subclavian, coronary, pulmonary and brain arteries, vena cava, and lung and kidney blood vessels in autopsy specimens of WS patients. Histological sections were stained with hematoxylin-eosin, Victoria blue-van Gieson and Masson's trichrome. An immunohistochemical study using anti-hLIMK1 was performed according to Ishiyama et al.[13] with slight modification.

References

1. Ewart AK, Morris CA, Atkinson D, et al. Hemizygosity at the elastin locus in a developmental disorder, Williams syndrome. *Nat Genet* 1993;5:11-16.

2. Hirota H, Matsuoka R, Kimura M, et al. Molecular cytogenetic diagnosis of Williams syndrome. *Am J Med Genet* 1996;64:473.

3. Nakayama T, Matsuoka R, Kimura M, et al. Hemizygous deletion of the HPC-1/syntaxin 1A gene (STX1A) in patients with Williams syndrome. *Cytogenet Cell Genet* 1998;82:49.

4. Osborne LR, et al. Williams Bevrev Syndrome: Unravelling the mysteries of a microdeletion disorder. *Mol Genet Metabol* 1999; 67:1–10.

5. Tassabehji M, Metcalfe K, Fergusson WD, et al. LIM-kinase deleted in Williams syndrome. *Nat Genet* 1996;13:272.

6. Osborne LR, Martindale D, Scherer SW, et al. Identification of genes from a 500-kb region at 7q11.23 that is commonly deleted in Williams syndrome patients. *Genomics* 1996;36:328.

7. Peoples R, Perez-Jurado L, Wang YK, et al. The gene for replication factor C subunit 2 (RFC2) is within the 7q11.23 Williams syndrome deletion. *Am J Hum Genet* 1996;58:1370.

8. Wang YK, Samos CH, Peoples R, et al. A novel human homologue of the *Drosophila frizzled* wnt receptor gene binds wingless protein and is in the Williams syndrome deletion at 7q11.23. *Hum Mol Genet* 1997; 6:465.

9. Meng X, Lu X, Morris CA, et al. A novel human gene *FKBP6* is deleted in Williams syndrome. *Genomics* 1998;52:130.

10. Li DY, Toland AE, Boak BB, et al. Elastin point mutations cause an obstructive vascular disease, supravalvular aortic stenosis. *Hum Mol Genet* 1997;6:1021.

11. Tassabehji M, Metcalfe K, Donnai D, et al. Elastin: Gnomic structure and point mutations in patients with supravalvular aortic stenosis. *Hum Mol Genet* 1997;6:1026.

12. Matsuoka R, Kimura M, Scambler PJ, et al. Molecular and clinical study of 183 patients with conotruncal anomaly face syndrome. *Hum Genet* 1998;103:70.

13. Ishiyama S, Hiroe M, Nishikawa T, et al. Nitric oxide contributes to the progression of myocardial damage in experimental autoimmune myocarditis in rats. *Circulation* 1997;95:486.

Index

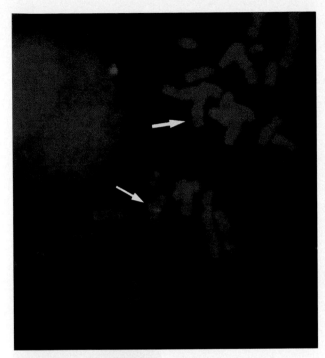

Figure 7-1. Metaphase spread of a cell derived from the heterotaxy patient, probed with y775-h-1 mapped on 11q13. Bold arrow and the thin arrow indicate inv(11)(q13,q25) and normal chromosome 11, respectively. FISH analysis was carried out, as described previously.[5]

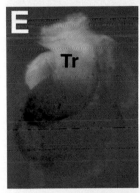

Figure 17-1. E. Hearts infected with adenovirus expressing lacZ at stage 17 and then harvested 48 hours later show labeling throughout the heart segments except the newly formed truncus. **F.** Labeling site on a stage 15 heart tube at the distal myocardial tip next to the body wall using a red fluorescent dye (mitotracker). **G.** Labeled heart shown in F) after 24-hour incubation shows labeling in the forming conotruncus. RHF, right heart field; LHF, left heart field; AV, atrioventricular segment; PTRV, primitive trabeculated right ventricle; PTLV, primitive trabeculated left ventricle; PI, primitive inlet; RA, right atrium; LA, left atrium; Tr, truncus; OT, outflow tract; RV, right ventricle; Ct, conotruncus.

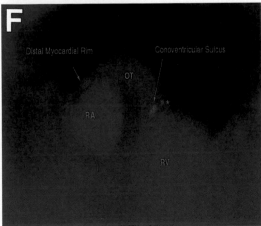

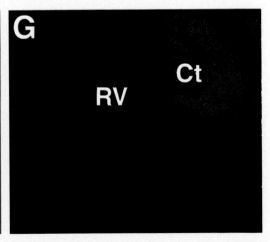

1

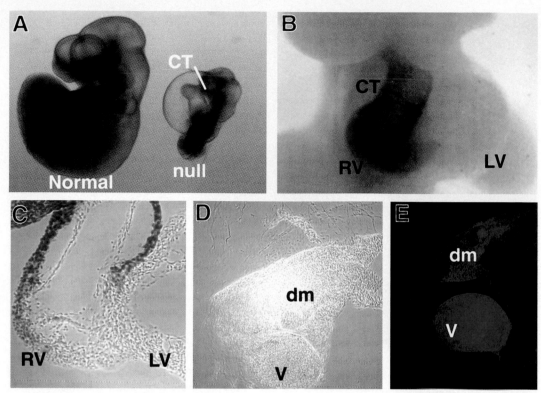

Figure 17-2. A. Comparison of a normal day 10.5 post coitus (p.c.) embryo with a homozygous *hdf* embryo (Cspg2/versican null). The Cspg2 null embryo displays impaired conotruncal (CT) formation. **B.** LacZ expression in a day 10.5 p.c. *hdf* hemizygous heart shows a segmental expression pattern associated with the conotruncus and RV development. **C.** Transgenic lacZ expression in a heterozygous BMP4/LacZ knock-in heart shows a segmentally restricted pattern associated with conotruncus development. **D.** Phase-contrast image of an explanted piece of the dorsal mesocardium (dm) dissected from a stage 12 embryo and co-cultured on a collagen gel with the distal tip of a stage 12 ventricular (V) explant. Within 24 hours of co-culture the dm began to beat spontaneously and express the MF20 muscle marker. CT, conotruncus; RV, right ventricle; LV, left ventricle.

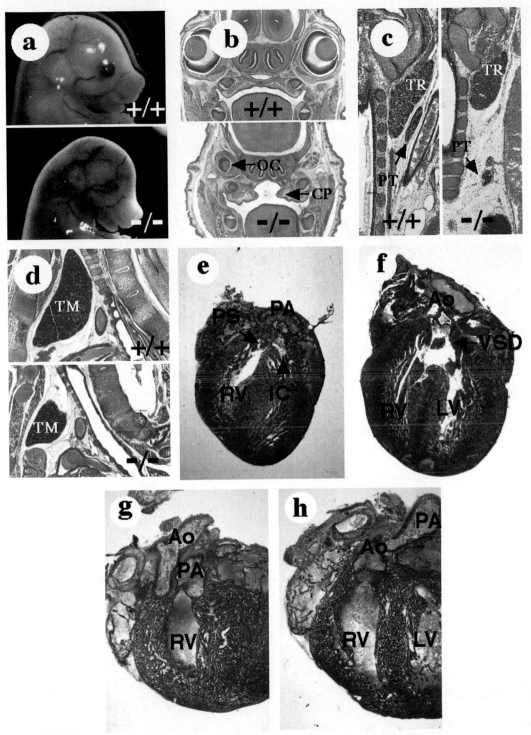

Figure 18-1.

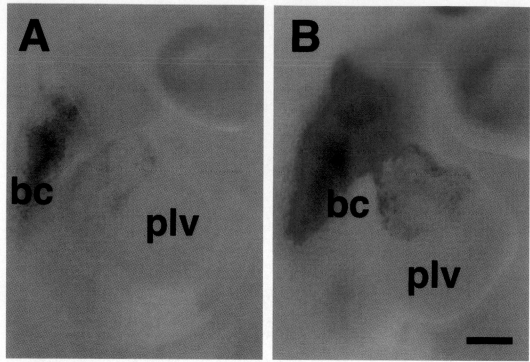

Figure 19-1. Abnormal morphology of the bulbus cordis of the *jmj* mutant embryo. Lateral views of hearts of heterozygous (**A**) and homozygous embryos (**B**) at E9.5. Embryos were stained with X-gal. Note that *jmj* is expressed in the bulbus cordis (bc) (**A**) and the proximal region of the bulbus cordis of mutant embryos appeared swollen (**B**). plv, primitive left ventricle. Bar, μm.

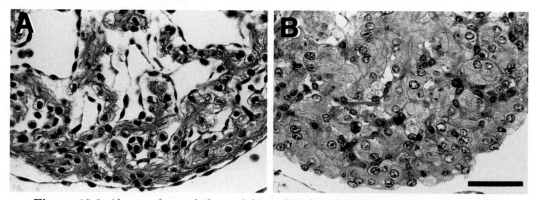

Figure 19-2. Abnormal morphology of the trabeculae of the *jmj* mutant embryo. Transverse sections of left ventricles of wild type (**A**) and homozygous (**B**) embryos at E11.5. Note that the ventricles of mutant embryos are occupied by trabecular myocytes. Bar, μm.

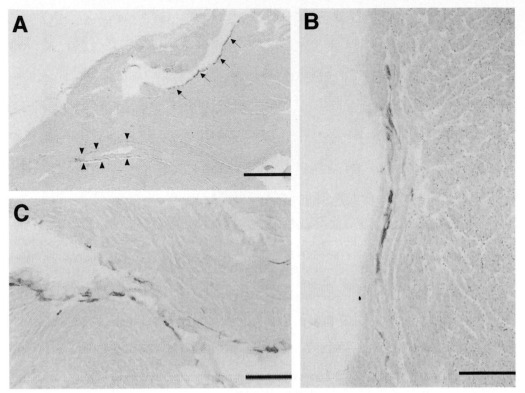

Figure 21-2.

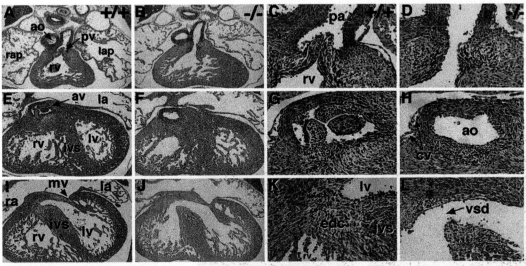

Figure 27-1.

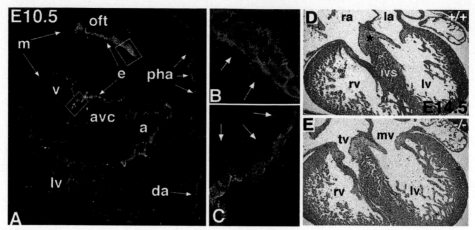

Figure 27-2. Dual-immunofluorescent confocal photomicrographs (**A–C**) of a sagittal section through the heart of an E10.5 embryo utilizing a monoclonal antibody to PECAM-1 (green, FITC-labeled secondary antibody) in combination with a monoclonal antibody to NFATc1 (red, Cy5-labeled secondary antibody). NFATc expression is restricted to the endocardium of the heart (a, ventricle; avc, atrioventricular canal; v, ventricle; oft, outflow tract) and was not detected in endothelial cells outside the heart (lvr, liver; da, dorsal aorta; pha, pharyngeal arch). A higher-power magnification of the oft (**B**) and avc (**C**) documents the nuclear localization of NFATc in the endocardium and the down regulation of NFATc in endothelial cells that have undergone mesenchymal transformation (arrows). Photomicrographs through the mitral (mv) and tricuspid (tv) valve region of an E14.5 wild type (**D**) and null mutant (**E**) embryo demonstrating no qualitative defects in valve formation. (ra, right atrium; la, left atrium; rv, right ventricle; lv, left ventricle).

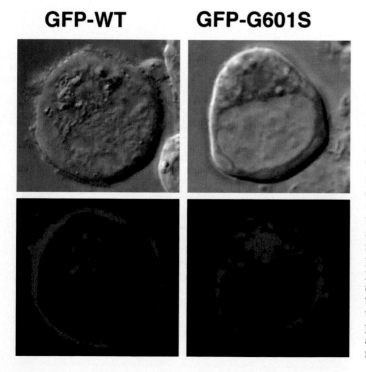

GFP-WT   **GFP-G601S**

Figure 60-2. Electrocardiogram and QaT/RR slope of long QT syndrome patients (**a**). Confocal imaged GFP-tagging of G601S and wild-type HERG channels (**b**). The upper panels exhibit merged images of Nomarski with GFP fluorescence; and the lower panels, GFP fluorescence images. A wild-type HERG protein (GFP-WT) signal was present intracellularly in the endoplasmic reticulum and perinuclear space, and in the plasma membrane. The unstained region within the cell is the nucleus. For the G601S mutation (GFP-G601S), the signal was present, intracellularly, but with a reduced plasma membrane signal.

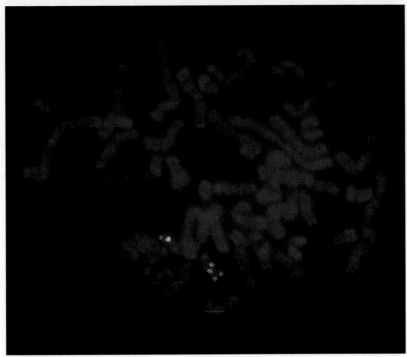

Figure 64-2. Definition of the candidate region and genes for CHD in DS. A graphic summary of molecular analyses from eight individuals with partial trisomy 21 and CHD defines the region. Solid lines indicate regions of known duplication; dotted lines indicate regions of duplication inferred from cytogenetic findings; white open box indicates one deleted region. *Symbols for genes mapping in the region are listed and descriptions are available through http://www.expasy.ch/cgi-bin/lists?humchr21.txt. Superscripts indicate published studies.

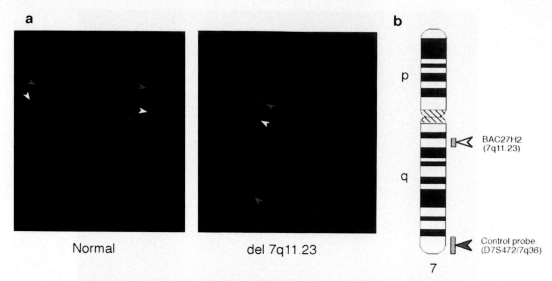

Figure 65-3. Fluorescent in situ hybridization study on the human chromosomes. **a.** FISH analysis on human lymphocytes was carried out.[18] The hybridization signals were viewed with a confocal laser microscope. The chromosomes are shown in blue. Red points indicate the signals of the chromosome 7 marker (D7S472, green arrow heads) or the HPC-1 probe (BAC27H2, white), respectively. All the No.7 chromosome have HPC-1 signal in the normal control (left), but a No.7 chromosome without HPC-1 signal is present in WS (right, del7q11.23), indicating hemizygous deletion of HPC-1 (STAX1A) gene in WS. **b.** Schematic representation of localization of genome probes on No.7 chromosome.

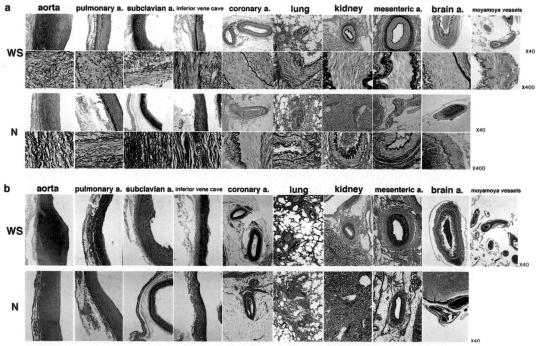

Figure 67-2. a. Photomicrographs of Victoria blue-van Gieson stained histological sections. In WS the thickening of the media was observed with intimal proliferation and the media shows a marked disarray of elastic fibers. **b.** Photomicrographs of Masson's trichrome-stained histological sections. In WS shows hypertrophied smooth muscle. WS, histological sections from a patient with WS; N, histological sections from normal control.